Contents

CONTENTS

Preface

"Carry a small notebook which will fit in your waistcoat pocket" advised Sir William Osler as he counselled students to spend their days at the bedside and their nights in the library. Succeeding generations of student practitioners have confirmed his conviction that "to study medicine without books is to go to sea without a chart, while to study medicine only from books is not to go to sea at all."

Drs. William Grace, Richard Kennedy, and Frank Flood used Osler's advice some years ago when they devised a way to help young physicians face the biotechnological tide that often seemed to inundate them. They prepared brief summaries of timely information and packaged them in a small notebook that could be carried in the modern version of the waistcoat, the short white coat of the resident physician. Three editions of the *Medical Resident's Manual* have shown the value of this approach; the authors were close to preparing the fourth edition when sudden illness led to the premature death of Dr. William Grace, Director of Medicine at Saint Vincent's Hospital and Medical Center in New York City. We agreed to assist his colleague of long standing, Dr. Richard Kennedy, in the preparation of the fourth edition; work had scarcely begun when Dr. Kennedy also became ill and died a short time later.

Drs. Grace and Kennedy, like Sydenham, Osler, and many other physician-teachers, were deeply concerned with clinical education—the transmutation of knowledge into action, the leap from textbook to patient care. Saint Vincent's Hospital with its large number of public beds became a model for the Oslerian approach to bedside teaching. At a time when university hospitals seemed to replace city-operated hospitals as a suitable environment for clinical education, these men showed what a few inspired professors working with a mix of private and public patients could achieve. We miss both of them and hope they would have enjoyed this fourth edition.

The present edition, completely rewritten, follows the approach summarized in the preface of the first edition. Sometime between initial work-up of each patient and the morning of the following day, the resident physician is expected to read extensively enough so that the patient may be presented in an arena known variously as "morning report" or "morning work rounds." These events are traditional in most institutions and a good presentation by the resident goes a long way towards establishing a reputation. Ideally, the early morning literature perusal would include textbooks of medicine, pathophysiology, clinical pharmacology, and treatment, as well as several selected key papers from recent journals. Because time is the constant enemy of the physician, a portable compilation of pertinent facts seems essential.

Those much sought after "pearls" of medical wisdom have been culled from many sources and compacted for early morning reading. Each section begins with a brief review of normal and disordered physiology, since intelligent analysis of a series of problems is impossible unless fundamental principles are recalled. A discussion of common manifestations, laboratory studies, treatment, and new developments relating to specific disease processes follow. *Key symptoms, signs, and laboratory abnormalities are shown in bold type in the index so that several presenting problems can be rapidly reviewed; the index is intended to be a table of differential diagnosis.*

Facts and their interrelationships are emphasized in an effort to free the student from the rote memorization of bits of unrelated information. Freed from that bondage, precious early morning hours can be spent in creative reflection and constructive synthesis. Obsession with recall of facts frequently leads young physicians to forget their primary purpose. Decisions must be ethically right as well as medically correct; only time spent with the patient can provide answers for the right decision for that particular patient at that particular time. This modern version of Osler's waistcoat notebook should provide time for talking with patients and understanding their needs.

This book draws liberally from a number of important sources including the textbooks of medicine edited by Harvey, Beeson, and Harrison; the cardiology text prepared by Braunwald; the review material developed by the American College of Physicians (Medical Knowledge Self-Assessment Program); and original articles from the medical literature. Particularly useful has been the textbook edited by Wilkins and Levinsky.

Many individual members of the Department of Medicine of Saint Louis University have served as reviewers and consultants. We especially thank Dr. Heinz Joist, Dr. Joseph Marr, and Dr. Alan Hopefl for their important contributions in specific sections of the text, and Anne Ramey and Jayma Mikes for their assistance in preparing the material for publication.

Preface to the First Edition

As characteristic of the medical resident as his curiosity, his questions, and his dedication is the loose-leaf notebook he carries. The book is his private medical text in which he notes clinical pearls, rules of thumb, diagnostic clues, seldom used and easily forgotten procedures that are of importance in emergencies, dosage of drugs, key references, summaries of his reading, and many unanswered questions that arise during his busy day. The notebook grows with time and experience, becoming more and more a reference source from which, after a careful history and physical examination, the vast number of problems encountered in resident practice are approached.

This manual is the outgrowth of many residents' notebooks. In it we endeavored to include the "heart of the matter" as it pertains to the resident in hospital practice. It is not intended to be a textbook but rather a *vade mecum* in which the resident may readily locate brief descriptions of clinical states, clues to diagnosis, and selected laboratory tests necessary to further substantiate a clinical impression arrived at by history, physical examination, logical reasoning, and experience. We have emphasized particularly those problems which from teaching experience have been found to offer difficulty. In the manual we have aimed to select and synopsize much material scattered in recent medical literature. Most topics are concluded with an up-to-date and readily available key reference that may be consulted for further study of a subject. Many commonly used abbreviations have been employed throughout the book for the sake of brevity.

We are grateful to the many members of the house and attending staff of St. Vincent's Hospital. Their encouragement and advice have been invaluable in the preparation of this manual.

FRANK B. FLOOD
RICHARD J. KENNEDY
WILLIAM J. GRACE

4
EDITION
Medical Resident's Manual

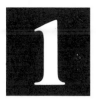

1
Cardiovascular System

CARDIAC STRUCTURE AND FUNCTION

The left ventricle, motive force of the entire cardiovascular system, may be visualized as a muscular blunt-tipped cone; the base of the cone gives rise to the atria and atrioventricular valves, and the longitudinal axis of the cone is directed downward but about 30° to the left and 30-45° anteriorly. Figure 1-1 is a cross-sectional diagram looking downward from the head and shows that the right ventricle and septum are close to the anterior chest wall. The *septum* accounts for about one third of the left ventricular wall, runs 30-45° to the left from back to front, and is bounded by the anterior and posterior descending coronary arteries. The remainder of the left ventricular circumferential wall is arbitrarily divided into *anterior* and *posterior walls* or segments; note that the anterior wall is really anterolateral. Since the apex is tipped forward, part of the circumferential wall rests on the diaphragm and is called the *inferior wall*.

These anatomic relationships are important for understanding radiographic, echocardiographic, and electrocardiographic phenomena. Figure 1-2 is a useful view obtained by rotating the left side of the chest 45° toward the observer. It looks down the septum and separates the left and right ventricles; radiographically, the left anterior oblique is suprisingly close to the echocardiographer's view of the heart. Note the conical left ventricle, septum, posterior wall, and papillary muscles. The two divisions of the left bundle terminate in the papillary muscles; since the

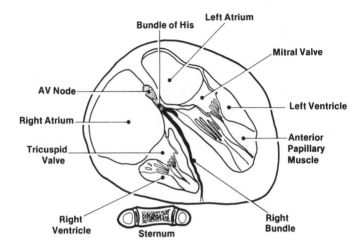

Figure 1-1. Cross-sectional view of heart looking downward from head.

anterior muscle is also superior and lateral to the posterior muscle, left anterior hemiblock produces a large R_1 and S_3 as depolarization moves superiorly and leftward.

Figure 1-3 shows that the left posterior chest rotated about 45° to the observer is the left posterior (or right anterior) oblique of the radiographer. Here one is looking at the septal wall (the view is 90°, or perpendicular to that in Figure 1-2). Note the conduction system with the His bundle penetrating the base of the heart (or cone), bifurcating at the membranous septum and giving rise to the longer right bundle and the anterior and posterior divisions of the left bundle. Note that the posterior division is related to the inflow segment, the anterior to the outflow segment.

Ventricular Function
The cardiac action potential changes sarcolemmic permeability so that sodium and calcium enter the cell rapidly; calcium is released from intracellular stores and initiates contraction by

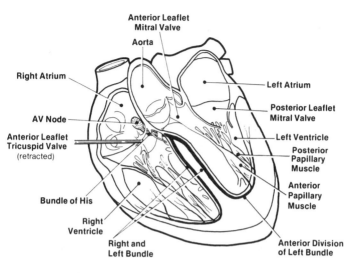

Figure 1-2. Rotating the left side of the chest 45° anteriorly separates the left and right ventricles. This view is the left anterior oblique radiographic position and is also close to the echocardiographers view of the heart.

relieving the inhibitory action of tropomyosin on actin and myosin union, and by hydrolyzing adenosine triphosphate, liberating energy. Ionized calcium is thus important for myocardial contraction. Catecholamines appear to increase contractility by augmenting calcium release from the intracellular sarcoplasmic reticulum; digitalis appears to act by inhibiting the sodium-potassium membrane pump, increasing intracellular sodium, and in some manner increasing intracellular calcium.

Stroke volume is directly related to the extent of myocardial fiber shortening and reduction in circumferential size. Diastolic inflow stretches muscle fibers, enhancing their extent of shortening (*preload*), while systolic pressure decreases their ability to shorten (*afterload*). *Contractility* implies the velocity and extent of shortening with preload and afterload held constant. About

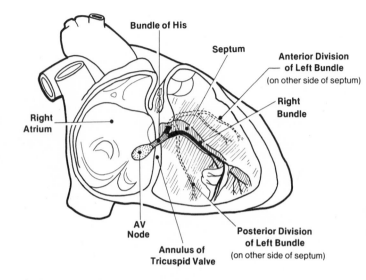

Figure 1-3. Posterior rotation of 45° provides a frontal view of the ventricular septum and conducting system. Orientation of illustration is right anterior oblique.

40-50 ml of blood remain in the ventricle after systolic ejection (residual volume). Sixty to 75 ml flow in during diastole and are ejected as the stroke volume. Ventricular dysfunction is characterized by increase in fiber length and chamber size; initially stroke output is maintained by the increase in preload associated with the increase in diastolic volume; as contractility continues to fall, stroke volume also falls.

End-diastolic pressures, measured by central venous or Swan-Ganz catheters, are used to estimate diastolic volumes. Although their use in constructing a Frank-Starling diagram provides a reasonable guide, especially when changes following fluid loading are measured, direct measurement of volume by radionuclide ventriculography shows that ventricular stiffness (compliance) complicates the relationship. The stiff ventricle of acute myocardial infarction may have a normal volume but a high pressure, while the dilated ventricle of cardiomyopathy may have a high volume but a normal pressure. Table 1-1 shows residual volumes, end-diastolic volumes, ejection fractions, and end-diastolic pressures for several typical situations.

Increasing afterload by increased systemic vascular resistance and systolic pressure decreases stroke output; the effect is minimal in the normally contractile heart but may be precipitous in individuals with poor contractility. Vasodilator therapy exploits this relationship by decreasing arterial resistance, allowing an increase in stroke output. Since arterial blood pressure is the product of cardiac output times systemic vascular resistance, it is possible for the decrease in resistance to be exactly balanced by an increase in output so that blood pressure is unaltered. In practice this ideal is rarely achieved, and some fall in blood pressure occurs.

Myocardial Oxygen Consumption

Ischemic heart disease results from an imbalance between oxygen need and oxygen availability. Coronary blood flow through rigid arterial segments is largely determined by pressure, so that a decrease in perfusion pressure must be avoided. Agents that increase systolic blood pressure, heart rate, or contractility increase oxygen consumption, and the product of heart rate and systolic pressure is commonly used as an index of this consumption. The actual tension generated by the ventricular wall is the product of systolic blood pressure and chamber diameter (Laplace law). Decreasing chamber size by use of an inotropic agent may actually decrease wall tension and oxygen consumption, even though contractility is increased. In addition, norepinephrine may improve oxygenation by increasing perfusion pressure even though increased systolic pressure increases oxygen consumption.

Treatment of Ventricular Failure

As the left ventricle dilates and fails, stroke output falls and left ventricular end-diastolic and left atrial pressure rise. This pressure rise is reflected backward to the pulmonary vascular bed. When

TABLE 1-1—LEFT VENTRICULAR VOLUMES AND PRESSURE IN DISEASE

	Residual Volume	End-Diastolic Volume	Stroke Volume	Ejection Fraction	End-Diastolic Pressure
NORMAL	40 ml	110	70	0.64	10 mm Hg
DECREASED CONTRACTILITY (EARLY)	85	140	55	0.39	18 mm Hg
DECREASED CONTRACTILITY (LATE)	210	240	30	0.13	25 mm Hg
SLIGHTLY DECREASED CONTRACTILITY WITH DECREASED VENTRICULAR COMPLIANCE	50	105	55	0.52	18 mm Hg

Ejection fraction = stroke volume divided by end-diastolic volume. Note that similar end-diastolic pressures are found with end-diastolic volumes of 140 and 105. The latter volume suggests decreased ventricular compliance.

left atrial pressure is much above 20 mm Hg, fluid accumulates in the interstitial space and ultimately in the alveoli, causing acute pulmonary edema. Pulmonary artery pressure rises in response to the increased vascular pressure within the lung, and right ventricular failure with systemic venous hypertension may follow. Clinical syndromes include congestive heart failure (left and right ventricular failure), pulmonary edema, and shock.

Many consequences of ventricular failure may be explained by the ubiquitous neurohumoral stress response. A falling aortic pressure and tissue ischemia lead to catecholamine release; decreased renal blood flow leads to renin, angiotensin, and aldosterone generation. The net effect is an increase in arterial resistance that increases afterload, an increase in venous resistance that increases fluid filtration to the tissues and favors accumulation of lung water, and an increase in salt and water retention by the kidney.

Treatment of ventricular failure includes: (1) control of underlying cause where possible, (2) enhancement of contractility, (3) reduction in arterial or venous resistance, (4) reduction of total body salt and water, and (5) reduction of body oxygen requirements by decreased activity.

Many drugs can be best understood and monitored by use of the Frank-Starling diagram, considering the problems relating end-diastolic pressure to volume. Figure 1-4 shows that nitroprusside, amrinone (a nonglycosidic inotrope), and captopril (an angiotensin-converting enzyme inhibitor) decrease left atrial pressure and increase stroke output, but by different names. Nitroglycerine, primarily a venodilator, decreases pressure but does not increase output, since it decreases preload but not afterload. Ambulatory patients should be treated with diuretics, an inotropic agent like digitalis, and a vasodilator such as prazosin, hydralazine, or captopril.

Acute pulmonary edema should be treated initially by agents that decrease lung water. Oxygen administered by mask with retard or continuous positive airway pressure (CPAP) improves systemic oxygenation and may decrease pulmonary-vascular permeability. Intermittent positive pressure breathing (IPPB) with or without retard appears to decrease venous return and

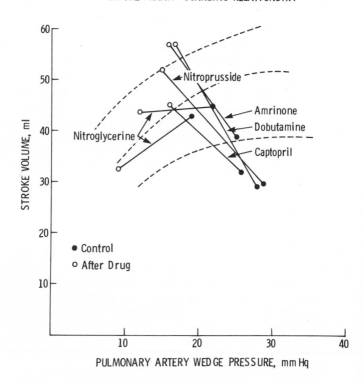

Figure 1-4. The Frank-Starling diagram with pressure instead of stroke output on the vertical axis and a group of regions or "domains" where certain pharmacologic agents are useful.

enhance lung expansion. Morphine (an alpha blocking agent) and rotating tourniquets decrease venous return. Furosemide enhances excretion of salt and water; it is also a vasodilator, decreasing lung water. Inotropic support with digitalis is useful but should be done with caution to avoid toxicity. Overly enthusiastic use of diuretics can produce hypovolemic shock.

Selection of drugs for treatment of low-output syndromes after adjustment of vascular volume to optimal levels requires consideration of underlying disease, the status of coronary arteries, permeability of microcirculation, and arterial blood pressure (coronary perfusion pressure). Table 1-2 shows the effects on key variables of a pure vasoconstrictor (angiotensin), a vasodilator (nitroprusside), a group of catecholamines, and intraaortic balloon counterpulsation (IACP). Arrows show the direction of effect; the numbers of arrows show the magnitude.

Dopamine at low doses (under 4-6 $\mu g/kg/min$) lowers vascular resistance and increases peripheral blood flow, particularly splanchnic and renal. At higher doses, its beta agonist effect becomes more important, and tachycardia is prominent. Doses high enough to raise blood pressure frequently produce tachycardia (increasing beta agonist activity), so that it is advisable to add norepinephrine to the dopamine infusion rather than increase the dopamine dosage. Norepinephrine and higher doses of dopamine increase left atrial pressure, increasing pulmonary vascular congestion; dobutamine increases cardiac output and decreases left atrial pressure. Nitroprusside may decrease blood pressure and thus decrease coronary blood flow. In general, dopamine is used when there is microcirculatory damage (septic shock), dobutamine when reduced myocardial contractility is present. Figure 1-5 shows that the Frank-Starling diagram may be used to predict physiologic indications for specific therapeutic agents. IACP increases cardiac output, decreases left atrial pressure, and increases coronary blood flow—a constellation of effects not achieved by any pharmacologic agent. Mean aortic pressure rather than cardiac output is shown since it may be measured continuously at the bedside.

ISCHEMIC HEART DISEASE
Ischemic heart disease, coronary artery disease, and atherosclerotic heart disease are all synonyms for the common form of heart disease that is the greatest cause of death in the developed

TABLE 1-2—EFFECTS OF PHARMACOLOGIC AGENTS ON KEY CARDIOVASCULAR MEASUREMENTS

	Heart Rate	Stroke Output	Wedge Pressure	Systemic Resistance	Blood Pressure	Coronary Flow
ANGIOTENSIN	○↓	↓↓	↑↑	↑↑	↑↑	↑
NOREPINEPHRINE	○↓	↑	↑	↑↑	↑↑	↑↑
ISOPROTERENOL	↑↑	↑↑	↓↑	↓↑	↓	↑
DOPAMINE—LOW	○↑	↑↑	○	↓↑	○↑	—
DOPAMINE—HIGH	↑↑	↑↑↑	↑	↓↑	↑	—
DOBUTAMINE	○↑	↑↑↑	↓↓	↓↑	○↑	—
NITROPRUSSIDE	↓	↑↑	↓↓↓	↓	↓	—
IACP	↓↓	↑↑	↓↓	↓	↑↑	↑↑

Measurements obtained in patients with low cardiac outputs, high wedge pressures and varying arterial blood pressures. IACP = intraaortic balloon counterpulsation. 1 symbol = moderate, 2 = substantial, 3 = striking.

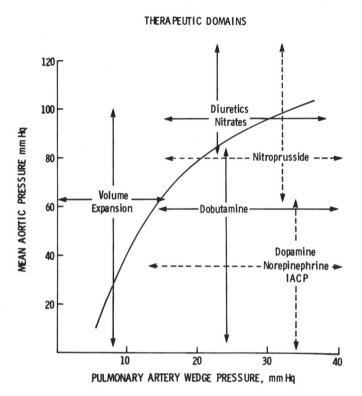

Figure 1-5. Action of a group of drugs including inotropic agents, venodilators, and arterial vasodilators on filling pressure and stroke output.

countries of the world. In the United States, about one million people die each year from cardiovascular diseases, primarily atherosclerosis. About 700,000 of these deaths are from ischemic heart disease, 200,000 from cerebrovascular disease, and 100,000 from other peripheral vascular involvement or hypertension.

Elimination of atherosclerosis would reduce mortality in the United States by almost 50%.

Atherosclerosis is a form of arteriosclerosis characterized by the local occurrence of fatty streaks and fibrous or complex plaques in many arteries, particularly the aorta, coronary and cerebral arteries, and the arteries of the lower extremity. Other forms of arteriosclerosis include: (1) age-related rigidity of arteries, (2) hyalinization, fibrous and elastic hyperplasia, and necrosis of smaller arteries, especially in hypertension (arteriolosclerosis), and (3) localized medial calcification (Monckeberg's in lower extremities and Fahr's in extracranial cerebral arteries).

Causes of Atherosclerosis

The importance of hyperlipidemia and hypertension as major risk factors suggests they play causal roles in the development of atherosclerosis. Presumably, endothelial injury due to hypertension, arteritis, or other factors invites the entry of cholesterol and other lipids into the arterial wall. Smooth muscle cells migrate to areas of injury and absorb cholesterol and triglycerides, forming foam cells that may initiate plaque formation. Platelets attempting to stanch endothelial tears aggregate and release vasoconstrictor agents such as thromboxane A2 and serotonin, reducing blood flow and providing a focus for the subsequent entry of lipid.

Lipoproteins. Blood lipids are heterogenous complexes of triglycerides, cholesterol, phospholipids, and free fatty acids, all bound to plasma proteins. Termed lipoproteins, they may be classified on the basis of their relative densities on ultracentrifugation or on the electrophoretic mobility of their apoproteins.

Chylomicra, the lightest lipoproteins, are composed mostly of triglyceride and do not migrate electrophoretically. They transport lipid from the gut to the liver, adipose tissue, and any tissue containing an active lipoprotein-lipase enzyme system.

Very low-density lipoproteins (VLDL) are the next lightest, have a high concentration of triglyceride with smaller amounts of cholesterol and phospholipid, and migrate with the pre-beta plasma proteins. They transport lipids that are synthesized by the liver.

Low density lipoproteins (LDL) transport most of the plasma cholesterol and migrate with the beta plasma proteins. They enter cells via an LDL receptor and are able to turn off subsequent synthesis of cholesterol by a negative feedback mechanism. A decrease in receptors leads to a back-up of plasma cholesterol and an increase in synthesis because of the absence of negative feedback.

High-density lipoproteins (HDL) are rich in phospholipid and migrate with the alpha plasma proteins. They appear to reduce entry of cholesterol into tissue, in part by transferring an unsaturated fatty acid group to LDL cholesterol.

Abnormalities of blood lipids appear to be important risk factors for atherosclerosis. They may arise from genetic or dietary factors; usually a combination of both is operative. *Hypercholesterolemia* in the presence of normal or moderately elevated triglyceride is due to an increase in LDL and is termed type II hyperlipoproteinemia. The familial form is associated with xanthomata and corneal arcus. *Hypertriglyceridemia* with a slightly increased cholesterol concentration indicates an increase in VLDL and is the most common type of hyperlipoproteinemia. While it may be genetic, it is commonly related to hormonal, emotional and dietary factors. The Fredrickson classification is presented in Table 1-3. In most individuals, measurement of cholesterol and triglycerides together with inspection of the serum is sufficient for diagnosis.

Therapy is based on the type of lipoprotein present in excess. An increase in VLDL (hypertriglyceridemia) is treated by weight reduction and decrease in alcohol and carbohydrate consumption, the major precursors of VLDL. Drugs that decrease lipoprotein synthesis such as nicotinic acid and clofibrate are useful; nicotinic acid is the only available agent that will also increase HDL, clofibrate must be used with caution in other situations since it may increase the concentration of LDL.

An increase in LDL (hypercholesterolemia) is treated by reducing dietary cholesterol to below 300 mg each day and adherence to a diet with a polyunsaturated to saturated fat ratio

TABLE 1-3—CLASSIFICATION OF THE HYPERLIPIDEMIAS

	I	II
LIPOPROTEIN, CHOLESTEROL (C), AND TRIGLYCERIDE (TG) ABNORMALITIES	Dietary excess causes increase in TG-rich chylomicra	Increased LDL C; type A has normal TG; type B has slight increase
CAUSE	Deficiency of lipoprotein lipase; familial predisposition	Deficiency of LDL receptor. Dominant trait but also with myxedema, nephrosis, and liver disease
SERUM APPEARANCE	Milky	Clear
PAPER ELECTROPHORESIS	Chylomicrons increased, all others decreased	Beta markedly increased, pre-beta slightly increased or normal
CLINICAL FEATURES	Xanthomas, lipemia retinalis, abdominal pain, hepatosplenomegaly	Xanthomas, corneal arcus
ORIGIN	Genetic	Genetic (dominant), sporadic
FREQUENCY	Rarest	Relatively common

III	IV	V
C esters and TG	Increased VLDL TG; slight increase in C	Increased TG; normal C
Deficiency of apoprotein EIII of VLDL, recessive trait	Unknown	Perhaps increased hepatic synthesis of VLDL and decreased chylomicra clearance. Seen with diabetes, pancreatitis, nephrosis, alcoholic liver disease
Turbid	Turbid	Turbid or milky
Broad beta, pre-beta slightly increased or normal	Pre-beta markedly increased	Chylomicrons present, pre-beta increased
Xanthomas, glucose tolerance decreased	Glucose tolerance decreased	Abdominal pain
Genetic (recessive), sporadic	Genetic, sporadic	Probably genetic
Relatively uncommon	Most common	Uncommon

of 2:1. Cholestyramine, colestipol, and D-thyroxine increase lipoprotein catabolism and will reduce LDL. The former two drugs are bile acid sequestrants that may increase the concentration of VLDL.

Mixed abnormalities are treated by combined therapy.

Clinical Presentation
RISK FACTORS
The Framingham study demonstrated important correlations among ischemic heart disease, and hypercholesterolemia, hypertension, diabetes, and cigarette smoking. Recent studies have pointed to a protective effect of HDL; exercise and the moderate use of alcohol seem to increase HDL. HDL is 20% lower in men than in premenopausal women, and, in some studies, is an accurate predictor of atherosclerosis. Oral contraceptives increase the risk of ischemic heart disease, particularly when associated with cigarette smoking. Estrogens appear to increase thrombogenicity but also increase HDL; progestins, in contrast, decrease HDL. A strong family history in the absence of other risk factors also predicts the development of ischemic heart disease.

CLINICAL SYNDROMES
Coronary artery disease is found in more than 75% of autopsies and is severe in more than half of these. Angina pectoris is not a sensitive indicator of its presence, occurring in less than one third of those found to have coronary artery disease at autopsy. The clinical expression may be seen in the modes of death observed in an autopsy study of more than 1000 individuals dying in Rochester, Minnesota, between 1947 and 1952; the autopsy rate was 73%. In those individuals with coronary disease identified at autopsy, the following syndromes were observed: sudden death, 45%; acute myocardial infarction, 39%; congestive heart failure, 14%; thromboembolism, 4%. Sudden cardiac death in individuals without recognized angina is the most common expression of coronary artery disease.

Diagnosis

Asymptomatic but high-risk individuals or those with chest pain.
While classic angina pectoris is not a sensitive indicator of
coronary artery disease, it is reasonably specific. Proudfit et al.
found that 94% of patients with "typical" angina and 65% of
those with "atypical" angina had significant coronary disease
identified at arteriography; 96% of those thought to be normal
and 81% of those listed as probably normal had relatively normal
coronary arteries.

An exercise test with achievement of a heart rate that is 90% of
predicted is useful if integrated with other clinical data. An ST
segment depression of 1 mm or more, horizontal or downsloping
in appearance and lasting for 0.08 seconds after the J point, is
commonly used as a positive end-point. Even more useful may be
the workload required to produce ST segment depression, the
appearance of typical ischemic chest pain, and the persistence of
ST segment depression for several minutes. Normal individuals
increase blood pressure with exercise; a decrease in pressure
suggests abnormal left ventricular function and the presence of
multiple vessel disease. A recent multiinstitutional study showed
that a positive test defined as 1 mm depression yielded the
following results in more than 2000 individuals later evaluated by
coronary arteriography: sensitivity, 80% in males and 76% in
females; specificity, 74% in males, and 64% in females. In almost
all studies, sex is an important predictive factor.

In individual patients, thallium imaging provides important
additional information. This isotope accumulates in normal
myocardial cells in a manner similar to that of potassium. When
injected during exercise just before maximal exertion, it identifies
ischemic regions or "cold spots." Several hours later, redistribution of tracer occurs and thallium now enters previously ischemic
areas; a persistent thallium defect suggests a fibrotic scar rather
than acute ischemia. False-negatives occur in 10-40% of individuals with proved coronary artery disease; false-positives are
unusual.

The data in Tables 1-4 and 1-5 from 65 patients with suspected
coronary artery disease studied by Holman et al. demonstrates

TABLE 1-4—POSITIVE EKG STRESS TEST

Thallium positive	66%	
Arteriography positive		100%
Thallium negative	34%	
Arteriography negative		80%

TABLE 1-5—NEGATIVE EKG STRESS TEST

Thallium negative	62%	
Arteriography negative		77%
Thallium positive	38%	
Arteriography positive		75%

the advantage of combining exercise electrocardiography with exercise thallium imaging.

A combination of a positive EKG plus thallium stress test was 100% successful in predicting coronary artery disease; a negative EKG plus thallium test was only 77% successful in predicting the absence of coronary disease.

Since the presence of risk factors including sex are much more predictive than either EKG or thallium testing, it is probably prudent to limit screening to males over 40, females over 50, and others with significant risk factors. Coronary arteriography is indicated in patients with typical angina, patients following acute myocardial infarction (4-6 weeks later), those with atypical chest pain but positive stress tests, and probably those who are asymptomatic but have both positive EKG and thallium tests.

Presumed ischemic pain for 30 minutes or more suggests a group of patients variously labeled as the intermediate syndrome, crescendo angina, or unstable angina. Usually ST segment abnormalities are visualized. Such patients should be monitored electrocardiographically to eliminate the possibility of transmural or subendocardial infarction. Most of these patients should be studied by coronary arteriography, although some will have normal coronary arteries. In general, prolonged ischemic-type chest pain suggests either severe disease or no coronary disease at all.

Variant (Prinzmetal) angina. Ischemic chest pain, occurring mainly at rest, not precipitated by exertion or emotional stress, associated with ventricular arrhythmias and conduction disturbances, exhibiting ST segment elevation instead of depression, and responding to nitroglycerine is thought to be due to coronary arterial spasm. Spasm may occur either in patients with severe coronary arterial stenoses or in those with normal coronary arteries. The administration of ergonovine maleate during angiocardiography will frequently provoke coronary arterial spasm.

Coronary arterial spasm may also occur in patients with typical angina pectoris. Humoral vasoconstrictor agents or alpha adrenergic stimulation may be responsible, although proof of the precise mediators is absent. Propranolol may unmask alpha adrenergic activity by blocking beta activity and may provoke spasm in some individuals. Nitroglycerine and calcium inhibitors appear to be useful agents for coronary spasm.

Acute myocardial infarction. Diagnosis is based on a typical history with electrocardiographic changes and typical appearance and disappearance of abnormal concentrations of CPK, SGOT, and LDH enzymes. SGOT and CPK reach peak levels in 24-48 hours and fall to normal in 3-4 days. LDH rises during the first 24 hours, peaks at 3-4 days, and falls to normal in 14 days. CPK is most specific, since it is found only in heart and skeletal muscle and in the brain. GOT is found in heart, skeletal muscle, liver, and red blood cells; the extremely high levels found in acute myocardial infarction with shock are due to centrilobular hepatic necrosis. A small infarction will sometimes increase enzyme concentrations two- or threefold without reaching the upper limit of normal. A typical rise and fall is highly suggestive of infarction even if levels are not particularly high. CPK isoenzymes are useful in patients with skeletal muscle or brain damage; the MB isoenzyme is found only in the myocardium.

Electrocardiographic evolution with ST segment elevation shortly followed by the appearance of pathologic Q waves and later by ST segment depression and T wave inversion indicate a transmural myocardial infarction. Enzyme abnormalities together with ST-T segment changes but without Q waves suggest a subendocardial myocardial infarction. While many of these patients do not appear as sick as those with transmural infarction, the ultimate mortality is about the same.

Scanning with Technetium-99m stannous pyrophosphate is useful when the electrocardiographic diagnosis is obscured by conduction defects such as left bundle branch block. Since the tracer is attracted to areas of necrosis or fibrosis, a positive finding ("hot" spot) is not specific for acute infarction.

Ischemic cardiomyopathy. Evidence of significant left ventricular failure without a moderately large Q wave area in the electrocardiogram usually suggests diffuse cardiomyopathy—not ischemic disease. Occasionally, diffuse abnormalities may occur, especially in diabetics, without angina pectoris or a typical electrocardiogram. Echocardiography or radionuclide ventriculography may reveal segmental dysfunction, distinguishing ischemic left ventricular failure from that due to other causes.

Treatment

Angina pectoris. Sublingual nitroglycerine is the mainstay of pharmacologic therapy, and there is no evidence that sublingual isosorbide dinitrate or erythrityl tetranitrate are superior. The two latter preparations are also available in oral preparations, but gastrointestinal degradation makes prediction of blood levels unreliable. Nitrates produce arterial and venous dilatation; venous dilatation decreases venous return to the heart and reduces diastolic size and filling pressure. Blood flow is redistributed to ischemic areas and to the subendocardium. This effect may be due to a direct action on collaterals and to a decrease in transmural pressure related to a decrease in diastolic chamber pressure. Nitroglycerine deteriorates so that fresh supplies should be available for optimal activity. Patients should be encouraged to use nitroglycerine *before* engaging in physical activity that might produce chest pain. Propranolol or other beta adrenergic blocking agents are frequently given together with nitrates and appear to have an additive effect (see autonomic changes, p. 7).

Accumulating evidence suggests that aortocoronary bypass surgery markedly improves the quality of life by increasing tolerable activity; it also probably increases life expectancy. Increasing left ventricular dysfunction increases operative mortality, but successful surgery also seems to improve left ventricular function. Overall mortality is below 2% in many centers, and graft patency above 85%. Recent published reports have emphasized that the number of procedures performed in a given institution have a direct effect on operative mortality, the lowest mortality rates occurring with centers performing more than 200 bypass procedures yearly.

Acute myocardial infarction. The ischemic and necrotic regions of the myocardium produce electrical instability leading to dysrhythmias and loss of contractile tissue leading to ventricular dysfunction. Therapy has evolved dramatically over the past two decades, and the introduction of the coronary care unit reduced inpatient mortality from 30 to 15% by the early recognition and treatment of dysrhythmias. Continuing changes in therapy can best be evaluated by understanding a group of principles that underlie development of treatment techniques.

Early and vigorous treatment is necessary, since 65% of deaths occur in the first hour of infarction and 85% within the first 24 hours. Acute myocardial infarction is not a homogenous disease; mortality rates and treatment vary with age, status of coronary arteries, ventricular function, location of infarction, underlying autonomic status, and associated diseases. The Killip clinical classification (Class I, no left ventricular (LV) failure; Class II, evidence of LV dysfunction with rales less than one third of lung fields; Class III, pulmonary edema; Class IV, shock) is useful but not specific for subsequent events, even though group mortality rises from under 3% in Class I to over 90% in Class IV. Hemodynamic, myocardial metabolic, and ventriculographic studies reveal a variety of abnormalities that do not predict clinical class but have important consequences for short- and long-term mortality and morbidity. For many individuals, the episode of infarction is but one event in the continuing process of chronic ischemic heart disease; it is an episode that has important implications for subsequent function because of its destruction of ventricular tissue.

Treatment directed to one problem may aggravate another, so that priorities must be continually and explicitly stated. Problems requiring priority setting include: (1) life-threatening dysrhythmias, (2) oxygen requirements of the myocardium as determined by heart rate, blood pressure, contractile state, and ventricular dimensions, (3) pulmonary venous hypertension with accumulation of lung water, and (4) perfusion of vital structures such as brain, liver, splanchnic bed, and kidneys. Note that the last two problems reflect ventricular dysfunction.

The routine use of either intramuscular lidocaine (300 mg) or multiple boluses every 5 minutes until ventricular ectopy is controlled appears effective. All patients should receive oxygen by face mask or nasal cannula (flow rate, 5 liters/min) for 4 or 5 days, because hypoxemia is common and an index of pulmonary congestion. In spite of certain studies suggesting cost-ineffectiveness, patients should be admitted to a coronary care unit for continuous electrocardiographic monitoring. A catheter should be introduced through a peripheral vein into intrathoracic veins for administration of drugs, and the patient should be placed in bed. If ventricular dysfunction is not present, several periods of chair rest may be introduced early in the hospital course. Oxygen requirements should be kept at a minimum by avoiding unnecessary exertion; assistance with feeding and bathing and the use of a bedside commode are important. Pain should be controlled by frequent, small intravenous doses (2 mg) of morphine; propranolol reduces increased sympathetic activity and is probably indicated if left ventricular function is clinically normal, asthma and diabetes are not present, and the pulse rate is above 75 beats per minute. Anticoagulants have not been shown to reduce mortality but do reduce the incidence of thromboembolic complications and are indicated during the initial 2 weeks in patients with left ventricular failure, poor cardiac output, and pulmonary congestion or edema (Killip Classes III and IV).

Cardiac dysrhythmias in acute myocardial infarction. Tachyarrhythmias must be treated quickly because they increase myocardial oxygen requirements; conduction disturbances are potentially lethal because they may reflect extensive myocardial damage. The more remote the infarct area from the conduction system (as in anterolateral infarction), the larger the area of ischemia if the patients manifest conduction defects. In general, ventricular dysrhythmias reflect an irritable myocardium while atrial dysrhythmias, particularly in anterolateral myocardial infarction, reflect left ventricular and left atrial dilatation. For details of treatment see page 35.

Ventricular failure in acute myocardial infarction. Although electrical instability is more obvious clinically, almost all patients have some evidence of ventricular dysfunction, usually left ventricular. Left ventricular ejection fractions are reduced by more than 30% even in Killip Class I patients. The modifying factor in acute myocardial infarction is the tendency of pharmacologic agents that increase contractility to increase myocardial oxygen requirements also. Oxygen requirements are related to aortic blood pressure and ventricular dimensions by the LaPlace law: the larger the ventricle, the greater the wall tension and the oxygen required. Inotropic interventions that reduce ventricular size may reduce oxygen requirements, emphasizing the need for early attention to ventricular dysfunction in acute myocardial infarction. Intraaortic balloon counterpulsation is an ideal approach because it increases cardiac output, reduces myocardial oxygen requirements, and increases coronary blood flow (see ventricular function, page 9).

Other complications. Although not a complication, *right ventricular infarction* (diagnosed by finding a high right atrial pressure and a lower wedge pressure) produces right ventricular failure. *Thromboembolism* may occur in up to 25% of patients. Preventive measures include anticoagulation with coumadin derivatives or low-dose heparin and regular active contraction of leg muscles while in bed or early chair rest. *Cardiac rupture* occurs during the early days of infarction and is more common with increasing age. *Septal perforation* is diagnosed by an increase of oxygen concentration in the pulmonary artery due to a left to right shunt. *Acute mitral regurgitation* is caused by necrosis of the mitral valve apparatus and diagnosed by a suddenly appearing apical systolic murmur without a pulmonary artery oxygen step-up, require immediate cardiac surgery. Since both imply considerable left ventricular damage, prognosis may be determined more by surviving ventricular tissue than by the hemodynamic insult of ventricular septal defect or mitral regurgitation.

Three synovial syndromes may occur during the course of acute myocardial infarction. *Pericarditis* with friction rub may occur within the first few days and produce characteristic pain, which may be confused with ischemic pain. *Dressler's syndrome* occurs 1 to 6 weeks after infarction and is probably an autoimmune pericarditis, pleuritis, and pneumonitis. Anticoagulants should be avoided in both forms of pericarditis. The *shoulder-hand syndrome* occurs at a variable time and is of uncertain etiology. Early mobilization decreases its incidence, suggesting it may be due to inactivity; reflex vascular changes in the region of referred cardiac pain or autoimmune synovitis could also play a role.

Treatment after Acute Myocardial Infarction

Acute myocardial infarction serves to identify a large population of individuals with symptomatic coronary artery disease. A structured post-infarction treatment program should include:

1. Classification of status by 24-hour electrocardiographic monitoring and submaximal stress testing.
2. Dietary control directed to overall weight and to lipid abnormalities.
3. Graded exercise program based on results of electrocardiographic testing.
4. Control of hypertension if present.
5. Use of drugs such as propranolol, sulfinpyrazone, or aspirin.

Unfortunately, the value of pharmacologic intervention is not yet settled, but considerable new information suggests specific agents may be useful. Several studies showed that beta blockade might be useful in reducing postinfarction mortality in several situations; suprisingly, mortality was reduced in anterolateral but not in inferior wall infarctions, and in patients under but not over 65 years of age.

Sulfinpyrazone, a uricosuric agent used for the treatment of gout, was randomized with placebo to 1558 patients. The drug was begun soon after recovery from acute myocardial infarction and exhibited a striking effect in reducing sudden cardiovascular deaths, particularly in the first 6 months. Total cardiovascular deaths were 10.3% for placebo and 5.0% for drug at 6 months; an additional 4.1% of placebo patients and 3.7% of drug patients died within the subsequent 18 months. There was no difference, however, in deaths from acute myocardial infarction. The drug inhibits platelet aggregation, but the effect on the reduction of sudden death rather than death from acute myocardial infarction suggests that some other effect on electrical stability might be operative.

The aspirin data are less clear. Earlier studies showed that aspirin protected against stroke in men but not in women. Elwood et al. administered 300 mg per day of aspirin or placebo to a randomized group of individuals soon after myocardial infarction (a design similar to the sulfinpyrazone study) and demonstrated a decrease in mortality and readmission to the hospital with aspirin in nonfatal myocardial infarction. The recently reported study of the Aspirin Myocardial Infarction Study Group (AMIS) failed to identify improved survival with aspirin; at 6 months, the total mortality was approximately 2%, and at 24 months, 6%. The substantially lower mortality in placebo patients compared to the sulfinpyrazone placebo group is probably related to the experimental design, which permitted admission of patients up to 8 months after infarction. It is likely that the AMIS study "missed" the high mortality period of the first 6 months and actually analyzed the lower mortality observed in the subsequent 30 months. The incidence of nonfatal infarction was reduced by aspirin.

While both aspirin and sulfinpyrazone may be effective in reducing mortality after acute myocardial infarction, the mechanisms of action are not clear. Aspirin does produce significant side effects including gastrointestinal bleeding, while the complications associated with sulfinpyrazone therapy appear trivial.

CARDIOMYOPATHIES

Biventricular failure, conduction disturbances, and dysrhythmias
are characteristic manifestations of disease mainly affecting the
myocardium. In an earlier era, they were diagnosed as chronic
myocarditis or coronary artery disease. Diagnostic evaluation
usually shows global ventricular dysfunction, normal coronary
arteries, and physical findings of akinetic heart activity without
striking murmurs but with S3 and S4 cardiac sounds.

The cardiomyopathies may be classified etiologically or functionally. Primary cardiomyopathies indicate a cardiac abnormality without other systemic disease, while secondary cardiomyopathies indicate the cardiac manifestations of systemic disease.
Pathologic findings may include: (1) infiltration of some cellular
or acellular material, (2) destruction of myocardial muscle, or (3)
abnormal structure or function of myocardium, perhaps from
genetic or acquired problems with protein synthesis. Functional
classification is based on the predominant hemodynamic abnormality: ventricular dilatation with congestive consequences
(congestive cardiomyopathy), restrictive cardiomyopathy, or outflow track obstruction (obstructive cardiomyopathy). A variety
of primary and secondary factors may produce congestive cardiomyopathy. Obstructive cardiomyopathy is typified by the
genetically determined syndrome with asymmetric septal hypertrophy and myocardial fiber disarray, although other diseases
can produce a similar syndrome. Restrictive cardiomyopathies
overlap the other two types, but isolated restriction—a situation
resembling constrictive pericarditis with impaired filling, normal
early but elevated late diastolic pressures, and normal systolic
ejection—is limited to conditions such as Loeffler's eosinophilic
endocarditis and nontropical endomyocardial fibrosis. Isolated
restrictive disease implies either endocardial or pericardial rigidity with normal myocardial contractility.

Etiologic Considerations

While etiologic diagnoses are often ignored, the distribution of
causes is probably similar to that reported by Brigden in his
classic description of the "noncoronary cardiomyopathies" in

1957. Of 42 patients in whom diagnosis was possible, 7 had familial heart disease, 8 had infectious myocarditis, 3 were postpartum, 7 had primary amyloidosis, and 13 were severe alcoholics. One had acromegaly, emphasizing that many diseases can produce cardiomyopathy. The use of endomyocardial biopsy for evaluation of these patients should lead to more precise etiologic diagnosis.

Viral agents. These may produce direct myocardial damage (more than one-third of individuals dying during an influenza pandemic have myocarditis) or, following a lag period, produce damage by an immunologic mechanism. The Stanford cardiology group described ten patients with round-cell inflammatory changes found by endomyocardial biopsy; a number of these were dramatically improved by immunosuppressive drugs. The possible importance of an abnormal immune response is suggested by the finding that patients with cardiomyopathy following a viral-like illness had abnormalities of suppressor cell function so that a cytotoxic or "killer" T cell might emerge following viral stimulation.

One of the most common viral agents is coxsackie B virus; members of the B group (easily cultured and identified serologically compared to the A group) produce an acute illness with fever, chest pain, cardiomegaly, and elevation of sedimentation rate that may mimic rheumatic carditis and may be prolonged or produce chronic cardiac manifestations. Other infective agents include influenza A_2 virus, arbovirus, adenovirus, echovirus, and *Mycoplasma pneumoniae.* Toxoplasma and aspergillus myocarditis are found in immunosuppressed patients. Infectious mononucleosis can produce a syndrome that mimics acute myocardial infarction, and conduction defects have been observed to persist after infection with that agent. In Central and South America, Chagas's disease (*Trypanosoma cruzi*) commonly produces chronic myocarditis; diphtheria produces a severe myocarditis that may be fatal.

Drugs. A number of drugs produce myocardial depression. Cyclophosphamide, daunorubicin, and adriamycin are cancer chemotherapeutic agents known to be cardiotoxic; since radiation therapy in excess of 4000 rads produces pericardial and myocardial changes, combined therapy must be monitored with care. The problem of developing heart disease in the cancer patient is further complicated by the frequency of myocardial involvement in Hodgkin's disease (25%), the leukemias (37%), malignant melanoma (60%), and metastatic disease, particularly of the breast and lung.

Other cardiotoxic drugs include alpha methyl dopa, the amphetamines, tricyclic antidepressants, phenothiazines, and emetine. Many of these are either sympatholytic or sympathomimetic, suggesting that a change in catecholamine activity may play an important role in determining drug toxicity. Isoproterenol produces myocardial necrosis when given experimentally; beta blockade produces ventricular depression in individuals with preexisting cardiovascular disease.

Alcoholism. Alcoholism is a causal factor in up to one third of individuals with cardiomyopathy. Although it is directly toxic to the myocardium, its effects were confused with those of nutritional deficiency, leading to the term "occidental beri-beri." True thiamine deficiency does occur in alcoholics and leads to severe high-output failure that responds to thiamine administration. More common is the cardiomyopathic low-output failure that is seen in alcoholics with relatively normal nutritional state. Alcoholics can also drink other cardiotoxic materials either added by the manufacturer or obtained from other sources during binge drinking. The cobalt beer-drinkers syndrome of the mid-1960s resulted from the use of cobalt as a foam stabilizer and led to a substantial number of deaths in Quebec, Omaha, and Minneapolis; it is no longer added to beer.

Alcoholics without evidence of heart disease exhibit abnormalities at cardiac catheterization or by noninvasive testing, emphasizing that cardiomyopathy may be latent for varying periods of time; abnormalities in systolic time intervals are more common in male alcoholics, suggesting a sexual predilection. Administration of one cocktail increased cardiac output in normal subjects but decreased output in patients with heart disease of varying etiology. Histologic abnormalities are found in the hearts of 90% of alcoholics randomly studied at autopsy. Dogs deriving one third of their total daily calories from alcohol for 7-33 months developed bradycardia, prolongation of H-V intervals, and myocardial accumulation of glycoprotein and lipid. Biochemical studies show that alcohol interferes with calcium binding by the sarcoplasmic reticulum and with mitochondrial function. Even severe forms of alcoholic cardiomyopathy can be reversed by complete abstention from alcohol.

Relationships with skeletal myopathies. Since striated muscle is found in both cardiac and voluntary muscle, such relationships have been observed. Abnormalities involving enzymes, mitochondria, or contractile proteins could affect both types of muscle. Cardiomyopathy is found with muscular dystrophy, myotonic dystrophy, Friedreich's ataxia, Refsum's disease, and spinal atrophy; in Refsum's disease, the common problem is the accumulation of an abnormal lipid (phytanic acid) throughout the body. In Friedreich's ataxia, there is both neural and myocardial degeneration, and in the others there may be shared abnormalities in contractile protein function. Smith et al. demonstrated that most patients with hypertrophic cardiomyopathy had electromyographic or morphologic abnormalities in skeletal muscle. Occasionally, rhabdomyolysis of skeletal muscle and acute cardiomyopathy may be seen with alcoholism.

Hypertrophic Cardiomyopathy

Known also as idiopathic hypertrophic subaortic stenosis (IHSS), patients with this form of disease share striking myocardial abnormalities with disarray of myofibrillar architecture and the presence of hypertrophied and bizarre muscle cells. Since the disease is frequently familial, abnormal protein synthesis due to faulty DNA coding may be responsible. There is marked left ventricular hypertrophy, particularly of the septum with a normal or small ventricular cavity; the cavity may obliterate almost completely with systole, leading to outflow or midventricular obstruction. While some patients have hypertrophy without outflow obstruction, the disease is probably similar to subaortic stenosis. In the latter, histologic abnormalities are most obvious

TABLE 1-6—COMPARISON OF CLINICAL FINDINGS—HYPERTROPHIC MUSCULAR SUBAORTIC STENOSIS (IHSS) VS. VALVULAR AORTIC STENOSIS (AS)

	IHSS	AS
DOUBLE APICAL IMPULSE	Characteristic	Infrequent
PROMINENT JUGULAR A WAVE	Frequent	Infrequent
SYSTOLIC THRILL	Less frequent	Common
PARADOXICAL SPLITTING	More frequent	Less frequent
SINGLE SECOND SOUND	Less frequent	More frequent
ATRIAL GALLOP	Frequent	Infrequent
SYSTOLIC EJECTION MURMUR	At left sternal border or apex, increased by Valsalva M	At base or neck Decreased or unchanged by Valsalva M
SYSTOLIC EJECTION SOUND	Unusual	Common unless valve is calcified

DIASTOLIC MURMUR	Usually absent	Frequent
ARTERIAL PULSE	Rapid rise and bifid	Slow rise
PULSE PRESSURE	Increased or normal	Decreased or normal
X-RAY—INTRACARDIAC CALCIFICATION AND AORTIC DILATATION	Usually negative	Frequently positive
ELECTROCARDIOGRAM	Evidence of biatrial and biventricular hypertrophy, Frequent delta waves and abnormal Q waves	Mainly left ventricular hypertrophy with ST and T wave abnormalities
ANGINA AND SYNCOPE	Onset soon after exertion	Onset during exertion

in the septum, and the free wall of the left ventricle may be
relatively spared. The unusual ventricular architecture leads to
systolic anterior motion of the mitral valve, impairment of
ventricular filling, and mitral regurgitation.

Electrocardiographic evidence of left ventricular hypertrophy
and a basal systolic ejection murmur may lead to confusion with
valvular aortic stenosis. Differential characteristics are shown in
Table 1-6.

Angina, syncope, sudden death, and left ventricular failure are
common in both forms of outflow obstruction, so that differentiation is important.

The diagnosis may be further supported by maneuvers that
increase the outflow gradient and the systolic murmur. Inotropic
agents such as isoproterenol, vasodilators like amyl nitrate, and
hypotension from any cause increase the gradient. A Valsalva
maneuver increases while a Mueller maneuver decreases the
gradient.

Identification of outflow track obstruction in patients with
cardiomyopathy has important implications for therapy. Vigorous diuresis, digitalis, nitroglycerine, and isoproterenol must be
avoided. Beta blockade with propranolol and restriction of
activity are useful if symptomatology is present. Surgical intervention with septal myotomy and myectomy produces symptomatic relief, but the global obstructive myopathy persists and life
may not be extended.

Prognosis is difficult to ascertain because of the wide variability
in symptomatology. A normal electrocardiogram suggests an
excellent prognosis, while evidence of left ventricular hypertrophy
indicates elevation of left ventricular end-diastolic pressure, presence of a substantial outflow gradient, anterior mitral valve
movement in systole, mitral regurgitation, and papillary muscle
hypertrophy. Significant Q waves are common and reflect septal
hypertrophy but may mimic myocardial infarction. Studies from
Goodwin's group estimated total mortality at 15% at 5 years,
35% at 10 years, and 56% at 15 years. Patients die from either
congestive failure or sudden death associated with ventricular
arrhythmias.

Cardiomyopathy and Systemic Disease

Occasionally, left ventricular failure, arrhythmias, or conduction defects may be the first evidence of generalized disease.

Primary amyloidosis. This may account for 5-10% of patients with cardiomyopathy. Termed an acquired systemic beta fibrillosis by Glenner, it produces conduction disturbances and either a restrictive or congestive cardiomyopathy, peripheral neuropathy, autonomic disturbances, arthropathy, macroglossia, isolated factor X deficiency, and carpal tunnel syndromes. It may also produce pulmonary hypertension from vascular deposits, valvular abnormalities, arrhythmias, and conduction disturbances. Most but not all patients have monoclonal immunoglobulins present. The Congo red uptake test is unreliable, and diagnosis is best made by biopsy of rectal submucosal tissue (positive in 75-85%), gingiva, or skin. Secondary amyloidosis follows chronic infection or rheumatoid arthritis. Myocardial involvement is rare, and the amyloid is deposited in liver, spleen, and kidneys. Fifty percent of individuals over the age of 90 have infiltration of the myocardium by an unusual amyloid substance that produces electrocardiographic abnormalities and ventricular failure—senile cardiac amyloidosis. See page 292.

Sarcoidosis. Rarely, sarcoidosis may involve the heart and produce cardiomegaly, congestive failure, arrhythmias, conduction disturbances, and sudden death. Pulmonary hypertension from severe pulmonary disease may produce cor pulmonale.

Hemochromatosis. Like amyloidosis and sarcoidosis, hemochromatosis may infiltrate the myocardium and produce the findings of cardiomyopathy. Cardiac involvement occurs in 15% of patients, and the diagnosis should be considered when cardiomyopathy occurs together with hepatomegaly, skin pigmentation, diabetes, arthritis, and evidence of gonadal atrophy. Elevated plasma iron, transferrin saturation, serum ferritin, and urinary excretion of iron following administration of an iron chelating agent (desferrioxamine, 0.5 gm I.M.) support the diagnosis, which may be confirmed by a liver biopsy showing extensive deposits of parenchymal iron. Alcoholic cirrhosis may also be associated with iron deposition and may present with cardiomyopathy; the distinction is sometimes difficult, but the greater the iron deposition relative to the degree of fibrosis, the more likely the diagnosis is hemochromatosis.

Collagen diseases. These may involve the myocardium extensively without causing cardiomegaly, congestive failure, or QRS and T wave abnormalities in the electrocardiogram. Fifty to 80% of patients with systemic lupus have cardiovascular abnormalities, and more refined studies have shown ventricular dysfunction in individuals without obvious clinical evidence of heart disease.p Decreased coronary vascular reserve has been demonstrated and may be due to vasculitis or to perivascular infiltration. Pericarditis is common, and endocardial involvement may produce aortic or mitral disease.

A group of unusual infiltrative diseases may produce cardiomyopathy: Whipple's disease with infiltration of PAS-positive laden macrophages, Hunter-Hurler syndrome with mucopolysaccharide, and Pompe's disease with glycogen deposition due to acid maltase deposition.

Diagnosis of Cardiomyopathies

Echocardiography reveals diminished septal and posterior left ventricular wall motion, while usually some segment of ventricular wall moves normally in individuals with ischemic cardiomyopathy. Usually both walls visualized are equal in size; asymmetric septal hypertrophy is diagnosed when the ventricular septum is 1.3 times or more greater in thickness than the posterobasal ventricular wall. Thallium radionuclide ventriculography is superior to blood pool scanning for the evaluation of hypertrophic cardiomyopathy, since it visualizes myocardial muscle, while the latter technique is a useful way to distinguish the global dysfunction of cardiomyopathy from the segmental dysfunction of ischemic disease. Both echocardiography and thallium scanning have shown that concentric left ventricular hypertrophy produces similar but increased thickness of septal, basal, and midposterior ventricular walls, while an increase in septal size relative to other left ventricular wall measurements suggests outflow obstruction. In nonobstructive hypertrophic cardiomyopathy, the basal portion is thinner than other segments, suggesting that it hypertrophies in response to increased outflow resistance. Echocardiography appears to be a valuable technique for the study of preclinical cardiomyopathy; Boreret al. found major abnormalities in 19 patients with diseases known to produce restrictive myopathy (amyloid, idiopathic hypereosinophilic syndrome, iron overload from blood transfusions). All but five of these were normal clinically in terms of heart disease.

CARDIAC ARRHYTHMIAS

Electrophysiologic studies on isolated and intact cardiac tissue together with pharmacologic studies on animals and humans provide a rational approach for treating cardiac arrhythmias. Although trial and error is still necessary, understanding of physiologic principles minimizes the use of agents with little chance for success.

Look at the electrocardiogram shown in Figure 1-6 and imagine the multiple action potentials shown above that are responsible for its generation. While the sodium-potassium AT-Pase pump maintains intracellular concentrations by pumping potassium in and sodium out, changing permeability of the sarcolemma produces the characteristic action potential. During diastole, potassium leaks out through potassium "gates" that are open (increased potassium permeability); the outward current accompanying potassium leakage produces a resting or membrane potential with the inside of the cell −90 mv relative to the outside (phase 4). A sudden activation of sodium channels in the sarcolemma opens sodium "gates" that carry in sodium ions, leading to a rapid inward current that produces the rapid upstroke of the action potential (phase 0). As these gates close, opening of another set of calcium-sodium gates leads to a slow inward current that maintains the plateau characteristic of phase 2. (Phase 1, not labeled, is the sudden drop following phase 0 and may be due to chloride influx.) Opening of the potassium gates initiates the outward potassium current, which leads to repolarization of the cell and return to the resting state.

These permeability changes create the characteristic properties

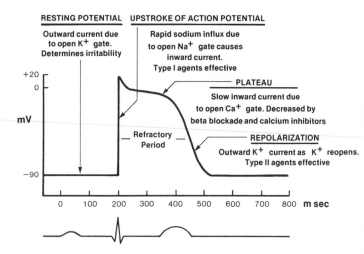

Figure 1-6. The cardiac action potential, obtained from a single fiber, and the surface electrocardiogram. Different classes of anti-arrhythmic drugs appear to work on different phases of the cycle.

of cardiac muscle. The *resting potential* makes the muscle cell excitable, since a stimulus leads to depolarization by opening the sodium gates. The lower the resting potential, the closer to threshold and the more excitable the cell. Adjacent cells depolarize in sequence, conducting an impulse through the myocardium; the rate of *conduction* is determined by the action potential amplitude, its rate of rise, the excitability of adjacent cells, and the resistance of adjacent structures. *Refractoriness* to excitation occurs when the cell is already depolarized and prevents conduction of impulses in that region.

Sinus node cells, cells in the His-Purkinje fibers, and certain others spontaneously depolarize during diastole, demonstrating *automaticity.* In health, only the SA node depolarizes spontaneously, initiating the integrated sequence of cardiac excitation and contraction. Arrhythmias are due to either increased *automaticity* of other regions, producing an ectopic focus, or to short-circuiting of the original propagated impulse, causing a *reentrant premature contraction or tachycardia.* Factors that slow conduction, leading to decremental conduction and unidirectional block, and those that decrease refractoriness produce areas of excitable tissue that become redepolarized, producing reentry. Reentry may occur in the AV node, in anatomic tracks such as the bundle of Kent, or in other areas where conduction and refractoriness vary. More than half of supraventricular tachycardias arise from reentry; drugs that supress ectopic foci may actually tend to maintain arrhythmias due to reentry.

Therapeutic Considerations

Correction of underlying factors. *Myocardial ischemia* leads to decreased activity of the sodium-potassium pump; the decreased intracellular potassium concentration that results produces a decrease in resting potential and an increase in slow inward currents, setting the stage for reentrant arrhythmias. *Catecholamine* release increases automaticity, decreases action potential and refractory period duration, and increases slow inward currents. These changes are nonuniform, particularly in the diseased heart, setting the stage for reentrant arrhythmias. *Hyperkalemia* decreases conduction by decreasing rapid sodium currents and produces peaked T waves by enhancing repolarization. The decrease in conduction leads to AV block and to severe arrhythmias. *Hypokalemia* produces decreased T wave amplitude and prolongation of the Q-T interval by prolonging the action potential and slowing the rate of depolarization, situations leading to decremental conduction. *Hypercalcemia* increases the amplitude of the action potential and accelerates repolarization, producing a short Q-T interval; *hypocalcemia* has the opposite effect, prolonging the action potential, decreasing its amplitude, and prolonging the Q-T interval. *Acidosis* has an effect resembling that of hyperkalemia, *alkalosis* that of hypokalemia.

ANTIARRHYTHMIC DRUGS

Almost all antiarrhythmic drugs have membrane-stabilizing or "local anesthetic" effects, which reduce the fast inward sodium current, decreasing automaticity and conduction velocity while prolonging refractory period. Quinidine, procainamide, and diisopyramide act mainly by this mechanism, tend to prolong PR, QRS, and QT intervals particularly at higher doses, and are sometimes called *type I agents.* Lidocaine and phenytoin have somewhat different properties, probably because they increase outward currents as well as reduce the fast inward current. These *type II drugs* appear to have a lesser effect on the fast inward current, so that conduction is less retarded while refractoriness is increased, particularly in ischemic tissue. Type II drugs have little effect on electrocardiographic intervals, generally do not impair impulse conduction, and may have less effect on contractility. Since decreasing conduction may produce reentrant arrhythmias as well as abolish them, the reduced effect of type II drugs on conduction makes them useful alternatives in ischemic disease or when a type I agent has been ineffective. Probably the classification of two types of agents is an oversimplification.

Propranolol. This drug seems to be in a class of its own, since it decreases the arrhythmogenic action of catecholamines as well as exerts a direct effect by increasing outward currents and thus stabilizing membranes. Newer, more specific beta blocking agents may have the former action without the latter. All three type I agents have a vagolytic effect that is most marked with diisopyramide; quinidine has an alpha blocking activity.

Bretylium tosylate. This prevents the release of norepinephrine from sympathetic nerve terminals and also increases refractory periods without decreasing conduction. It increases the ventricular fibrillation threshold and decreases the heterogeneity of refractory periods, particularly in ischemic muscle. At present, its use is limited to severe and resistant ventricular arrhythmias.

Verapamil. Verapamil inhibits the slow inward calcium current and appears useful in certain reentrant arrhythmias due to prolongation of this current; it also slows AV nodal conduction.

ELECTRICAL THERAPY
Direct current cardioversion is indicated whenever there is a rapid tachyarrhythmia causing hemodynamic deterioration; it is also indicated when drug therapy has been unsuccessful. Ideally, elective cardioversion should be preceded by quinidine adminis-

tration for at least 24 hours and anticoagulation for at least 2 weeks. Digitalis should be withheld for 24-48 hours before conversion.

Electrical stimulation of the heart can terminate certain arrhythmias by capturing an automatic ectopic focus or by altering the electrophysiologic properties of tissues so that a reentrant loop is interrupted.

Specific Cardiac Arrhythmias

Atrial premature beats (APB). APBs occur early, the P wave morphology differs from the sinus-initiated beats, the PR interval is prolonged, and the pause is not compensatory because depolarization of the sinus node resets its rhythmicity. Very early APBs find the AV node refractory and are not conducted; somewhat later, beats may experience partial refractoriness and conduct in an aberrant way, usually producing a right bundle branch block (RBBB) configuration. Frequently, treatment is not indicated. They may be ablated by use of a type I agent, propranolol, or digitalis if left ventricular failure is present. Right atrial APBs and a variety of other atrial arrhythmias may be seen in chronic pulmonary disease because of elevation of right atrial pressure.

Paroxysmal supraventricular tachycardias (PST). Atrial or nodal in origin, these tachycardias are frequently due to reentry within the AV node, may be seen with the Wolff-Parkinson-White syndrome, and have a rate between 150-250 per minute. Abnormal P waves may occur but are usually buried, and ST segment depressions are common. R-R intervals are regular; if irregular, atrial flutter or fibrillation should be considered. AV block may occur with disease or digitalis; the classic digitalis toxic form has an atrial rate of 150-180 with a ventricular response of 75-90. Preexisting bundle branch block or aberrant conduction will produce an arrhythmia mimicking ventricular tachycardia. Electrocardiographic and clinical separation is shown in Table 1-7.

Direct current (DC) cardioversion is indicated in the presence of heart disease with hemodynamic deterioration. In other pa-

TABLE 1-7—DIFFERENTIATION OF SUPRAVENTRICULAR TACHYCARDIA WITH ABERRANCY FROM VENTRICULAR TACHYCARDIA

1	Irregular cannon waves in neck suggest VT
2	Fusion (Dressler) beats suggest VT
3	SVT with aberrancy are suggested by the following: Preceding P wave RBBB contour Triphasic contour in Vl and V6 Initial vector identical with conducted beats

Modified from Marriott HJL: Practical Electrocardiography. Baltimore, Williams and Wilkins, 1972.

tients, carotid sinus massage or the Valsalva maneuver should be attempted both before and after administration of digitalis. Digoxin, 0.75-1.0 mg I.V. frequently converts this arrhythmia by stimulating the vagus. Intravenous propranolol, 1 mg I.V. every 10 minutes, may be added if needed, but the possibility of left ventricular failure must be carefully excluded. Type I agents like quinidine and procainamide are also useful but are generally reserved for prevention of paroxysmal tachycardia.

Nonparoxysmal atrioventricular nodal (junctional) tachycardia. This form of tachycardia (Fig. 1-7) is a relatively slow, nonparoxysmal tachycardia arising from a junctional focus that depolarizes at a rate below 120-130 per minute. Since automatic cells have not been found in the AV node proper but are located in the His bundle and the junction between AV node and bundle, junctional is probably a more accurate description. The P wave may precede, be buried in, or follow the QRS complex, depending on the relative rates of antegrade and retrograde conduction. This arrhythmia almost always results from increased automaticity of the junction due to myocardial infarction, digitalis toxicity, or myocarditis. It should be distinguished from the escape rhythm, AV nodal rhythm, which usually has a rate below 60 per minute. Specific treatment is usually not necessary.

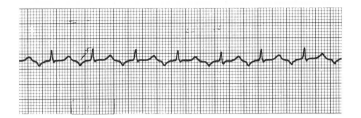

Figure 1-7A. Junctional rhythm with antegrade delay of conduction. This would be termed "upper nodal rhythm" in the older classification.

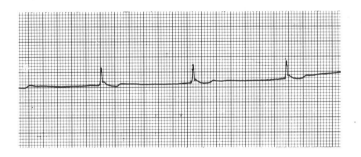

Figure 1-7B. Junctional rhythm with balanced antegrade and retrograde conduction. This would be called "middle nodal rhythm" in the older classifixation. (*Continued*)

Atrial flutter. Prinzmetal suggests that atrial flutter differs only by a rate greater than 250 per minute from supraventricular tachycardia. Flutter classically occurs in older patients with heart disease, has an atrial rate greater than 300, and is associated with 2:1 block. Atrial flutter has a regular rate; when irregularly irregular in certain leads, it is sometimes called flutter-fibrillation but should usually be treated like fibrillation. Digitalis or type I

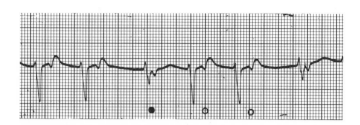

Figure 1-7C. Junctional rhythm with delayed retrograde conduction. Beats indicated by open circle clearly represent retrograde conduction with an inverted P wave following the QRS complex. This would be termed "lower nodal rhythm" in the older classification. The beat indicated by the solid circle probably represents nodal escape but also suggests delayed retrograde conduction.

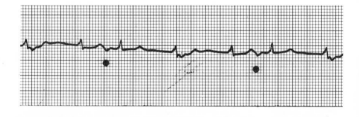

Figure 1-7D. Junctional rhythm with varying delay in retrograde conduction. Certain P waves, indicated by dots, reveal marked retrograde conduction delay and are able to reenter the conduction system and produce a reciprocal beat (three to two Wenckebach).

agents may be used to treat flutter; conversion to atrial fibrillation or normal sinus may occur. Conversion is usually difficult with drugs, easy with cardioversion.

Atrial fibrillation. This generally occurs with diseased hearts, sometimes with normal hearts. Junctional rhythm due to digitalis should be suspected when the ventricular response is regular and low. APBs with aberrancy may be seen and mistaken for ventricular premature beats (VPBs); VPBs would suggest digitalis toxicity, so differentiation becomes important. Atrial fibrillation may be imitated clinically by frequent ectopic beats, atrial tachycardia, or flutter with varying block, sinus rhythm with varying block, gross sinus arrhythmia, or wandering pacemaker.

Control of ventricular rate by digitalis administration is usually preferable to conversion for those with chronic atrial fibrillation. If ventricular rate cannot be slowed adequately without evidence of toxicity (common in patients with hyperthyroidism or fever), propranolol or verapamil may be added. Electrical conversion is indicated for individuals with recent onset or with hemodynamic deterioration because of uncontrollable rate. Maintenance therapy with quinidine is necessary to prevent reversion. In one study, pretreatment with dicumarol reduced embolism from 6.8% to 1.1%.

Ventricular premature beats (VPB). VPBs should be treated if there is evidence of serious underlying heart disease such as ischemic heart disease, cardiomyopathy, mitral valve prolapse, or hypertrophic subaortic stenosis. The classic concept of treating multifocal, three or more consecutive, or early VPBs to prevent ventricular fibrillation in patients with acute myocardial infarction has given way to the general use of intravenous lidocaine for all patients with acute myocardial infarction (AMI). Epidemiologic studies show that VPBs decrease life expectancy, but this finding probably relates to the associated occurrence of coronary artery disease.

Parasystole. As seen in Figure 1-8, parasystole results from an autonomous ectopic ventricular focus firing at its own rate. The beats occur later than premature ventricular beats, which are usually seen in the supernormal period of repolarization in the area of the EKG u wave. Parasystolic beats show variable coupling times, with the time between the previous beat and the ectopic beat a function of the rates of each pacemaker. An additional aid in separation from VPBs is that the time between ectopic beats is equal to or a multiple of the shortest interectopic beat interval.

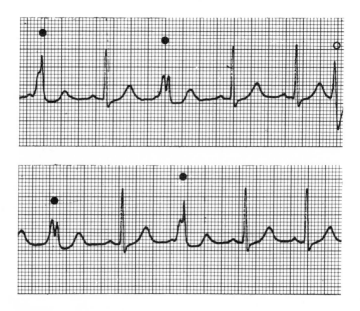

Figure 1-8. Premature ventricular contractions with varying coupling due to a parasystolic focus. The open circle denotes the parasystolic focus which appears in multiples at a rate of 83. The black circles denote fusion beats which are diagnostic of parasystole.

Ventricular tachycardia (VT) and accelerated idioventricular rhythm (AIVR). Both are seen in the patient with acute myocardial infarction; the former may be seen in ambulatory individuals and in those with other forms of heart disease; it is occasionally seen in normal individuals. VT usually occurs at rates of 100-200 per minute; AIVR of 50-90 per minute. Ventricular tachycardia early in the course of infarction appears due to increased automaticity; that in chronic ischemic disease with or without ventricular aneurysm, to reentry. AIVR is seen in up to

25% of patients with AMI, is thought to be benign, but may be associated with VT. DC conversion should be initiated immediately if the diagnosis is VT. Lidocaine, procainamide, and bretylium may be used for treatment and prophylaxis of VT.

Conduction Disturbances

Conducting tissue may be affected by ischemic, myopathic, infiltrative, or degenerative disease. The sinus node is supplied by a special artery that arises from either the right (60%) or the left circumflex (40%) coronary artery. The artery to the AV node arises from the right coronary in 85% of people.

Atrioventricular (AV) block. In this form of conduction disturbance, sinus impulses have difficulty in reaching the ventricle. In first-degree block (prolonged PR interval), they are merely delayed; in second-degree block, some are prevented from entering the ventricle; in third-degree block, all are prevented from entering and there is AV dissociation. AV dissociation is a generic term. When due to block, the ventricular rate is slower than the atrial. When due to supression of atrial pacemakers or to ventricular myocardial irritability, ventricular rate is faster than atrial rate. Mobitz confused generations of students when he introduced the term interference-dissociation to describe an arrhythmia associated with rheumatic carditis and digitalis toxicity. It is better termed AV dissociation due to an ectopic ventricular pacemaker with occasional capture or fusion beats.

Second-degree AV block may be fixed or variable. Wenckebach in 1899, using a jugular venous tracing, noted progressive prolongation of the AV interval followed by a dropped beat; 7 years later he observed dropped beats with constant AV intervals. Twenty years later Mobitz proposed that these two types be called types I and II. The Wenckebach (Mobitz I) (Fig. 1-9) is characterized by increasing PR intervals until an impulse is completely blocked. Usually the first PR interval after the dropped beat is close to normal, the second much more prolonged, and subsequent ones each prolonged slightly more than its predecessor. The longest R-R interval, of course, is that with the dropped beat, but it is always less than twice that of the

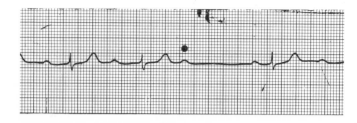

Figure 1-9. Wenckebach (Mobitz Type I) block with variable A-V conduction delay. While interesting historically, the use of degrees of block is flawed since anatomic site of block, atrial rate at which block is manifest, effective ventricular rate, and underlying disease process determine treatment and prognosis.

shortest R-R interval. The R-R intervals shorten progressively because of the smaller and smaller lengthening of the PR intervals. Wenckebach A-V block is due to reversible problems in the AV node; Mobitz type II or fixed second-degree block (Fig. 1-10) implies a more serious problem, usually distal to the AV node.

Third-degree AV block is frequently symptomatic due to the low ventricular rate. The defect is usually distal to the AV node; it is generally proximal to the His bifurcation when congenital and either bilateral bundle or trifasicular when acquired. The QRS complex is generally normal when the pacemaker is above the His bifurcation but prolonged and slurred when distal to it. The atrial mechanism may be sinus or any other, such as fibrillation or flutter.

Bundle branch and hemiblocks. These may be fixed, transient, or exhibit Wenckebach conduction abnormalities. Figure 1-3 shows the 1-2 cm His bundle entering the region of the membranous septum, adjacent to the aortic valve ring, and dividing into the right bundle which follows the right septal surface. The left bundle is broad and short, dividing early. An anterior division traverses anterior septum and anterior wall to reach the anterior papillary muscle; the posterior division crosses posteriorly and

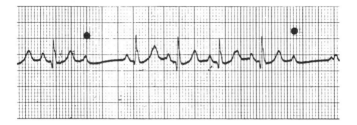

Figure 1-10. Mobitz Type II block is an example of periodic failure of conduction; the PR intervals are constant. When this type of block occurs with atrial rates below 90, or when two or more consecutive ventricular impulses are blocked at rates below 130-140, the term "high grade A-V block" is considerably more meaningful than the conventional "second degree heart block."

enters the posterior papillary muscle. Note that the anterior division crosses near the outflow tract, the posterior division near the inflow tract.

The EKG patterns for the hemiblocks are characteristic (see Fig. 1-11). With left anterior hemiblock (LAH), a small Q_1 and R_3 denote early activation of the posterior wall; a large and prolonged R_1 and S_3 denote later activation of anterior wall (initial and later vectors are 180° separated). With left posterior hemiblock (LPH), a small R_1 and Q_3 denote early anterior wall activation, while a later and broad S_1 and R_3 denote posterior wall activation. These patterns appear as left and right axis deviations, respectively.

Etiology of blocks. The anatomic relationships of the conduction system make involvement in diverse disease processes likely. The left bundle has a double blood supply, so that ischemic block requires involvement of both right coronary and anterior descending arteries. The right bundle is relatively long, supplied by the right coronary at its origin but by the anterior descending during its long septal course; an anteroseptal infarction may produce RBBB. The anterior division is supplied by the anterior

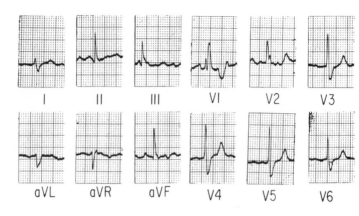

Figure 1-11A. Left anterior hemiblock associated with right bundle branch block indicating bifasicular block.

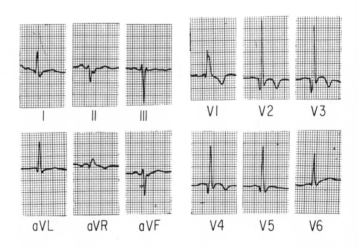

Figure 1-11B. Left posterior hemiblock and right bundle branch block.

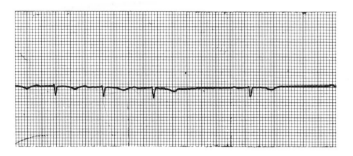

Figure 1-12. Sinoatrial block; the pause is twice the duration of the PR interval.

descending, while the posterior division has a dual supply like the left bundle. Less than 10% of individuals with acute infarction have complete heart block, and it is permanent in only 10% of these. Transient complete block is common in inferior wall infarction because of transient ischemia of the artery supplying the AV node.

The right bundle, because of its long course and vulnerable position, is involved in many disease processes; the left posterior division appears most resistant to injury. Most chronic blocks are probably not due to coronary artery disease. Lenegre's disease is a progressive fibrosis of both bundles, producing RBBB and LAH initially, followed by complete AV block. It is seen in middle-aged and older people and may produce syncopal episodes. Lev's disease is sclerosis and calcification of the left cardiac skeleton including mitral annulus, membranous septum, and periaortic region. It is not as progressive as Lenegre's, usually does not involve the posterior division, but at times may involve both bundles.

Sick sinus syndrome (SSS). The syndrome embraces a series of situations characterized by problems with SA node impulse formation. SA block is shown in Figure 1-12. A pause that is twice the duration of a normal R-R interval occurs at regular intervals. It may be followed by nodal or ventricular escape beats as well as by resumption of normal sinus rhythm. The *bradycardia-tachycardia syndrome* is a variant of sinus node failure where runs of atrial tachyarrhythmias follow periods of bradycardia. Atrial fibrillation can also develop as a result of sinus node failure; attempts at electrical conversion could lead to cardiac arrest unless AV pacemaker activity appears. Since AV nodal dysfunction is common in individuals with SA node problems, a slow ventricular rate in the undigitalized patient may be a clue to the presence of SA disease and atrial fibrillation. This syndrome illustrates that arrhythmias can result from *default* when another pacemaker replaces an ineffective sinus pacemaker or from *usurpation* when another pacemaker appears because it has a more rapid rate and steals the action from the SA node. Treating the latter with suppressive agents makes sense but could be disastrous in the default situation.

Wolf-Parkinson-White syndrome (WPW). When the PR interval is less than 0.12 and the QRS complex greater than 0.10 because of early activation of the ventricle by an accessory pathway, the WPW syndrome is diagnosed. In type A, the early QRS inscription or delta wave is positive in precordial leads, suggesting a left-sided connection; in type B, it is negative in V1-V3, suggesting a right-sided connection. Reentrant arrhythmias are common. *The Lown-Ganong-Levine syndrome* is a variant where an accessory AV tract produces a short PR interval but a normal QRS interval. Reentrant tachyarrhythmias may occur but are less common than in the WPW syndrome.

Long QT syndrome. This is a familial disorder that should be suspected when ventricular tachyarrhythmias occur in individuals with a corrected QT interval greater than 0.45 second. Abnormalities in ventricular repolarization, perhaps due to abnormal autonomic influences, may be responsible.

PACEMAKER TREATMENT OF CONDUCTION DISTURBANCES

Pacemaker technology has improved dramatically, and lithium-powered programmable demand pacemakers may be used with few complications. Atrial pacing with positioning in coronary

sinus or right auricular appendage has become more popular for
SA node dysfunction with intact AV conduction. The major
problem is that of indication. Level and degree of block, symptomatology, and disease process should all be considered. Patients with second- or third-degree infra-His block with or
without symptoms should have pacemakers. Those with bifasicular block should be considered if HV prolongation is associated
with syncope not due to other causes.

Indications in acute myocardial infarction are controversial,
but since complete AV block can be devastating and prophylactic
insertion is relatively simple, it is frequently considered. It seems
indicated with second-degree His or infra-His block (perhaps
suggested by Mobitz type II appearance or by electrophysiologic
study) or by third-degree block. Third-degree block in the AV
node is frequently transient, and pacemaker therapy is usually
not indicated. Both RBBB and LBBB appearing with the infarct
require a pacemaker. RBBB with anteroseptal infarction or with
left anterior hemiblock is an important indication. The indications for pacemaking are based not only on the conduction defect
but on an estimate of the ischemic damage and a prediction of
what additional conduction problems might ensue.

ACUTE AND CHRONIC RHEUMATIC
HEART DISEASE

Acute rheumatic fever is an inflammatory process of unknown
cause, closely related to streptococcal infection, which involves
the heart, skeletal muscle, joints, and brain. At one time, 40% of
all patients with heart disease were considered rheumatic, but
there has been a dramatic decrease in incidence and it is now
diagnosed in less than 0.5% of school children. Its predilection
for attacking myocardium and valves, however, makes it continue
to be a major health problem.

It is virtually certain that infection with type A beta-hemolytic
streptococcus initiates rheumatic fever, and multiple studies have
demonstrated the importance of early recognition and treatment
of such infections. A purified streptococcal membrane antigen
that cross-reacts with myocardial sarcolemma has recently been
identified and appears to be different from the type-specific M

protein, suggesting the possibility of a vaccine. Whether the cross-reactivity thesis is the sufficient explanation for the pathogenesis of this disease is not clear.

Diagnosis is made by finding evidence of streptococcal infection together with one major and two minor, or two major, revised Jones criteria. Major Jones manifestations are: carditis, polyarthritis, chorea, erythema marginatum, or subcutaneous nodules. Minor manifestations are fever, arthralgia, previous rheumatic fever or heart disease, elevated acute phase reactants such as CRP or ESR, and prolonged PR interval. Sydenham's chorea alone is diagnostic of rheumatic fever. The incidence of these manifestations has changed dramatically. In 1921-31, carditis was present in 65%, arthritis in 41%, and subcutaneous nodules in 9%; in 1954-64, arthritis was present in 97%, carditis in 23%, and nodules were rare.

Streptococcal infection may be confirmed by identifying antibodies to one or more bacterial components (antistreptolysin 0, antihyaluronidase, antistreptokinase, and others). If tested for one antibody within the first week, 80% will be positive; if two antibodies are tested for, one will be found in 90%; if three are evaluated, at least one will be found in virtually all. A commercially mixed antigen has been used for screening (antistreptozyme or ASTZ test) and is extremely sensitive. Anti-DNAase B remains elevated longer than others and together with ASO is used most generally for diagnosis.

Treatment with steroids or salicylates has not been shown to prevent development of chronic valvular deformity. Steroids appear to reverse the inflammatory phase more rapidly than salicylates and may be better tolerated than large doses of salicylates. They should not be used for extended periods of time and most would begin with high doses such as 40-60 mg/day of prednisone and taper rapidly. Rebounds occur during tapering, and therapy should be reinstituted.

Rheumatic Heart Disease

The pancarditis of acute rheumatic fever produces chronic deformity of the cardiac valves and may also produce chronic myocarditis. Valvular stenosis, insufficiency, or both cause striking physical signs and produce characteristic syndromes. A study in 1940 showed the following incidence of abnormalities in 779 patients with rheumatic heart disease studied at autopsy: mitral, 37%; aortic, 13%; mitral and aortic, 28%; mitral aortic and tricuspid, 7%; mitral and tricuspid, 4%. Cournand and his group showed more than 25 years ago that certain patients had myocardial failure, since cardiac surgery did not help significantly but symptoms responded to digitalis.

The diagnosis is suspected by history and confirmed by the identification of characteristic murmurs. The murmur of mitral stenosis is sometimes difficult to hear, especially when the valve is extremely tight or if the patient is fibrillating. An opening snap, however, is almost always present unless the valve is heavily calcified. Mitral insufficiency is unusual in the absence of a typical apical holosystolic murmur; the intensity of the murmur is an indicator of the severity of the mitral leak. Aortic insufficiency produces a soft decrescendo diastolic murmur at the left sternal border, which may be difficult to hear. The presence of a forceful apical impulse suggests left ventricular hypertrophy due to mitral insufficiency or aortic disease; a forceful left parasternal impulse indicates right ventricular hypertrophy due to mitral stenosis with pulmonary hypertension. Tricuspid murmurs may be heard to the left of the lower sternum and are accentuated by inspiration (Rivero Carvallo's sign).

Mitral stenosis produces a large left atrium, pulmonary venous hypertension, Kerley B lines and redistribution of blood flow on the radiograph, exertional dyspnea and orthopnea, and acute pulmonary edema. Fatigue may be more common with mitral insufficiency. Aortic stenosis is asymptomatic for long periods of time and may present with angina or syncope; dyspnea suggests left ventricular failure. Tricuspid disease produces jugular venous distension, hepatomegaly, edema, and ascites. Insufficiency secondary to pulmonary hypertension is the most common form of tricuspid disease. Tricuspid stenosis may be isolated but is commonly associated with mitral stenosis.

Echocardiographic studies of mitral and aortic valve function confirm clinical diagnosis. Cross-sectional echocardiographic measurements correlate closely with calculations of mitral valve area made at cardiac catheterization in patients with stenosis or insufficiency. Cardiac catheterization is probably necessary for precise evaluation of pulmonary vascular resistance. The decision for surgery should be based on symptomatology and knowledge of natural history of valvular lesions. Progressive left ventricular deterioration and rising pulmonary vascular resistance must be avoided. Surgery is indicated whenever patients cannot live a reasonably rewarding life—certainly before they become housebound or bedridden. The results of valvular replacement are suprisingly satisfactory. A recent study of 159 patients undergoing noncardiac surgery at varying periods of time after valve replacement revealed that 10% had experienced thromboembolic phenomena. Oral anticoagulants were stopped 1-3 days before surgery and resumed 1-7 days afterward. There was no evidence of thromboembolism during this period, but some bleeding complications with surgery were observed. Another study showed that 68% of patients compared to 12% preoperatively denied any limitation of activity; three quarters of men were capable of working, and three quarters had returned to their usual employment. Starr et al. reported a 4% operative mortality for isolated mitral valve replacement using a cloth-covered prosthesis; 76% were alive at 5 years, 58% at 10 years; 76% of those living more than 6 years were in functional class I or II. Cohn et al. reported similar good results but observed reduced long-term mortality and thromboembolism with the Hancock porcine xenograft compared to the Harken prosthetic disc valve.

NON-RHEUMATIC VALVULAR DISEASE
Mitral prolapse. This may occur in more than 5% of normal individuals and is the most common cause of mitral insufficiency. It may be an autosomal dominant trait with enhanced expressivity in women. Many individuals with echocardiographic evidence are asymptomatic, but others have chest pain, palpitations, dyspnea, dizziness, and syncope. One study showed that transient ischemic attacks in younger people were frequently associated with mitral prolapse. Paroxysmal supraventricular tachycardias are common, and electrophysiologic studies have shown atrio-

ventricular bypass tracts. It has become recognized as a major cause of infective endocarditis.

Ruptured chordae tendineae. Ruptures may be spontaneous, associated with heavy exertion, traumatic, or occur with endocarditis. A sudden holosystolic murmur radiating to the back with anterior leaflet rupture and to the aortic area with posterior leaflet tears is characteristic. A suddenly developing holosystolic murmur in a patient with acute myocardial infarction indicates *papillary muscle rupture* but must be distinguished by intracardiac blood sampling from *ventricular septal rupture.*

Other processes causing mitral insufficiency include cardiomyopathy with migration of papillary muscles, annulus or cuspal calcification due to degenerative disease, Ehlers-Danlos syndrome, Hurler's and Marfan's syndromes, and Ebstein's anomaly with corrected transposition of the great vessels. Mitral regurgitation occurs as part of the ostium primum type of atrial septal defect (cleft mitral valve); mitral valve prolapse is seen in 20% of individuals with ostium secundum.

Isolated aortic valvular disease. Called in adults calcific aortic stenosis, this usually results from the fusion and calcification of a congenitally bicuspid aortic valve. Many patients have associated coronary artery disease. Up to 2% of the population have bicuspid valves; many appear to develop progressive obstruction, and a significant number develop endocarditis. Aubrey Leatham's group has shown that an aortic ejection sound may be the earliest sign of bicuspid aortic valves.

Aortic insufficiency. Possible causes are aortic dissection, ascending aortic aneurysm or aneurysm of the sinus of Valsala due to cystic medial necrosis (either as Marfan's syndrome or an isolated phenomena—forme fruste), trauma, or endocarditis. Syphilis was once a common cause, is still seen occasionally, and is suggested by calcification of the ascending aorta.

INFECTIVE ENDOCARDITIS

Infective endocarditis is a febrile illness caused by bacterial or fungal infection of either valvular or mural endocardium. The introduction of antibiotics, corticosteroids, immunosuppressive drugs, and cardiac surgery and the increasing prevalence of narcotic addiction have resulted in significant changes in the clinical presentation of the disease. Infective endocarditis was formerly divided into acute and subacute (subacute bacterial endocarditis), depending on survival beyond 8 weeks. Uwaydah and Weinberg emphasized that acute endocarditis was associated with hectic fever, leukocytosis, extreme toxicity, and rapid deterioration of cardiac function. Sixty-nine percent of the subacute cases were due to alpha-hemolytic streptococci, while 53% of the cases were due to *Staphylococcus aureus*. In addition, 37% of patients with acute endocarditis did not have evidence of predisposing heart disease, while only 5 % of those with the subacute form had clinically normal hearts before the development of endocarditis.

Many patients with subacute infective endocarditis have a prior history of rheumatic endocarditis. Predisposing congenital lesions include ventricular septal defect (Fallot's tetralogy), bicuspid aortic valve, pulmonic stenosis, patent ductus arteriosus, peripheral arteriovenous fistula, and coarctation of the aorta. Recent studies have shown a significant prevalence of endocarditis in individuals with prolapse of the mitral valve. Infection of prosthetic aortic valves remains a continuing problem. Infection of vessels, usually at the site of arterial disease, is properly termed *infective endarteritis.*

The consequences of subacute infective endocarditis are strikingly different from those of the acute form because of sustained antigenemia and the formation of immune complexes. Weinstein and Schlesinger pointed out that four mechanisms were responsible for the subacute infection: (1) previously damaged cardiac valve or a hemodynamic situation where blood flowing from high to low pressure produces a "jet" effect, (2) a sterile platelet-fibrin thrombus, (3) bacteremia, sustained or transient, and (4) a high titer of agglutinating antibody, which appears to produce a sticky infective plug that adheres to damaged valvular tissue.

CLINICAL FEATURES

Infective endocarditis, particularly the subacute variety, has been frequently underdiagnosed because of the up to 20% incidence of negative blood cultures and its subtle presentation. Rabinovich et al. observed the following incidence of physical signs: fever, 100%; murmurs, 96.4%; petechiae, 47.5%; splenomegaly, 43.2%; hematuria, 28.3%; albuminuria, 26.2%; arthralgia, 25.1%; retinal abnormalities, 17.0%; clubbing, 14.9%; Osler nodes, 11.3%; changing murmur, 9.9%; Janeway lesions, 4.9%. The Osler node is a painful, red, indurated area found in the pads of either fingers or toes and lasting up to several days. It is composed of endothelial swelling and is probably nonbacterial. Janeway lesions are painless, hemorrhagic, nodular lesions found on the palms and soles and believed to be embolic. Petechiae are most frequently found in the mucous membranes of the mouth, the conjunctiva, around the neck, or about the wrists and ankles. Splinter hemorrhages are nonspecific and may be seen in a variety of disease states (trichinosis, rheumatic fever, following commissurotomy, infectious mononucleosis) or associated with trauma. A variety of retinal lesions, including hemorrhagic areas with white centers (Roth spots), flame-shaped hemorrhages, petechiae, retinal thrombosis, segmental filling defects, and papilledema may be seen.

Endocarditis may rarely present without fever. The following syndromes have been described and make diagnosis difficult: (1) neurologic syndrome, (2) hematologic syndrome with anemia, (3) peripheral vascular disease with sudden vascular occlusion, (4) renal disease, (5) left upper quadrant pain due to splenic infarction, (6) congestive heart failure, and (7) bone disease with abcess.

DIAGNOSTIC APPROACHES

While recent reports have stated that 12-23% of patients with infective endocarditis have negative blood cultures, failure to culture organisms is usually due to prior antibiotic therapy or inadequate duration of agar plate culture that fails to provide fastidious organisms with sufficient time to thrive. Bacteremia is usually persistent; Tompsett found that only 6 of 168 cultures from 48 patients who had not been given antibiotics were negative. Usually, four to five blood cultures are sufficient to identify bacteremia if present. Rabinovich et al. found that 82% of positive cultures were positive on the first culture; in 50% of patients, every culture was positive.

Bacteremia alone does not provide positive evidence for infective endocarditis, although persistent bacteremia certainly makes it likely. Positive rheumatoid factor (20-50% of patients), cryoglobulins (up to 90%), and circulating immune complexes (up to 97% in one study) suggest sustained antigenemia and support the diagnosis. Antibodies to staphylococcal teichoic acid appear early in the course of *S. aureus* endocarditis and decline during convalescence. Immune complexes and teichoic acid antibodies can also be found in nonendocarditic bacteremia, but concentrations are usually lower. Clinical evidence of immune complex disease (glomerulonephritis, arthritis-arthralgia, Janeway lesions, and Osler nodes) also support the diagnosis of infective endocarditis.

Echocardiography may reveal mitral and aortic vegetations. Vegetations less than 5 mm in size cannot be identified, so that false negatives are common; usually not more than 50% of patients exhibit positive findings on echocardiography. Rarely, myxomatous degeneration of valve tissue may present as a false-positive.

Prosthetic Valve Endocarditis (PVE)
Less than 1% per year of patients with prosthetic heart valves developed infective endocarditis; the incidence of early endocarditis (less than 2 months postoperative) has been reduced by the use of prophylactic antibiotic therapy. Clinical presentation varies, but acute endocarditis syndromes are more frequent in the early postoperative cases. Staphylococci or gram-negative and fungal organisms cultured from the environment are found early; streptococci, staphylococci, and a variety of other organisms that produce transient bacteremia appear responsible for late prosthetic valve endocarditis (LPVE). Blood cultures are almost always positive except when caused by certain fungi. Mortality rates from early PVE are from 68-88%; they are from 36-53% in LPVE.

Certain pathologic differences from endocarditis on native valves have been observed. Invasion of the perivalvular tissue with formation of ring abcesses are common. Hemodynamic abnormalities are frequent; aortic PVE almost always causes valve regurgitation, while mitral PVE frequently causes obstruction. Invasion of the myocardium occurs in a high percentage of patients and may lead to valve dehiscence, disruption of AV conduction system, or produce fistulas into the right heart or pericardium. These complications are much less common with native valves.

Early surgical intervention should be considered in view of the poor results with medical therapy and late reoperation. The presence of nonstreptococcal etiology, new regurgitant murmurs, hemodynamic deterioration, or evidence of myocardial invasion all favor early valvular replacement.

Bacteriology and Treatment

Mortality remains disquietingly high. Rabinovich et al. found an immediate mortality rate of 30%; it rose to 51% in patients followed for 5 years. Finland and Barnes found the mortality to be 40% with either *S. viridans* and *S. albus,* but 93% with all other agents.

The protection of microorganisms within valvular vegetations prevents attack by phagocytic cells and makes the use of bactericidal agents rational. Principles of treatment include selection of an agent that produces an in vitro serum bactericidal at a dilution of 1:8 or greater and treatment duration of 4-6 weeks with sensitive streptococci but 6 weeks with other microbial agents.

S. viridans and other penicillin-sensitive streptococci. Penicillin G, 1,000,000 units every 3 hours for 4 weeks. Cephalothin, 1 gm I.V. every 3 hours for 4 weeks, may be used in penicillin-sensitive individuals. *S. viridans* is still the most commonly isolated microbial agent in infective endocarditis.

Penicillin-sensitive S. aureus or albus (epidermidis). Penicillin G, 2,000,000 units every 3 hours for 6 weeks. Finland and Barnes reported that survival with *S. albus* was similar to that with *S. viridans,* and it is not clear whether to treat these patients with the *S. viridans* program or with the *S. aureus* program.

Penicillinase-producing S. aureus or albus. Methicillin or oxacillin, 2.0 gm I.V. every 3 hours for 6 weeks. Cephalothin, 2 gm every 4 hours for 6 weeks in penicillin-sensitive individuals.

Enterococci. Penicillin G, 2,000,000 units I.V. q3h for 6 weeks plus streptomycin, 1.0 gm I.M. twice daily for 3 weeks and 0.5 gm twice daily for the remaining 3 weeks. Gentamycin, 3-5 mg/kg in three divided doses, appears more effective than streptomycin since more strains are sensitive to it; ampicillin, 6-12 gm per day for penicillin G; vancomycin, 0.5 gm q4h 4 hours for 3 days followed by q6h for 21 days may be used in the penicillin-sensitive individual.

Enterococcal (*S. faecalis*) endocarditis emerged following the introduction of penicillin and streptomycin therapy. It is more common in the older individual and has a very high mortality. The use of two agents demonstrates antimicrobial synergism; penicillin injures the mucopeptide of the cell wall, facilitating entry of the aminoglycoside, which inhibits protein synthesis by binding to ribosomes. One-quarter of the minimum bactericidal concentration of each drug alone kills enterococci when used together. This information suggests that the combined use of penicillin and an aminoglycoside might permit reduction of therapy in *S. viridans* endocarditis from 4-6 weeks to as little as 2 weeks. Evidence is unclear as to the efficacy of this approach at present, however, and it should only be considered if a long duration of therapy is impossible.

Surgical treatment. If there is evidence of hemodynamic deterioration, peripheral embolization, or uncontrolled sepsis, surgical valvular replacement should be strongly considered. Boyd et al. describe the indications for surgery in 54 patients. None of eight patients who had surgery within 10 days of the onset of embolization or heart failure died. Nine of 10 patients with persistent sepsis who were not operated upon died; 10 of 12 patients with persistent sepsis who had early surgery survived even though organisms were present in valvular tissue and blood.

Prophylaxis of endocarditis. The presence of high levels of antibiotic agents is required at the time of dental or surgical procedures. The most recent recommendations of the American Heart Association are shown in Table 1-8.

TABLE 1-8—PROPHYLAXIS FOR BACTERIAL ENDOCARDITIS

For Dental Procedures and Surgery of the Upper Respiratory Tract

Aqueous crystalline penicillin G (1,000,000 units intramuscularly) *mixed with* Procaine penicillin G (600,000 units intramuscularly). Give 30 min to 1 hr prior to procedure and then give penicillin V (formerly called phenoxymethyl penicillin) 500 mg orally every 6 hrs for 8 doses.

or

Penicillin V (2.0 gm orally 30 min to 1 hr prior to the procedure and then 500 mg orally every 6 hrs for 8 doses.)

For patients allergic to penicillin:
Erythromycin (1.0 gm orally 1 ½-2 hrs prior to the procedure and then 500 mg orally every 6 hrs for doses.)

or

Vancomycin (1 gm intravenously over 30 min to 1 hr). Start initial vancomycin infusion ½ to 1 hr prior to procedure; then *erythromycin* 500 mg orally every 6 hrs for 8 doses.

For Gastrointestinal and Genitourinary Tract Surgery and Instrumentation

Aqueous crystalline penicillin G (2,000,000 units intramuscularly or intravenously)

or

Ampicillin (1.0 gm intramuscularly or intravenously)

plus

Gentamicin (1.5 mg/kg, not to exceed 80 mg) intramuscularly or intravenously)

or

Streptomycin (1.0 gm, intramuscularly). Give initial doses 30 min to 1 hr prior to procedure. If gentamicin is used then give a similar dose of gentamicin and penicillin (or ampicillin) every 8 hrs for 2 additional doses. If streptomycin is used then give a similar dose of streptomycin and penicillin (or ampicillin) every 12 hrs for 2 additional doses.

For patients allergic to penicillin:
Vancomycin (1.0 gm intravenously given over 30 min to 1 hr) *plus Streptomycin* (1.0 gm intramuscularly). A single dose of these antibiotics begun 30 min to one hr prior to the procedure is probably sufficient, but the same dose may be repeated in 12 hrs.

From the American Heart Association.
These dosages are guidelines and must be modified for individual patients.

HYPERTENSION

Average systolic blood pressure increases about 25% during the first two decades of life, plateaus between the ages of 20 and 50 years, and rises at about the same rate observed in youth thereafter; the later adult increase is due to increased stiffness of aorta and large arteries. Pressures above 165/95 are clearly hypertensive in adults; recent studies suggest that reduction of arterial pressure to 140/90 will reduce the incidence of stroke and heart disease and will increase life expectancy. Hypertension is more frequent and more severe in blacks than in whites; strokes are two to three times and heart failure twice as common in blacks as in whites.

Pathophysiology of Hypertension

Frequent use of the term "essential" to classify hypertension emphasizes ignorance and may encourage therapeutic nihilism but is ingrained in medical parlance. The best usage might specify "hypertension, etiology undetermined" or "hypertension, presumably initiated by . . . ," adding specific pathogenetic factors such as renovascular disease, renal parenchymal abnormalities, or endocrine malfunction.

Arterial blood pressure is related to arteriolar resistance and cardiac output; cardiac output is related to blood volume via the Frank-Starling effect on ventricular preload. Epidemiologic observations, studies in genetically hypertensive rats, and the identification of increased red cell sodium concentration in hypertensives and their nonhypertensive relatives suggest that both environmental and genetic factors may be operative in most patients. Hypertension is not observed in underdeveloped nations with low sodium intake but appears when individuals from those areas increase sodium intake as they become Westernized.

Either abnormal circulatory control or decreased sodium excretion relative to intake might initiate hypertension. Since sodium excretion is sensitive to neuroadrenergic tone, the former appears more likely. Either increased central sympathetic output or decreased afferent activity from carotid and aortic baroreceptors could "reset" the baroreceptor reflex arc and lead to an increased peripheral vascular resistance. Renal sympathetic stimulation decreases sodium excretion directly and also activates juxtaglomerular cells to produce renin. The resultant increases in angiotensin II and aldosterone concentrations increase vascular resistance and further decrease sodium excretion. The amplifying effect of positive feedback control is demonstrated by the effect of circulating angiotensin II to increase release of norepinephrine from sympathetic endings and to enhance the vasoconstrictor effect of norepinephrine on vascular tissue. Increased blood pressure and sodium retention make vessel walls stiffer than normal and appear to stimulate proliferation of smooth muscle and collagen, making reversal of hypertension more difficult with the passage of time.

Prostaglandins are another group of constrictor and dilator agents that may be important in the pathogenesis of hypertension. Both PGI_2 and PGE_2, produced by the intima and outer layers of vascular wall respectively, are vasodilators and antagonize the constrictor effects of norepinephrine and angiotensin II. The syndrome of severe hyperaldosteronism without hypertension or edema but with hypokalemia, alkalosis, and increased plasma renin activity (Bartter's syndrome) is associated with juxtaglomerular cell hyperplasia. Both PGI_2 and PGE_2 have been shown to stimulate renal renin production, and indomethacin, an inhibitor of prostaglandin synthetase, lowers renin and corrects hypokalemia in these patients.

Blood pressure, cardiac output, vascular resistance, and blood volume are interrelated, complicating the identification of primary causal agents. About one-third of borderline hypertensive patients have increased cardiac outputs, suggesting that sodium retention and increased blood volume are important factors. Reduction of cardiac output by atropine and beta adrenergic blockade reduces cardiac output, but borderline hypertension remains because of an increase in vascular resistance. Such data suggest that enhanced sympathetic activity affects cardiac output, systemic resistance, and sodium excretion simultaneously; the dominant physiologic abnormality is probably a function of duration of disease, status of end-organ, and measurement technique. Measurement of peripheral vein renin or catecholamine concentration and studies of sodium excretion describe segments of this abnormal control network and are probably not useful in determining therapy.

Secondary Hypertension

Specific abnormalities involving kidney, sympathetic nervous system, or endocrine organs may produce hypertension. While a search for these specific factors is frequently undertaken, they are identified in less than 2% of hypertensive individuals. The younger the individual and the more severe the hypertension, the more vigorous the search for a dominant causal factor. Understanding of the pathophysiology of these causal factors, however, enhances understanding of the regulation of blood pressure in all individuals.

Adrenal cortical hypersecretion. Hypersecretion of either cortisol (Cushing's disease) or aldosterone produces hypertension by reducing sodium excretion. Primary aldosteronism is twice as common in women as in men and may be due to either unilateral adrenal adenoma or bilateral hyperplasia. Hypertension due to an adenoma generally responds to surgical removal, while that due to hyperplasia is resistant and best treated with spironolactone. It should be considered in hypertensive patients without edema who exhibit hypokalemia and hypersecretion of aldosterone that does not suppress with volume expansion.

Renovascular disease. Caused by fibromuscular hyperplasia in younger individuals and atherosclerosis in older ones, this produces hypertension by increasing renin and angiotensin II production. Peripheral vein renin concentrations are neither sensitive nor specific enough for routine screening. The diagnosis is strengthened by identification of normal renin concentrations in renal vein blood from the uninvolved kidney and of concentrations 1.5 or more times higher in renal vein blood from the involved kidney. A significant decrease in blood pressure following the administration of saralasin, a competitive antagonist of angiotensin II, in the volume depleted patient provides important confirmation.

Renal parenchymal disease. Hypertension is produced by reduction of sodium excretion and increase of renin secretion because of decreased sodium delivery to the macula densa of the juxtaglomerular apparatus. Since long-standing hypertension can lead to nephrosclerosis and secondary parenchymal disease, separation between cause and effect is important. Generally, proteinuria and other abnormalities in urinary sediment together with major reductions in creatinine clearance suggest that renal abnormalities are of primary responsibility.

Pheochromocytomas. Hypertension is produced when norepinephrine, epinephrine, or dopamine is secreted into the circulation. Occurring in less than 0.1% of hypertensive patients, pheochromocytomas should be suspected by the clinical manifestations of paroxysmal hypertensive episodes, excessive sweating, orthostatic hypotension, or evidence of a hypermetabolic state. The diagnosis is confirmed by identifying increased urinary excretion of catecholamines or their metabolites, vanillymandelic acid (VMA), or the metanephrines.

Increased hepatic production of renin substrate. This is the cause of hypertension commonly seen in young women taking oral contraceptives. Glucocorticoids may also increase the concentration of renin substrate, providing an additional explanation for the hypertension of Cushing's disease.

The hypertension of toxemia of pregnancy. Both sodium-retaining and vasoconstrictor influences are operative. Estrogen, progesterone, and mineralocorticoid activity lead to mild hypertension. In certain individuals, a hypoxic placenta liberates vasoactive polypeptides, which produce renal arteriolar constriction with subsequent release of renin and production of angiotensin II.

Consequences of Sustained Hypertension

Sustained hypertension implies vasoconstriction and medial hypertrophy of systemic arterioles. Barotrauma to large and medium-sized arteries that are proximal to the resistance vessels produces intimal thickening and accelerated atherosclerosis. Intimal injury due to barotrauma may produce immunologic damage, leading to generalized or regional vasculitis. The kidney shares the burden of hypertension as well as serving as a fundamental cause. About 10% of patients with hypertensive disease develop enough nephrosclerosis to produce renal insufficiency. Intimal hyperplasia and necrosis of preglomerular arterioles are found in rapidly progressive or "malignant" hypertension. Renal arteriolosclerosis is common in hypertensive patients but also occurs in patients without hypertension.

Sustained hypertension leads to left ventricular hypertrophy and also to acceleration of coronary artery disease. In addition, increased left ventricular systolic and diastolic pressures compress subendocardial vessels, leading to myocardial ischemia, and also decrease cardiac output by the effect on ventricular afterload.

The vessels of the optic fundi provide a mirror for changes in blood vessels throughout the body. Vasoconstriction and structural abnormalities of the vessels go on simultaneously; arteriolosclerotic changes reflect the duration of hypertension, while hypertensive changes reflect its severity. Retinal arteriosclerosis can occur, as it can anywhere in the body, without the presence of hypertension.

Most of the retinal arteries except those close to the disc are arterioles; increased light reflex (copper and silver wiring) and arteriovenular crossing abnormalities more than one disc diameter from the disc reflect arteriolosclerosis and are similar to those found in other vascular beds such as the kidney. Decrease in the arteriole-venule ratio from 3:4 indicates arteriolar constriction; focal spasm is of particular diagnostic value. Hemorrhages, exudates, and papilledema indicate vascular, injury, vasculitis, or increased intracranial pressure.

Kirkendall and Armstrong used the following modification of the classification suggested by Scheie which separates arteriolosclerotic from hypertensive retinal changes. They noted that treatment frequently reversed angiospastic abnormalities but had little effect on those associated with arteriolosclerosis Table 1-9.

Treatment

Knowledge of the pathophysiologic determinants of hypertension provides a rational framework for the understanding and selection of antihypertensive agents.

TABLE 1-9—KIRKENDALL-ARMSTRONG
CLASSIFICATION OF RETINAL VASCULAR CHANGES

Stages	Arteriolosclerotic	Hypertensive
I	Thickening of vessel with slight depression of veins at A-V crossings	Narrowing in terminal branches
II	Definite A-V crossing changes and moderate local sclerosis	Narrowing general and severe with local constrictions
III	Invisibility of vein beneath arteriole and severe local sclerosis with segmentation	Above plus hemorrhages and exudates
IV	Above plus venous obstruction and arteriolar obliteration	Above plus papilledema

Diuretics. Since they reduce sodium retention and volume expansion, these are the first line of management. Most diuretics also have a direct vasodilating effect on vascular smooth muscle.

Sympatholytic agents. Different agents act at different levels in the neurohumoral control network. Reserpine depletes norepinephrine from vesicles within sympathetic nerve endings, while guanethidine blocks its release. Clonidine and alpha methyl dopa stimulate centrally located alpha adrenergic receptors and decrease sympathetic neural activity. *Beta blocking agents* act centrally to decrease sympathetic activity, inhibit renin release by the kidney, and decrease both heart rate and myocardial contractility. In some individuals, especially those with pheochromocytoma, beta blockade may unmask alpha adrenergic activity and increase arterial blood pressure. *Alpha blocking agents* such as prazosin, phentolamine, and dibenzyline reduce alpha adrenergic stimulation and produce vasodilatation.

Smooth muscle relaxants (direct vasodilators). These include hydralazine, diazoxide, and minoxidil.

Agents that interrupt the renin-angiotensin axis. Saralasin is a competitive inhibitor of angiotensin II, and captopril is an inhibitor of the angiotensin I converting enzyme. The converting enzyme activates the decapeptide angiotensin I by cleaving two terminal amino acids and transforming it into an octapeptide; the same enzyme inactivates bradykinin by cleaving two terminal amino acids from the active form. Converting enzyme inhibitors produce vasodilatation by decreasing angiotensin II and increasing bradykinin concentrations.

Antihypertensive drugs act at specific locations in the control network and may induce reciprocal responses at other locations that reduce their effectiveness. The vascular contraction related to diuresis may stimulate renin production, while the vasodilatation produced by hydralazine produces a tachycardia as well as increasing renin secretion. The use of two or more drugs acting at different locations prevents such deleterious reciprocal responses.

Indications and Results of Treatment

A number of large-scale national trials have shown that reducing blood pressure improves life expectancy. A recent trial conducted by the National Heart, Lung and Blood Institute followed over 10,000 individuals divided into three levels of blood pressure elevation. Since it was considered unethical to compare treated and untreated patients, half were treated by a formalized "stepped" program while the remainder were randomly treated according to physician preference. The "stepped" care was as follows, each individual advancing an additional step if diastolic pressure was not reduced below 90 mm Hg.

- Step 1: Diuretic (chlorthalidone or other) alone
- Step 2: Diuretic plus reserpine (or methyldopa)
- Step 3: Diuretic, reserpine plus hydralazine
- Step 4: Diuretic, reserpine, hydralazine, plus guanethidine

(The study was initiated prior to the general availability of beta blocking agents. These could be inserted as step 2 agents).

Since the treated group was compared against another less structured treatment group rather than an untreated control group, the improvements in mortality shown below are particularly striking. The data (Table 1-10) also show the importance of treating mild hypertension.

The greater improvement in life expectancy shown with the milder hypertensive group is a strong argument for early treatment.

PERICARDIAL DISEASE

Etiologic factors are listed in Table 1-11. These may cause acute pericarditis, pericardial effusion, or constrictive pericarditis.

Acute pericarditis. Frequently, acute pericarditis is termed viral pericarditis or benign idiopathic pericarditis; neither of these terms is sufficiently complete. Many viral agents, including coxsackie B, influenza, and Ebstein-Barr viruses, have been implicated; recent studies have implicated *Mycoplasma pneumoniae*. The syndrome is characterized by fever, generalized constitutional symptoms typical of a viral illness, evidence of pleurisy, and typical pericardial chest pain. The characteristic three-component rub (presystole, systole, and diastole) occurs early in the disease and is best heard at the left sternal border with the patient sitting forward and holding his breath in deep expiration.

Most cases subside spontaneously, and the major problem in management is distinguishing it from acute myocardial infarction. The possibility of tuberculous or septic pericardtis, espe-

TABLE 1-10—FIVE YEAR MORTALITY RATES ALL CAUSES (Percent)

Diastolic Blood Pressure Group	Random Care	Stepped Care	Percent Change
90-104 mm Hg	7.4	5.9	20.3
105-114	7.7	6.7	13.0
115 and higher	9.7	9.0	7.2

TABLE 1-11—ETIOLOGY OF PERICARDIAL DISEASE

I. Nonspecific or idiopathic
II. Infectious
A. Viral
B. Bacterial
C. Fungal
D. Rickettsial
E. Protozoal
III. The collagen-vascular group, including rheumatic fever, rheumatoid arthritis, systemic lupus erythematosus, and other diseases
IV. Sensitivity states, including serum sickness, autoimmune states, and other allergic reactions
V. Inflammations of contiguous structures, such as myocardial infarction, pulmonary embolism, dissecting aneurysm, esophageal disease, and pulmonary disease
VI. Neoplastic
VII. Metabolic disorders, including uremia and myxedema
VIII. Traumatic
IX. Miscellaneous, e.g., infectious mononucleosis, sarcoidosis

cially in an immunosuppressed or debilitated patient, must be kept in mind, and pericardiocentesis is indicated if the diagnosis is not clear. Since these conditions may produce uneven collections of pleuropericardial loculated material, thoracic computed tomography may be useful. Marked eccentricity of the pericardium might suggest pericardial neoplasm. Rarely, viral pericarditis leads to persistent pericardial effusion or constrictive pericarditis.

Pericardial effusion may occur with heart failure or with any of the conditions listed in Table 1-10. Echocardiography has revolutionized the identification of effusions. In one study, effusions were found in 15% of 1225 routine echocardiograms and were substantial in 9.7%. In two-thirds they were unsuspected. Congestive heart failure or multiple explanations were most common. Less common were uremia, metastatic carcinoma, systemic lupus, viral pericarditis, rheumatoid arthritis, and hypothyroidism. Rarely, the pericardial fluid is creamy and contains numerous cholesterol crystals. While the etiology of cholesterol pericarditis is not clear, it is possible that the appearance of cholesterol crystals is in some way related to the duration of the effusion.

Chronic constrictive pericarditis. The gradual appearance of hepatomegaly, venous congestion, ascites, and ankle swelling suggests this disease. It is insidious and frequently confused with portal cirrhosis or some form of cardiomyopathy. While tuberculosis was the major cause in the past, many patients at present have unresolved viral pericarditis. Recently, constrictive pericarditis has been reported in association with rheumatoid arthritis. While small hearts are classic, many patients have associated myocardial disease or some pericardial effusion so that moderate cardiac enlargement is common. An early diastolic sound (pericardial knock) occurs later than an opening snap but earlier than an S_3 sound. A significant pulsus paradoxus of more than 10 mm Hg together with an increase in jugular venous pressure (Kussmaul's sign) is highly suggestive of pericardial restrictive disease but may also occur in restrictive cardiopathy, particularly amyloid. Pulsus paradoxus occurs in asthma and chronic pulmonary disease because of the marked negative intrathoracic pressure, but venous pressure also falls with inspiration. Since surgical treatment is curative, measurement of venous pressure is mandatory in any patient with hepatomegaly and ascites.

Cardiac tamponade. This should be suspected whenever dyspnea and hypotension occur in a situation predisposing to pericardial disease. The classic triad of a quiet heart, rising venous pressure, and falling arterial pressure is a late manifestation. Little rise in pericardial pressure occurs until at least 150-250 ml of fluid have accumulated; an increase above that volume produces steep increases in pressure and the development of tamponade. Pericardiocentesis, preferably by the subxiphoid approach, is necessary. Connecting the exploring needle to the chest lead of the electrocardiograph provides safety since ventricular premature contractions and elevation of the ST segment indicate contact with the myocardium.

ARTERIAL DISEASES

Abdominal Aortic Aneurysm

The identification of a palpable abdominal mass is the most common mode of identification. Almost all are atherosclerotic, are frequently associated with cerebral vascular disease, producing transient ischemic attacks, and are located below the origin of the renal arteries. Symptoms are late and result from aneurysmal expansion. They include persistent abdominal or back pain, frequently worse after meals. Radiation to the legs—usually the left—suggests expansion. Symptoms are nonspecific and frequently ignored, but rupture occurs within 1 year in 80% with symptomatic abdominal aneurysm. Size determines frequency of rupture; 25% of those larger than 4 cm and 60% of those larger than 10 cm rupture within 1 year.

Abdominal ultrasound examination confirms the diagnosis, and arteriography is indicated if extensive vascular disease suggests renal arterial involvement. Prophylactic surgery is necessary, since the risk electively is less than 4% while more than half of patients die if operated upon following rupture.

Dissecting Aortic Aneurysm

Dissecting aneurysm involving the ascending aorta (DeBakey types I and II) occurs in younger individuals without hypertension who frequently have either Marfan's syndrome or cystic medial necrosis (forme fruste). Immediate surgery is necessary because the coronary arteries and aortic valve are frequently involved.

Patients with dissecting aneurysm of the upper descending thoracic aorta are older, usually have hypertension and generalized atherosclerosis, and exhibit interscapular back pain. They are generally treated initially with propranolol (to reduce the increased shearing force of left ventricular ejection) and intravenous nitroprusside or trimethaphan (to reduce blood pressure). Pulse pressure should be reduced to 40 mm Hg, mean blood pressure to 90 mm Hg or lower if tolerated. Early mortality is reduced to 25% by this approach; many require elective surgery for enlarging aneurysm at a later date.

CONGENITAL HEART DISEASE (CHD)

Congenital lesions, undiagnosed during infancy or childhood, may lead to symptoms later in life. Many lesions correctable at one time may become inoperable as pulmonary arteriolar hypertension or ventricular failure supervene. The frequency of congenital lesions in adults varies from that seen in children for several reasons. Large ventricular septal defects, for example, (Table 1-12) may produce death in early life; small muscular septal defects may close and be undetectable in later life.

Cyanotic CHD is unusual in later life; most common lesions in young adulthood include tetralogy, transposition, and pulmonic stenosis with VSD. Later in adult life, cyanosis due to ASD with right ventricular failure and venoarterial shunting may be seen. Rarely, cyanosis due to either septal defects or ductus arteriosus with progressive pulmonary vascular hypertension occurs; the latter produces cyanotic lower but pink upper extremities ("blue toes") because the venoarterial shunt delivers poorly oxygenated blood into the thoracic aorta.

TABLE 1-12—INCIDENCE OF CONGENITAL HEART DISEASE IN ADULTS AND CHILDREN

	Adults (1960-70) (percent)	Children (1950-70) (percent)
ATRIAL SEPTAL DEFECT	46	5
VENTRICULAR SEPTAL DEFECT	23	19
PULMONIC STENOSIS	15	8
PATENT DUCTUS ARTERIOSUS	6	16
AORTIC COARCTATION	3	8
TETRALOGY OF FALLOT	2	6
OTHERS	5	29

TABLE 1-13—DIFFERENTIAL DIAGNOSIS OF LEFT STERNAL BORDER SYSTOLIC MURMUR

	Auscultation	Radiography	Electrocardiography
PULMONIC STENOSIS	Ejection murmur and sound S_2 widely split with decreased pulmonic component. Widest split in mild cases	Lung fields clear or decr. vascularity. Prominent main pulmonary artery. RVH	Systolic overload, peaked P wave. RVH pattern when RV systolic pressure exceeds 50 mm Hg
VENTRICULAR SEPTAL DEFECT	Holosystolic with normal split of S_2. Diastolic filling murmur and S_3 at apex reflecting increased mitral flow. Thrill common.	Arterial engorgement, LVH or biventricular hypertrophy, left atrial enlargement	Biventricular hypertrophy in young. LVH in adult.
HYPERTROPHIC SUBAORTIC STENOSIS	Ejection murmur which varies in intensity, increasing with amyl nitrate. S_3 at apex	LVH or biventricular hypertrophy	LVH with ST-T wave abnormalities

ATRIAL SEPTAL DEFECT	Ejection murmur may be soft. S$_2$ widely split and fixed	Characteristic appearance with RVH, right atrial enlargement, arterial engorgement with prominent main pulmonary arteries. Left atrial enlargement in some patients	Diastolic overload pattern. Peaked P wave. Atrial arrhythmias, Normal QRS axis with secondum, left axis with primum defects.
PATENT DUCTUS ARTERIOSUS	Usually continuous murmur heard below *left clavicle.* At times only systolic component, especially with pulmonary hypertension (loud S$_2$ and pulmonic insufficiency murmur) may be present also	LVH and arterial engorgement. Left atrial enlargement Rarely, calcified ductus present	Diastolic overload of LV. Broad and notched P waves
PRIMARY PULMONARY HYPERTENSION	Systolic murmur may be heard but usually LSB diastolic murmur, loud P$_2$ and right ventricular S$_3$ sound	Prominent main pulmonary arteries with attenuation of vessels in mid-lung field. RVH and right atrial enlargement; PA calcification rarely	Systolic overload of RV; peaked P waves

Auscultation. Ordinarily, auscultation is the first suggestion of CHD in the adult since systolic murmurs or changes in the second heart sound are almost always present. Errors of overdiagnosis or underdiagnosis are common. A systolic murmur of less than grade III intensity with normal chest radiography and electrocardiogram may be a functional murmur where reassurance is essential. Other evidence may lead to the diagnosis of mild pulmonic stenosis, bicuspid aortic valve, prolapsed mitral valve, or ventricular septal defect where prevention of endocarditis becomes the major recommendation. Almost always, careful integration of auscultatory, radiographic, and electrocardiographic data will suggest the correct diagnosis; confirmation by echocardiography or cardiac catheterization may be necessary.

Tips for diagnosis are found in Table 1-13. Certain hemodynamic deductions from the EKG are useful. *Diastolic overload of the RV* is indicated by an RsR' pattern in V1 and is due to later depolarization of the crista supraventricularis, not to RBBB. *Diastolic overload of the LV* produces large peaked T waves in the left precordium. *Systolic overload of either ventricle* may produce amplitude criteria for hypertrophy with or without a "strain" pattern.

ARTERIAL INSUFFICIENCY

Embolism, thrombosis or, injury (frequently catheter-related) may cause acute arterial occlusion, frequently in the superficial femoral or popliteal arteries. Coldness is immediate, loss of sensation occurs in about 1 hour; gangrene may develop in 6 hours so that immediate surgery is necessary.

Thromboangiitis obliterans (Buerger's disease) is probably a specific entity that differs from arteriosclerosis obliterans by its relationship to cigarette smoking, its occurence in young males, the appearance of early migratory nodular thrombophlebitis, Raynaud's phenomena, and development in smaller arteries of hand and feet with instep rather than calf claudication. Distal aortic occlusion due to arteriosclerosis may produce hip, thigh, and buttock claudication, and impotence—the Leriche syndrome.

REFERENCES

Structure and Function

Chatterjee K, Ports TA, Brundage BH, Massie B, Holly AN, Parmley WW: Oral hydralazine in chronic heart failure: sustained beneficial hemodynamic effects. Ann Intern Med 92:600, 1980.

Shine KI, Perloff JK, Child JS, Marshall RC, Schelbert H: Noninvasive assessment of myocardial function. Ann Intern Med 92:78, 1980.

Polese A, Fiorentini C, Olivari MT, Guazzi MD: Clinical use of a calcium antagonistic agent (Nifedipine) in acute pulmonary edema. Am J Med 66:825, 1979.

Benotti JR, Grossman W, Braunwald E, Davolos DD, Alousi AA: Hemodynamic assessment of amrinone. A new inotropic agent. N Engl J Med 299:1373, 1978.

Packer M, Meller J, Medina N, Gorlin R, Herman MV: Importance of left ventricular chamber size in determining the response to hydralazine in severe chronic heart failure. N Engl J Med 303:250, 1980.

Miller RR, Vismara LA, Williams DO, Amsterdam EA, Mason DT: Pharmacological mechanisms for left ventricular unloading in clinical congestive heart failure. Differential effects of nitroprusside, phentolamine, and nitroglycerin on cardiac function and peripheral circulation. Circ Res 39:127, 1976.

Ischemic Heart Disease

Luchi RJ, Chahine RA, Raizner AE: Coronary artery spasm. Ann Intern Med 91:441, 1979.

Thadani U, Davidson C, Singleton W, Taylor SH: Comparison of five beta-adrenoreceptor antagonists with different ancillary properties during sustained twice daily therapy in angina pectoris. Am J Med 68:243, 1980.

Weiner DA, Ryan TJ, McCabe CH, Kennedy JW, Schloss M, Tristani F, Chaitman BR, Fisher LD: Exercise stress testing. Correlations among history of angina, ST-segment response and prevalence of coronary artery disease in the coronary artery surgery study (CASS). N Engl J Med 301:230, 1979.

Slone D, Shapiro S, Rosenberg L, Kaufman DW, Hartz SC, Rossi AC, Stolley PD, Miettinen OS: Relation of cigarette smoking to myocardial infarction in young women. N Engl J Med 298:1273, 1978.

Eaton LW, Weiss JL, Bulkley BH, Garrison JB, Weisfeldt ML: Regional cardiac dilatation after acute myocardial infarction. Recognition by two-dimensional echocardiography. N Engl J Med 300:57, 1979.

Elwood TC, Sweetnam PM: Aspirin and secondary mortality after myocardial infarction. Lancet 2:1313, 1979.

Holman BL, Lesch M, Alpert JS: Myocardial scintigraphy with technetium-99m pyrophosphate during the early phase of acute infarction. Am J Cardiol 41:39, 1978.

Kaiser GC, Barner HB, Tyras DH, Codd JE, Mudd JG, Willman VL: Myocardial revascularization: a rebuttal of the cooperative study. Ann Surg 188:331, 1978.

A randomized, controlled trial of aspirin in persons recovered from myocardial infarction (AMIS Group). JAMA 243:661, 1980.

Sulfinpyrazone in the prevention of sudden death after myocardial infarction (The Anturane Reinfarction Trial Research Group). N Engl J Med 302:250, 1980.

Hillis LD, Braunwald E: Coronary-artery spasm. N Engl J Med 299:695, 1978.

Proudfit WL, Shirey EK, Sheldon WC, Sones FM Jr: Certain clinical characteristics correlated with extent of obstructive lesions demonstrated by selective cinecoronary arteriography. Circ 38:947, 1968.

Cardiomyopathy

Brigden W, Cantab MD: Uncommon myocardial diseases—the noncoronary cardiomyopathies. Lancet, December 14, 1957, p 1179.

Brigden W, Robinson J: Alcoholic heart disease. Br Med J, November 21, 1964, p 1283.

Goodwin JF: Congestive and hypertrophic cardiomyopathies—a decade of study. Lancet, April 11, 1970, p. 731.

Regan TJ, Levinson GE, Oldewurtel HA, Frank MJ, Weisse AB, Moschos CB: Ventricular function in noncardiacs with alcoholic fatty liver: role of ethanol in the production of cardiomyopathy. J Clin Invest 48:397, 1969.

Gould L, Zahir M, DeMartino A, Gomprecht RF: Cardiac effects of a cocktail. JAMA 218:1799, 1971.

Fowles RE, Bieber CP, Stinson EB: Defective in vitro suppressor cell function in idiopathic congestive cardiomyopathy. Circulation 59:483, 1979.

Mason JW, Billingham ME, Ricci DR: Treatment of acute inflammatory myocarditis assisted by endomyocardial biopsy. Am J Cardiol 45:1037, 1980.

Smith ER, Heffernan LP, Sangalang VE, Vaughan LM, Flemington CS: Voluntary muscle involvement in hypertrophic cardiomyopathy. A study of eleven patients. Ann Intern Med 85:566, 1976.

Borer JS, Henry WL, Epstein SE: Echocardiographic observations in patients with systemic infiltrative disease involving the heart. Am J Cardiol 39:184, 1977.

Glenner GG: Amyloid deposits and amyloidosis: the B-fibrilloses (first of two parts). N Engl J Med 302:1283, 1980.

Arrhythmias

Dreifus LS, Ogawa S: Quality of the ideal antiarrhythmic drug. Am J Cardiol 39:466, 1977.

El-Sherif N, Hope RR, Scherlag BJ, Lazzara R: Reentrant ventricular arrhythmias in the late myocardial infarction period. II. Patterns of initiation and termination of reentry. Circulation 55:702, 1977.

Arnsdorf MF, Bigger JT Jr: The effect of procaine amide on components of excitability in long mammalian cardiac Purkinje fibers. Circ Res 38:115, 1976.

Arnsdorf MF, Bigger JT Jr: Effect of lidocaine hydrochloride on membrane conductance in mammalian cardiac Purkinje fibers. J Clin Invest 51:2252, 1972.

Margolis JR, Strauss HC, Miller HC, Gilbert M, Wallace AG: Digitalis and the sick sinus syndrome. Circulation 52:162, 1975.

Hoffman BF, Rosen MR, Wit AL: Electrophysiology and pharmacology of cardiac arrhythmias. VII. Cardiac effects of quinidine and procaine amide. Am Heart J 89:804, 1975.

Rosen MR, Wit AL, Hoffman BF: Electrophysiology and pharmacology of cardiac arrhythmias. IV. Cardiac antiarrhythmic and toxic effects of digitalis. Am Heart J 89:391, 1975.

Conrad KA, Molk BL, Chidsey CA: Pharmacokinetic studies of quinidine in patients with arrhythmias. Circulation 55:1, 1977.

Leahey EB Jr, Reiffel JA, Drusin RE, Heissenbuttel RH, Lovejoy WP, Bigger JT Jr: Interaction between quinidine and digoxin. JAMA 240:533, 1978.

Nies AS, Shand DG: Clinical pharmacology of propranolol. Circulation 52:6, 1975.

Valvular Heart Disease

Devereux RB: Mitral valve prolapse. Am J Med 67:729, 1979.

Rippe JM, Angoff G, Sloss LJ, Wynne J, Alpert JS: Multiple floppy valves: an echocardiographic syndrome. Am J Med 66:817, 1979.

Tinker JH, Tarham S: Discontinuing anticoagulant therapy in surgical patients with cardiac valve prostheses: observations in 180 operations. JAMA 239:738, 1978.

Starr A, Grunkemeier G, Lambert L, Okies JE, Thomas D: Mitral valve replacement: a 10-year follow-up of non-cloth-covered vs. cloth-covered caged-ball prostheses. Circulation 54(Suppl 3):47, 1976.

Cohn LH, Sanders JH, Collins JJ Jr: Actuarial comparison of Hancock porcine and prosthetic disk valves for isolated mitral valve replacement. Circulation 54(Suppl 3):60, 1976.

Ross JK, Diwell AE, Marsh J, Monro JL, Barker DJP: Wessex cardiac surgery follow-up survey: the quality of life after operation. Thorax 33:3, 1978.

Mills P, Leech G, Davies M, Leatham A: Natural history of a nonstenotic bicuspid aortic valve. Br Heart J 40:951, 1978.

Harvey RM, Ferrer MI, Samet P, Bader RA, Bader ME, Cournand A, Richards DW: Mechanical and myocardial factors in rheumatic heart disease with mitral stenosis. Circulation 11:531, 1955.

Infective Endocarditis

Sande MA, Scheld WM: Combination antibiotic therapy of bacterial endocarditis. Ann Intern Med 92:390, 1980.

Uwaydah MM, Weinberg AN: Bacterial endocarditis—a changing pattern. N Engl J Med 273:1231, 1965.

Rabinovich S, Evans J, Smith IM, January LE: A long-term view of bacterial endocarditis—337 cases, 1924 to 1963. Ann Intern Med 63:185, 1965.

Tompsett R: Bacterial endocarditis—changes in the clinical spectrum. Arch Intern Med 119:329, 1967.

Boyd AD, Spencer FC, Isom OW, Cunningham JN, Reed GE, Acinapura AJ, Tice DA: Infective endocarditis: analysis of 54 surgically treated patients. J Thorac Cardiovasc Surg 73:23, 1977.

Kaplan EL, Anthony BF, Bisno A, Durack D, Houser H, Millard HD, Sanford J, Shulman ST, Stillerman M, Taranta A, Wenger N: Prevention of bacterial endocarditis. Circulation56:139A, 1977.

Finland M, Barnes MW: Changing etiology of bacterial endocarditis in the antibacterial era: experiences at Boston City Hospital 1933-1965. Ann Intern Med 72:341, 1970.

Weinstein L, Schlesinger JJ: Pathoanatomic, pathophysiologic and clinical correlations in endocarditis. N Engl J Med 291:832, 1122, 1974.

Hypertension

O'Malley K, O'Brien G: Management of hypertension in the elderly. N Engl J Med 302:1937, 1980.

Gifford RW Jr, Tarazi RC: Resistant hypertension: diagnosis and management. Ann Intern Med 88:661, 1978.

Lowenstein J: Clonidine. Ann Intern Med 92:74, 1980.

Kirkendall WM, Armstrong ML: Vascular changes in the eye of the treated and untreated patient with essential hypertension. Am J Cardiol 9:663, 1962.

Moser M, et al.: Report of the Joint National Committee on Detection, Evaluation, and Treatment of High Blood Pressure. A cooperative study. JAMA 237:255, 1977.

Pericardial Disease

Klacsmann PG, Bulkley BH, Hutchins GM: The changed spectrum of purulent pericarditis. An 86 year autopsy experience in 200 patients. Am J Med 63:666, 1977.

Riba AL, Morganroth J: Unsuspected substantial pericardial effusions detected by echocardiography. JAMA 236:2623, 1976.

Arterial Diseases

Slater EE, DeSanctis RW: The clinical recognition of dissecting aortic aneurysm. Am J Med 60:625, 1976.

Wolfe WG, Moran JF: The evolution of medical and surgical management of acute aortic dissection (editorial). Circulation 56:503, 1977.

Congenital Heart Disease in Adults

Alpert JS, Braunwald E: Congenital heart disease in the adult. In Braunwald E (ed): Heart Disease—A Textbook of Cardiovascular Medicine. Philadelphia, Saunders, 1980, p. 1057.

Abraham KA, Cherian G, Rao VD, Sukumar IP, Krishnaswami S, John S: Tetralogy of Fallot in adults. A report on 147 patients. Am J Med 66:811, 1979.

2

Respiratory System

INFECTIOUS DISEASES OF LUNGS AND AIRWAYS
Upper Respiratory Infections

The common cold. The cold is a self-limited infectious rhinitis exhibiting minimal constitutional symptoms and caused by a group of viral agents including influenza, parainfluenza, respiratory syncytial virus, coronaviruses, rhinoviruses, coxsackie A and B viruses, echoviruses, adenoviruses, and others. A specific virus is isolated in about 60% of patients. Bacterial complications are rare, treatment is symptomatic, and antibiotics are not indicated.

Acute or chronic sinusitis. Sinusitis may follow upper respiratory infections and is more common in individuals with nasal polyps or allergic rhinitis. Fever, pain in the sinus area, purulent nasal discharge, and tenderness over the affected sinuses suggest the diagnosis, which can be confirmed by radiography. Since the sphenoidal sinus is deep, it may present as headache and fever of undetermined etiology. The pneumococcus and *H. influenzae* are commonly present; anaerobes may be found in chronic sinusitis.

Treatment includes the use of appropriate antibiotics and agents designed to decrease nasal congestion. Mixtures of antihistamines and vasocontrictors and neutral saline lavage (Ocean Mist) are useful. Analgesics should be added if sinusoidal pain is present.

Acute pharyngitis. The etiology may be viral or streptococcal. The manifestations are identical—fever, chills, sore throat, lymphadenopathy, exudative pharyngitis—so that throat culture is necessary to determine treatment. Adenovirus pharyngitis is common in military populations; herpes simplex can cause an ulcerated pharyngitis as well as recurrent fever blisters; coxsackie A may cause herpangina in children, a syndrome characterized by punched-out ulcers and vesicles. Gonococcal pharyngitis is commonly asymptomatic but may resemble either viral or streptococcal disease. Infectious mononucleosis may sometimes present a similar picture.

Infection with group A streptococcus (*S. pyogenes*) produces a classical bacterial pharyngitis. Rhinorrhea and suppurative complications are rare. Mild to striking pharyngeal erythema with uvular edema and tonsillar swelling, soft palatal petechiae, and a punctate or coalescent thick creamy exudate are present. Prominent systemic symptoms may overshadow the pharyngitis; in other patients, the entire syndrome is subclinical. The M surface protein antigen appears responsible for virulence and stimulates the production of protective antibodies. Antibodies to the carbohydrate-containing C antigen are not protective but persist for long periods of time in patients with carditis and may have some relationship to its pathogenesis. At least three exotoxins may produce erythema (scarlet fever in young individuals), stimulate fever, damage the myocardium and liver, increase capillary permeability, and inhibit the immune system. Peak levels of an antibody to hemolysin O, ASO, occur 3-5 weeks after acute infection and may persist for weeks to months, occasionally as long as one year.

Treatment consists of (1) benzathine penicillin, 1.2 million units I.M. in one initial dose, or (2) penicillin V, 500 mg q.i.d. for 10 days. Erythromycin may be used in patients sensitive to penicillin. Sulfonamides do not eradicate streptococci or prevent rheumatic fever; up to 40% of group A streptococci are resistant to tetracycline.

Pneumonia

Close to 100,000 individuals die each year from pneumonia in the United States. Introduction of antimicrobial therapy and the prevalence of the immunologically comprised host have led to modification of the classic pneumonitides; both atypical partially treated pneumonia and pneumonia due to unusual organisms are as common as classic pneumococcal pneumonia.

Defense mechanisms of the lower respiratory tract include: (1) epiglottal reflex, (2) IgA containing sticky mucus of the respiratory tract to which airborne organisms adhere, (3) cilia, (4) cough reflex, (5) lymphatic drainage of terminal airways, (6) phagocytic cells such as alveolar macrophages, (7) opsonins and specific antibody, and (8) dry alveoli. Defective leukocyte activity predisposes to infections with the pneumococcus, streptococcus, *H. influenzae,* and a group of other gram-negative bacteria. Acquired defects in T cell function due to antineoplastic chemotherapy, Hodgkin disease, sarcoid, and other situations predispose to a group of pathogens against which cell-mediated immunity is important. These pathogens include viral infections such as vaccinia, herpes and cytomegalic disease; fungal infections; bacterial diseases such as tuberculosis and listeriosis; other infections such as toxoplasmosis, *Pneumocystis carinii,* and disseminated strongyloidiasis.

PATHOLOGY

Pneumonias may be lobar (air space or alveolar), lobular (bronchopneumonic), or interstitial. Since an outpouring of hemorrhagic edema fluid is common in viral interstitial edema, alveolar filling is present so that viral and bacterial pneumonitis are indistinguishable by radiography. Classic untreated pneumococcal pneumonia began with a central edematous area with floating of bacteria centrifugally, leading to a spreading lesion often confined within one lobe. The differential diagnosis of pulmonary infiltrates includes: (1) infection, (2) aspiration, (3) atelectasis, (4) infarction, (5) neoplasm, and (6) chronic diffuse alveolar damage.

BACTERIAL PNEUMONIAS

The manifestations of a teeth-chattering chill followed by fever, pleural type chest pain, cough productive of bloody or rusty sputum, and severe constitutional symptoms may not be seen in incompletely treated disease or in immunologically compromised hosts. Atypical presentation is also seen in alcoholics, the elderly, and in patients with chronic airways obstruction. At times, radiographic findings are minimal in the dehydrated patient and are only seen following rehydration.

Etiologic diagnosis is accomplished by examination of sputum smear and by culture. The ever-present mouth anaerobes make sputum samples unsuitable for anaerobic culture. When evaluating sputum, a mucopurulent fleck must be selected and is probably validated when polymorphonuclear leukocytes are present and epithelial cells are absent. Transtracheal or bronchoscopic aspiration, direct needle aspiration or biopsy of lung, or open biopsy may be necessary, particularly in extremely ill patients or in immunocompromised hosts. Since gram-negative organisms are rarely seen in normal sputum, their appearance in the Gram-stained specimen must be taken seriously.

A blood culture should always be obtained, since the Gram stain is only about 75% sensitive and up to half of patients with blood culture-proved pneumococcal pneumonia may have negative sputum cultures.

A community study several decades ago revealed the following frequency of bacterial organisms: pneumococcus, 98%; staphylococcus, 1%; *Klebsiella,* 0.6%; and *H. influenzae,* 0.3%. The incidence of pneumococcal pneumonia in hospitalized patients has fallen to 60-70%; gram-negative bacteria have replaced the staphylococcus as the second most common cause.

Biopsy studies in the immunocompromised host with pulmonary infiltrates have isolated *Pneumocystis carinii, Aspergillus, Coccidioides, Candida,* cytomegalovirus, and a group of bacterial agents. Fiberoptic bronchoscopy with brushing and washing has given yields as high as 88% with little morbidity and may be the method of choice in these patients.

Friedlander's pneumonia. This form (*Klebsiella pneumoniae*) is most common in alcoholic males between the ages of 40 and 60. It is common in the upper lobe, and the striking enlargement of that lobe frequently produces bulging of the tissues. Sputum is classically brick red or currant jelly in character; early cavitation and leukopenia are common. Mortality rates are 40-60%, compared to 5% for pneumococcus.

Staphylococcal pneumonia. This occurs in infants, patients with alterations in pulmonary defense mechanisms, and other hospitalized individuals. The sputum is thick and yellow; abscess formation and patchy areas of involvement on the radiograph are common. It is frequent during influenza epidemics, and the overall mortality is from 25-60%.

H. influenzae pneumonia. Prevalence may be increasing because treatment of childhood infections reduces protective antibody response. Common in the same group that contracts *Klebsiella,* the diagnosis may be made by blood culture and missed on sputum culture because poor technique in decolorization may lead to the erroneous diagnosis of pneumococcus. One important control technique is to include a bit of debris from your own teeth on the same slide; if gram-negative organisms are not seen, there is probably difficulty with the staining technique.

TREATMENT

Pneumococcus. Procaine penicillin, 600,000 units twice daily. Erythromycin 500 mg q 6 hours, or a cephalosporin may be used in the allergic patient.

Staphylococcus. Nafcillin or oxacillin, 500 mg q4h I.V. in 4-hourly intravenous doses. Nafcillin has the advantage of greater activity over the pneumococcus and staphylococcus; it may reach levels in bile one to 100 times that in serum.

Klebsiella. Gentamicin, 2 mg/kg I.V. initially, followed by 1-2 mg/kg I.V. every 8 hours if renal function is normal. Chloramphenicol succinate, 1 gm q6h I.V. may be added.

H. influenzae. Ampicillin 0.5 gm I.V. q6h or penicillin G, 1 million units I.V. q6h if sensitive (strain not beta lactamase-positive); chloramphenicol succinate, 1 gm q6h I.V. if resistant.

Pseudomonas, Proteus (non-mirabilis), and other gram-negative organisms. Gentamicin, as above. Carbenicillin, 2-3 gm q2h I.V. may be added. *Caution*: These two agents cannot be mixed in the same bottle.

See pages 556 and 552 for detailed discussion of these drugs.

Penicillin in bacterial pneumonitis. The beta-lactam ring antimicrobials (penicillins and cephalosporins) are useful in most pulmonary infections, in part because of their gram-positive spectrum, in part because their action on bacterial cell walls (nonexistent in human cells) makes them quite nontoxic. Beta lactamase (penicillinase) is produced by many staphylococci, making them resistant; recently, plasmids have been acquired by some strains of *H. influenzae* and the gonococcus, making them resistant to ampicillin and penicillin respectively. A few pneumococcal type 57 isolates from South Africa have been shown to be resistant to penicillin; patients have received high doses of penicillin, beta-lactamase was not identified, and the pneumococci were sensitive to tetracycline, erythromycin, and clindamycin.

Vaccination for pneumococcal pneumonitis. Austrian and associates developed a polyvalent vaccine containing pneumococcal capsular polysaccharides, which is effective in at least 80% of individuals. Mass immunization is not advised but it should be considered for closed populations such as nursing homes and for patients with cardiorespiratory, hepatic, renal, or immunologic disorders, including asplenia.

VIRAL AND MYCOPLASMAL PNEUMONIA
Respiratory syncytial virus (in infancy), parainfluenza and influenza viruses, adenoviruses, rhinoviruses, coxsackie virus, and a small pleuropneumonia-like organism, *Mycoplasma pneumoniae,* produce pneumonitis in man. The disease is usually insidious in onset, accompanied by nonspecific "viral" symptoms of myalgia, malaise, headache and fever, and a dry cough. The chest radiograph is frequently more involved than predicted from the physical examination. Leukocyte counts are normal, and polymorphonuclear leukocytes are not seen in the sputum. More than half of patients with *M. pneumoniae* exhibit a rising titer of cold agglutinins.

Bacterial and viral pneumonias may be distinguished from one another in the otherwise normal individual not treated with antibiotics. Prior treatment with antibiotics or an altered immune system may make them indistinguishable. The prognosis is excellent in many but may be poor in influenza, varicella, and rubeola. Pre-existing heart disease or pregnancy has been associated with high mortality.

Heitzman divided the radiographic findings in viral pneumonia into six groups:

1. Peribronchial, septal, and reticular.
2. Lobular air-space filling.
3. Localized hemorrhagic pulmonary edema producing lobar or segmental consolidation.
4. Generalized hemorrhagic pulmonary edema similar to pulmonary edema from any cause.
5. Pleural exudation with effusion.
6. Chronic interstitial fibrosis.

These patterns are explained by the pathologic sequence, which begins with destruction of bronchial and bronchiolar epithelial tissue, at times extending to the alveolar epithelium. These walls become edematous and infiltrated with mononuclear cells, which then extend into the interstitium.

Legionnaires' disease and mycoplasmal pneumonia should be considered when treating nonbacterial pneumonia, since specific antibiotic therapy may be useful. One hundred eighty-two individuals attending an American Legion convention in July 1976 developed a febrile pneumonitis syndrome with infiltrates that were frequently bilateral. The pneumonitis was progressive in many, and 29 died. Subsequently, a small, pleomorphic, gram-negative rod, visualized best by silver impregnation, was identified as the causal agent. At present, diagnosis may be made by serologic techniques, isolation of the organism, or tissue analysis with special stains. Mycoplasmal pneumonitis, in contrast, is frequently unilateral, predominantly in the lower lobes, and is perihilar. Tetracycline and erythromycin appear effective in mycoplasmal pneumonia, while erythromycin at this time is the agent of choice in Legionnaires' disease.

The adult respiratory distress syndrome may result from diffuse nonbacterial pneumonias. Two recent CPCs published in the *New England Journal of Medicine* describe respiratory failure with Legionnaires' disease and adenovirus type 21 pneumonia.

Specific treatment of certain nonbacterial pneumonias is becoming available. In a recent series in the immunocompromised host, the following organisms were identified: *Pneumocystis carinii,* 27.5%; *Candida,* 5%; bacterial agents, 3.7%; viral agents, 8.7%. Pentamidine isethionate, 300 mg daily for 12 days or cotrimoxazole (trimethoprim, 960-1200 mg, and sulfamethoxazole, 4,800-6,000 mg) appear effective in pneumocystis pneumonitis.

Two relatively nontoxic antiviral agents are undergoing trial. Amantadine 100 mg twice daily for 7 days was observed to lessen the clinical course of individuals with uncomplicated influenza A infection, an important observation since the agent had hitherto been reserved for the prevention of influenza. Adenine arabinoside appears effective in both herpes zoster and herpes simplex encephalitis.

Lung Abscess

Necrotizing pneumonitis and lung abscess are most common in the posterior segment of the right upper lobe; they also occur in the apical-posterior segment of the left upper lobe and the apical segments of both upper lobes. This location derives from the initial aspiration of infected material that leads to the infectious process. Alcoholism, altered consciousness from any cause, factors leading to regurgitation, surgery, pulmonary embolus, and bronchogenic carcinoma predispose to this condition. Anaerobic organisms are involved in 70-90% and are the exclusive cause in about two-thirds. Aerobic organisms include *Staphylococcus, Klebsiella,* and *Pseudomonas,* while anaerobics include *Bacteroides, Fusobacterium,* and various anaerobic cocci and streptococci. Transtracheal aspiration or lung biopsy is necessary for isolation of anaerobic organisms, since anaerobic cultures of sputum are almost always contaminated with mouth aerobes. Abscesses have been seen in bacterial endocarditis, particularly when there was a history of drug abuse and tricuspid lesions.

Differential diagnosis includes tuberculosis and mycotic lesions, carcinoma, granulomata such as Wegeners, infected lung cyst, bronchiectasis, and pyopneumothorax. A major complication is empyema with or without bronchopleural fistula.

Penicillin in high doses is the mainstay of treatment, although it is not effective for certain anaerobes such as *B. fragilis* and occasional strains of *Fusobacterium*; it is obviously not useful for most gram-negative aerobes. While the precise dose of penicillin is in dispute, many recommend up to 15-20 million units daily depending upon body weight. A conservative beginning is 1 million units aqueous penicillin every 6 hours IM. If a good response is noted, this may be changed to 1 million units procaine penicillin every 12 hours. Clindamycin has specific activity against anaerobes and may be given intravenously, 300 mg q4h, or orally, 450 mg q6h. Even when the penicillin-resistant *B. fragilis* is present, penicillin therapy is effective, suggesting the importance of the mixture of anaerobic organisms.

Postural drainage and bronchoscopy are important adjuncts. Prompt defervescence is common, although the abscess cavity may remain open for several months.

Aspiration Pneumonitis

Aspiration of gastric contents is commonly unobserved, so that the nature of the subsequent pneumonitis may be incorrectly diagnosed. Aspiration of large fragments of material produce obvious airway obstruction, small amounts of infected material may produce lung abscesses, and spraying of gastric contents high in hydrochloric acid injure the alveolar epithelium and produce diffuse interstitial and alveolar edema. Since the contents may be infected, the anaerobic organisms described above are frequently present. Toung et al. demonstrated in an animal model that acid aspiration led to fluid accumulation with venoarterial shunting; treatment with albumin and corticosteroids tended to reverse this damage. Clinical studies, in contrast, have failed to demonstrate improvement or have even shown deterioration following high-dose steroid administration. Since the aggravation produced by steroids may be due to altered defense against bacterial invasion, better results might be expected if acid rather than bacterial fragments were responsible and also if steroids were accompanied by high-dose penicillin therapy.

Pleural Effusion

Pleural effusion is an important manifestation warranting work-up, since it may indicate serious but treatable disease. Light's important series used a protein in pleural fluid-to-serum ratio of greater than 0.5, an LDH ratio of greater than 0.6, and a pleural fluid LDH of greater than 200 units as evidence of an exudate. In the series of 47 transudates, 39 had congestive heart failure, 5 cirrhosis, and 3 nephrosis. Of 103 exudates, 43 had malignancies, 26 pneumonia, 14 tuberculosis, and 20 other conditions.

Additional studies on pleural fluid may be indicated if the diagnosis is unclear. A pH in pleural fluid less than 7.2 in infective processes suggests the need for closed tube drainage, less than 7.3 suggests tuberculosis, and more than 7.4 suggests malignancy or heart failure. Cytology and chromosome analysis produce the correct diagnosis in about 80%. Pleural fluid amylase may be higher than blood amylase in pancreatitis, carcinoma of the lung, bacterial pneumonias, and esophageal rupture. Elevated rheumatoid factors are seen in rheumatoid disease, carcinoma, tuberculosis, and bacterial pneumonia; pleural biopsy with immunofluorescence studies may identify collagen vascular disease.

Possible causes for transudates include: heart failure, cirrhosis, Meig's syndrome, nephrosis, hypothyroidism, systemic lupus, asbestosis, and pleural mesothelioma.

Causes for exudates include: carcinoma of bronchus, breast, ovary, pancreas, uterus, stomach, and others; lymphomas and leukemias; bacterial and other infections. Other causes are trauma, pulmonary infarction, pancreatitis, postmyocardial infarction, rheumatoid disease, infectious hepatitis, sarcoidosis, uremia, rheumatic fever, periarteritis, scleroderma, Wegener's granulomatosis, systemic lupus, asbestosis, and pleural mesothelioma.

Tuberculosis

Tuberculosis is an artful masquerader and should always be considered in patients with undiagnosed pulmonary disease, prolonged fever, meningitis, abdominal syndromes, or bone disease. Since the prevalence of tuberculous infection (measured by tuberculin testing) has declined from 80% in the early 1900s to less than 5% at present, physicians occasionally fail to identify a potentially curable serious illness.

Inhalation of a small number of bacilli may lead to bacterial multiplication in a small focus located in the respiratory bronchioles, alveolar ducts, or alveoli. Little opposition is encountered locally, and the infection spreads to the hilar nodes and thence to the circulation; the bacteremia produces metastatic foci that may lead to clinical tuberculosis and also stimulates the production of sensitized T lymphocytes. These lymphocytes elaborate a group of lymphokines that activate macrophages, causing them to differentiate into epithelioid cells. This cell-mediated immunity attempts to contain bacterial multiplication and also protects against subsequent exogenous infection.

Usually, the primary and metastatic lesions remain quiescent following the development of cell-mediated immunity; a peripheral granuloma with regional hilar adenopathy (Ghon complex) may be seen on chest radiograph. In some individuals, however, initial infection produces hilar adenopathy with bronchial obstruction, pleural effusion, or a pneumonic process (progressive primary tuberculosis). Tuberculous effusions are exudates, contain large numbers of lymphocytes, and are usually self-limited. More than 50% of patients with effusions may develop pulmonary or extrapulmonary disease within 5 years. In a small group of younger individuals, early hematogenous dissemination produces miliary tuberculosis or meningitis.

Conditions in the superior and posterior regions of the lung favor bacterial multiplication and breakdown of immune defense at any time following primary infection and lead to secondary or reinfection tuberculosis. Almost all examples of reinfection disease are due to breakdown of latent foci that occurred during the initial hematogenous dissemination; actual exogenous reinfection is probably uncommon. These infections are most common in postpubertal women and in elderly males.

Single or coalescent infiltrates in the upper lung fields with or without cough, fever, nightsweats, and weight loss suggest tuberculosis or a fungal infection. A cavity makes the diagnosis even more likely. Cavities result from liquefaction of caseous material and rupture into the trachobronchial tree. Endobronchial spread is responsible for extension of tuberculosis and makes the patient infectious to others. Persistent cough with sputum production suggests cavity formation in patients with tuberculosis.

Tuberculin testing. The intermediate dosage (5 TU) is ordinarily used; the low dosage (1 TU) should be used in children and in those with eye involvement; the high dose (250 TU) may be used when the intermediate dose is negative, but some cross-reactivity makes interpretation difficult. If anergy is ruled out by a positive test to *Candida* or mumps, a negative PPD in an afebrile, well individual tends to rule out tuberculosis. However, problems with the technique of administration and the association of other conditions such as Hodgkin's disease, sarcoidosis, certain viral diseases, carcinomatosis, and corticosteroid therapy account for up to 25% negative tests in individuals with proven tuberculosis.

The following data from the Center for Disease Control show the risk of tuberculosis in various groups:

1. Recent tuberculin converters: 3.3%.
2. Household contacts who are tuberculin positive: 3.3%.
3. Individuals with known but inadequately treated tuberculosis: 1.3%
4. Tuberculin reactors with abnormal chest radiographs: 0.8%.
5. Tuberculin-reactive adolescents with normal radiographs or parenchymal calcifications: 0.2%.
6. Tuberculin reactive-adults with normal radiographs: 0.08%.
7. Tuberculin-negative-individuals: 1 in 50,000.

Prophylaxis. Isoniazid (INH), 300 mg daily for 1 year, is strikingly effective in preventing symptomatic tuberculosis. Its use in all tuberculin reactors is tempered by hepatic toxicity characterized by elevation of SGOT and jaundice. Hepatotoxicity is age related: under 20 years, rare; 20-34 years, 0.3%; 35-49 years, 1.2%; 50 or older, 2.3%. It is more common in those who use alcohol daily and in the rapid acetylator phenotype.

INH prophylaxis is recommended for the following:

1. Household members and close associates of persons with recently diagnosed disease.
2. Tuberculin reactor with evidence of nonprogressive disease on chest radiograph.
3. Tuberculin conversion demonstrated within 2 years.

4. Tuberculin reactors in patients with Hodgkin's disease, diabetes, leukemia, silicosis, or previous gastrectomy or in those undergoing prolonged corticosteroid or immunosuppressive therapy.

Control of Tuberculosis in the Hospital. Respiratory isolation precautions until the patient has received 2-3 weeks of therapy are indicated. Tuberculin testing and chest radiographs should be obtained prior to employment in all personnel. Tuberculin testing should be repeated annually in nonreactors; every 6 months if they work in high-risk areas of the hospital. Annual chest radiographs should be obtained in reactors.

Treatment of pulmonary tuberculosis. Treatment is conveniently initiated in the hospital but in certain instances may be started at home. The three mainline drugs together with two others are described in Table 2-1. Resistance to INH is rare and, even when demonstrable, some in vivo effect is retained. Rapid reversal of infectiveness occurs in 95% of those treated for the first time; it is still as high as 90% in retreatment situations. Data from recent clinical trials indicate that the treatment period may be shortened from the previously recommended 18 months to as little as 9 months. This becomes particularly important with patient populations that tend to be relatively noncompliant.

Two or three drugs are recommended, depending upon the severity of the disease. In one program, INH (5-10 mg/kg per day as a single dose), SM (15 mg/kg per day IM), and EMB (15 mg/kg) are given for 3-4 months. If sputum becomes negative, the INH-EMB combination is then given for 18-24 months. A newer program that appears quite effective is the combination of INH as above with RMP (600 mg in a single daily dose). Each drug can be continued for 9 months or RMP can be changed to EMB in 4-6 months if the sputum becomes negative and the INH-EMB combination continued for 18-24 months. Retreatment usually includes RMP, pyrazinamide, and capreomycin for SM-resistant patients.

Corticosteroids (prednisone 5 mg/kg per day) may be used if disease is overwhelming and life-threatening, meningitis with subarachnoid block is present, or if there is hypersensitivity to one of the necessary antituberculous drugs.

TABLE 2-1—ANTITUBERCULOUS DRUGS

Agents	Dose (mg/kg/day)
Isoniazid (INH)	5-10, q.d., p.o.
Rifampin (RMP)	10, q.d, p.o.
Streptomycin (SM)	7-15, q.d., I.M.
Ethambutol (EMB)	15-25, q.d., p.o.
Para-aminosalicylic acid (PAS)	200 in 4 doses p.o.
Pyrazinamide (PZA)*	20-40 in 4 doses p.o.
Capreomycin (CM)*	15, q.d., I.M.

* Use Generally for Retreatment

Efficacy	Side Effects
Highly effective	Transient SGOT elevations in 10%; hepatitis in 1%; peripheral neuropathy
Highly effective	Rare jaundice but up to 25% when given with INH; serum sickness, thrombocytopenia
Highly effective (less than INH or RMP)	Vestibular and renal toxicity
Secondary drug; less effective	Optic neuritis
Less effective; poorly tolerated	Gastrointestinal irritation
Effective	Jaundice (3%); fatal hepatitis (1%); hyperuricemia
Moderately effective	Same as SM

EXTRAPULMONARY TUBERCULOSIS

Tuberculous meningitis. Once a disease of childhood but probably
more common today in adults, it results from direct extension of
a tubercle into the subarachnoid space, with extension and
allergic inflammatory response throughout the meningeal surfaces. Diagnosis is made by lumbar puncture. A mononuclear
response with high protein and low glucose is usual, although
neutrophils may be seen early. The tuberculin test is positive in
75%, pulmonary tuberculosis is present in about 50%, acid-fast
bacilli are seen on direct examination in less than 25%, and
cultures are eventually positive in 75%.

    Tuberculous peritonitis. This mimics almost any intraabdominal
process and, in alcoholics, may be confused with alcoholic
hepatitis, pancreatitis, or perforated peptic ulcer. Ascites, abdominal tenderness, and an abdominal mass with fever and weight
loss are common. Pulmonary lesions are found in less than 10%,
and the peripheral leukocyte count is generally normal. While
the peritoneal fluid is frequently exudative, transudates with low
protein content are found. Culture is frequently negative (up to
50%), so that laparotomy or peritoneoscopy with peritoneal
biopsy is necessary. For unknown reasons, the disease is most
common in black women.

    Tuberculosis osteomyelitis. The vertebrae (50%), hip (15%), and
knee (15%) are involved. Involvement may be multiple and also
include ankle, wrist, rib, shoulder, elbow, and sacroiliac joints.
Systemic symptoms are usually lacking, pulmonary disease is
absent in about half, and a history of antecedent trauma may be
present. The disease may present as localized arthritis, typical
osteomyelitis, back pain, a chronic draining sinus, or with
asymptomatic radiographic findings.

Pulmonary Disease Due to Fungi and Atypical Mycobacteria

Syndromes resembling infection with *M. tuberculosis* may be
produced by a group of indolent organisms; both pulmonary and
extrapulmonary manifestations are present. The differential
points are presented in Table 2-2.

TABLE 2-2—PULMONARY DISEASE DUE TO FUNGI AND ATYPICAL MYCOBACTERIA

	Epidemiology	Diagnosis and Therapy	Laboratory
HISTOPLASMOSIS	Widespread in North America. Up to 90% in Mississippi, Ohio, and St. Lawrence valleys. Infected by soil inhalation	Acute pneumonia, progressive disseminated or chronic cavitary resembling TB. RX: Amphotericin B	Skin test conversion or rising, fall or greater than 1:32 CF antibody titer. Serology negative in 25% with chronic cavitary form
BLASTOMYCOSIS	Throughout Americas but common in southeastern U.S. and Mississippi valley	Acute and chronic pneumonic, but calcification, cavitation and effusion rare. Bone (25%) skin and soft tissue lesions. RX: Amphotericin B best; 2-hydroxystilbamidine less toxic but less effective	Skin and serologic tests of no use. May show higher titers to *H. capsulatum*.

99

TABLE 2-2—PULMONARY DISEASE DUE TO FUNGI AND ATYPICAL MYCOBACTERIA (Cont.)

	Epidemiology	Diagnosis and Therapy	Laboratory
COCCIDIOIDOMYCOSIS	Southwestern U.S. and Mexico, Central America, South America. Soil particularly infective when hot and dry	"Valley fever" with pneumonitis, rash, erythema nodosum or multiforme. Hilar nodes and effusions common. Thin-walled cavities may remain. Also bones, soft tissues and meningitis. RX: Amphotericin B.	Skin test and precipitins positive early. CF antibodies appear later, rise with increased involvement may be found in CSF and joint fluid. CF negative in 40% with chronic cavities.
CRYPTOCOCCOSIS	Worldwide. More common with Hodgkin's lymphoma, sarcoid, leukemia, steroid therapy	Neurologic syndrome with low or absent fever, headache, ataxia, nuchal rigidity most common. Pneumonic lesions common; effusions, cavitation hilar adenopathy uncommon. Bone in 5%, skin in 10%	India ink reveals organism in CSF in 50%. Serologic studies positive in 90% with meningitis, much less with pulmonary disease

ASPERGILLOSIS	Sporadic and world-wide; frequently in decaying vegetation	Invasion in immuno-suppressed or those with granu-lomatous lung dis-ease. Circum-scribed enlarging lung mass or fun-gus ball in cavity. Also palate para-nasal sinuses and orbit. See asthma for discussion of al-lergic aspergillosis	Culture necessary. Serologic studies not useful
OTHER MYCOBACTERIA RUNYON GROUPS I-IV	No man-to-man trans-mission; found in soil, water, milk, normal oropharyn-geal secretions and as skin contaminant	M. kansasii and others produce TB-like syndromes but are of low virulence and usually colo-nize preexisting chronic lung dis-ease. Multiple thin-walled cavitation with little exudata-tion. Kansasii alone responds to INH and RMP. Resection freqently necessary	Bacteriologic identifi-cation required. Should be sus-pected with poor re-sponse to Rx or with highly drug-re-sistant strains

DIFFUSE ALVEOLAR DISEASE

Diffuse alveolar damage occurs whenever there is (1) primary injury to the alveolar lining cells (type I epithelial cells), (2) infiltration of the interstitial space, or (3) capillary leakage of plasma contents into the interstitial and alveolar spaces. Detailed histologic study made possible by the introduction of open and transbronchial lung biopsy suggests that the earliest response is proliferation of type II granular pneumocytes and appearance of lymphocytes, macrophages, and plasma cells as well as neutrophils and eosinophils in the interstitial space. While the appearance of proliferated type II cells was originally thought to be a specific form of damage (desquamated interstitial pneumonitis), sequential studies make it likely that it is an earlier cellular stage of a spectrum of diffuse damage leading from cellular proliferation to fibrosis. Focal or diffuse fibrosis is present in most biopsy specimens; frequently, the ratio of the more rigid type I collagen to the more compliant type III collagen is increased. The presence of granulomata within the interstitial space, arteritis, or evidence of minerals suggest relatively specific causes for diffuse alveolar damage.

A number of names have been used to describe diffuse alveolar damage, particularly when the cause is unknown. Hamman and Rich described four patients with progressive interstitial fibrosis. Interstitial pneumonitis and alveolitis emphasize cellularity rather than fibrosis; cryptogenic fibrosing alveolitis, an English term, suggests both fibrosis and cellularity of unknown etiology. Liebow suggested five subtypes: usual interstitial pneumonitis (UIP), desquamative interstitial pneumonitis (DIP), bronchiolitis obliterans, lymphocytic interstitial pneumonitis, and giant cell pneumonitis.

ETIOLOGY AND SPECIFIC DIAGNOSIS

Crystal et al. have suggested that classification is simplified if diffuse alveolar damage due to either known or unknown causes is considered.

Known causes. (1) Inert dusts such as silica and asbestos, (2) organic materials leading to extrinsic allergic alveolitis or chronic hypersensitivity pneumonitis, (3) drug responses, cytotoxic or hypersensitivity, (4) physical agents, (5) bacterial, viral and fungal disease, (6) chronic venous hypertension, and (7) maglinant disease.

Unknown causes. (1) Idiopathic diffuse alveolar damage, (2) associated with collagen-vascular disease, (3) associated with pulmonary arteritis, (4) sarcoidosis, (5) ankylosing spondylitis, (6) congenital and familial, (7) eosinophilic granuloma, (8) idiopathic pulmonary hemosiderosis, (9) alveolar microlithiasis, (10) Goodpasture's syndrome, and (11) alveolar proteinosis.

PATHOLOGIC PHYSIOLOGY
Increased cellularity, collagen deposition, and ratio of type I to type III collagen produce decreased pulmonary compliance. The work of breathing is increased; vital capacity and total lung capacity are reduced; residual volume is close to normal. While these abnormalities characterize a predominantly restrictive pattern, recent studies have shown evidence of small airway obstruction. A decrease in the diffusing capacity for carbon monoxide and varying degrees of arterial hypoxemia, almost invariably worsening with exercise, have been considered characteristic of the alveolar-capillary block syndrome. Recent studies have shown that mismatching of ventilation and perfusion may play an even more important role in the abnormalities of gas exchange. Carbon dioxide tension is normal or low until extremely late in the course of the disease. Vital capacity and resting diffusing capacity measurements show poor correlation, while measurement of lung mechanics and exercise determination of diffusing capacity and alveolar-arterial oxygen differences show good correlation with histopathologic abnormalities.

RADIOGRAPHIC DIAGNOSIS
Pulmonary roentgenologists frequently divide radiographic manifestations of diffuse disease into three patterns: *alveolar, interstitial,* and *nodular.* Great overlap and problems with histologic correlation exist, but the approach appears to improve diagnostic accuracy.

Alveolar. Lobar or segmental distribution of a homogeneous or ground-glass opacification; poor margination, areas of coalescence, and butterfly or batswing distribution.

Interstitial. Kerley A (radiating), B (horizontal), or C (reticular) lines, honeycombing, peribronchial cuffing, hilar haze.

Nodular. Large, small, or poorly defined nodularity. Ground-glass, localized linear, nodular, or other ill-defined densities suggest early alveolitis with substantial cellularity. As fibrosis increases, reticular and reticulonodular patterns appear; in later stages, honeycombing, coarse reticulation, and cystic changes are found. Pulmonary artery dilatation suggests pulmonary hypertension; pleural effusion, mediastinal displacement, or shift of tissues almost never occur.

CLINICAL MANIFESTATIONS

Symptomatology varies with the cause of diffuse alveolar injury. The following frequency of abnormalities is based on Crystal's data from 29 patients with idiopathic pulmonary fibrosis confirmed by open biopsy:

Dyspnea, 100%; cough, 86%; systemic manifestations, 48%; tachypnea, 46%; clubbing, 72%; abnormal ausculatory findings, 86%; increased pulmonic second sound, 70%; increased sedimentation rate, 94%; cryoglobulinemia, 41%; rheumatoid factor, 14%; ANA, 7%; increased IgA, 39%; increased alpha-2 macroglobulins, 22%; increased gamma globulins, 17%.

TREATMENT

Corticosteroids appear to be useful when biopsy studies show desquamation and increased cellularity; they seem to be of little use when fibrosis predominates. Dreisin et al. found that 13 of 16 patients with idiopathic damage and cellular histopathology exhibited circulating immune complexes; these patients appeared to respond to corticosteroids. Immune complexes were not found in patients with predominant fibrosis, and response to steroid administration was poor.

At present, it appears advisable to treat most patients with idiopathic alveolar damage with corticosteroids: prednisone, 1 mg/kg for 6 weeks, decreased by 0.05 mg/kg per week until 0.25

mg/kg is reached. If the disease is cellular, and particularly if lymphocytes or granulomata seem prominent or if clinical progression is rapid, azathioprine, 2.5 mg/kg per day, should be added. Therapy for specific varieties of alveolar damage may depend on the underlying condition.

SPECIFIC DIFFUSE ALVEOLAR DISEASES

Interstitial granuloma formation, developing as circulating monocytes and tissue macrophages evolve into epithelioid and multinucleated giant cells, is found in a variety of settings. Epithelioid granulomata are presumably immunologic in origin, while nonepithelioid granulomata result from foreign body reactions. Sarcoidosis, eosinophilic granuloma, and allergic alveolitis are three common pulmonary granulomata.

Sarcoidosis

Sarcoidosis is a multisystem granulomatous disease of unknown etiology. It is most common in American blacks and northern European whites; 90% of the patients are between the ages of 20 and 40 when first seen. Similar noncaseating granulomata may be observed in tuberculosis, fungal disease, leprosy, tertiary syphilis, foreign body reactions, allergic alveolitis, lymphomas, and in lymph nodes draining malignancies so that the sarcoid response may not result from a single exogenous agent. After ruling out known causes, a relatively homogeneous group of patients with "idiopathic" sarcoidosis emerges.

Hematogenous distribution of a causal agent seems likely, since microscopic granulomata may be found in almost every organ. Two-thirds of patients exhibit granulomata on conjunctival biopsy or liver biopsy, and similar microscopic foci may be found in radiographically normal areas of the lung.

Recent studies using lung lavage have shown the presence of large numbers of activated T lymphocytes within the lung. These cells secrete monocyte chemotactic factor which apparently recruits mononuclear cells to the lungs and leads to the development of epithelioid cells for granuloma formation. The presence of large numbers of T lymphocytes within the lungs leads to a peripheral T-lymphocytopenia.

CLINICAL MANIFESTATIONS

More than two-thirds of patients demonstrate pulmonary manifestations, although almost all patients reveal abnormalities at postmortem examination. Microgranulomata become confluent and may undergo fibrotic changes, producing interstitial fibrosis. Mediastinal lymph node involvement is common but not always clinically apparent, so that blind biopsy techniques such as mediastinoscopy may be useful. Clinically, about three-quarters of patients with pulmonary sarcoidosis have hilar adenopathy; two-thirds of this group have normal lung fields. Parenchymal disease is found in about half of the patients; half of this group have adenopathy. Interstitial fibrosis occurs in 10-15% of patients and is the major cause of death.

EXTRAPULMONARY MANIFESTATIONS

A variety of extrapulmonary manifestations are seen. Uveitis, conjunctivitis, keratoconjunctivitis sicca, retinal lesions, and lacrimal gland enlargement occur in 25% of patients. When associated with parotid gland enlargement and facial paralysis, the syndrome is termed uveoparotid fever. Erythema nodosum is common in European populations and suggests a good prognosis; other cutaneous lesions such as sarcoid plaques or disfiguring nodules indicate disseminated disease and suggest a poor prognosis. Muscle granulomata are found in more than half of biopsy specimens and may be associated with weakness and wasting. Skeletal lesions, either the classical cystic involvement of metacarpal and metatarsal bones or diffuse infiltration and cortical thinning, occur in about 15% of patients. Cardiac, neural, endocrine, and renal involvement is not uncommon. Usually, several organs are clinically affected, and the patient may experience systemic symptoms; occasionally, however, a single organ is involved, creating diagnostic confusion. (See Table 2-3.)

In addition, the angiotensin-converting enzyme is frequently elevated and may correlate with activity; exaggerated humoral responses to certain antigens have been observed, and alterations

TABLE 2-3—LABORATORY ABNORMALITIES IN SARCOIDOSIS

Hyperproteinemia	30%	Leukopenia	30%
Reversal of A/G ratio	88%	Eosinophilia	15%
Hypercalcemia	35%	Increased IgG	85%
Elevated alkaline		Rheumatoid factor	38%
phosphatase	30%		

in cell-mediated immunity may be identified by partial or complete anergy to skin testing. In a recent study, 10 of 21 patients with active disease had atypical lymphocytes, and there was a decrease in the absolute number of both total lymphocytes and T lymphocytes. The proliferative response of lymphocytes to phytoagglutinin was reduced.

TREATMENT
Although the use of steroids has been controversial, Johns et al. have presented convincing evidence for the long-term steroid therapy of symptomatic patients. Fifty-four % of patients had markedly reduced vital capacities before therapy. Vital capacity improved in 83% of that group; the maximum response occurred from 6 months to 3 years after onset of therapy. They recommended prednisone, 40 mg daily for the first 2 weeks, 30 mg for the second 2 weeks, 25 mg in a single morning dose for the third 2 weeks, and 15-20 mg each morning thereafter for 6 months. The dose was then tapered gradually unless relapse occurred. Relapses were not observed at the 15 mg/day dosage level.

Hypersensitivity Pneumonitis
A variety of diffuse alveolar damage of known etiology results from the inhalation of a group of organic dusts. A type III or Arthus reaction between the inhaled antigen and circulating precipitating antibody results in the deposition of immune complexes and complement within lung tissue. Acute symptoms resemble a viral or bacterial infection with chills, fever, dyspnea,

nonproductive cough, and systemic symptoms. The syndrome occurs 4-6 hours after exposure and subsides within 12-18 hours. A chronic form may be confused with idiopathic interstitial pneumonitis if the specific exposure is not identified. In these patients, gradually progressive pulmonary symptoms are experienced, and radiographs show pulmonary fibrosis with distinct linear fibrosis and honeycombing. A progressive restrictive defect, decreased compliance, diffusion limitations, and hypoxemia develop and cannot be reversed even if exposure to the offending organic dust is terminated. Histologic examination reveals granulomatous interstitial disease with fibrosis and airway obstruction.

Diagnosis of the less obvious types is possible only with considerable detective work on the part of the physician; the time relationships between exposure and symptomatology become less obvious in the more chronic situation. A careful environmental history, culture of the home and workplace for fungi, measurement of precipitating antibody, and challenge with antigens actually recovered from the environment will all lead to the correct diagnosis (See Table 2-4.)

Treatment. Prompt diagnosis and subsequent avoidance of the offending dust is the best treatment. Sodium cromolyn and corticosteroids are both useful in reversing the antigen-antibody reaction.

Eosinophilic Granuloma

Three diseases, Letterer-Siwe, Hand-Schuller-Christian, and eosinophilic granuloma, are grouped together in histiocytosis X. Of unknown origin, they differ only in age of onset, organs involved, and extent of involvement. Eosinophilic granuloma of the lung presents with malaise and fever or may be discovered on a routine radiograph. Dyspnea is not a prominent early symptom. Chest radiographs demonstrate small ill-defined nodules of varying size located mainly in the upper lung fields. Nodules composed of histiocytes and eosinophils are noted on lung biopsy. Diabetes insipidus is present in 20%, and 20% have lesions in the long bones. Spontaneous remission may occur, or the disease may

TABLE 2-4—HYPERSENSITIVITY PNEUMONITIS

Disease	Exposure	Specific Inhalant
Farmer's lung	Moldy hay	*Micropolyspora faeni Thermoactinomyces vulgaris*
Aspergillosis	*Aspergillus spores*	*Aspergillus fumigatus*
Bagassosis	Moldy sugarcane	*Thermoactinomyces vulgaris*
Humidifier lung	Fungal spores	*Thermophilic actinomycetes*
Detergent workers lung	Detergent manufacturing	*Bacillus subtilis**
Bird fanciers disease	Avian dust	Avian serum
(Occurs in people exposed to pigeons, parakeets, and budgerigars)		
Maple bark strippers disease	Moldy maple logs	*Cryptostroma corticale*

* Subsequently removed from detergents

Schlueter DP: Response of lung to inhaled antigens.
AM J Med 57:476, 1974.

terminate in pulmonary fibrosis, respiratory failure, and cor pulmonale.

Alveolar Proteinosis

The disease initially presents with dyspnea, malaise, and fever, and the chest radiograph exhibits characteristic fine coalescent nodules that radiate from the hilar region, producing a butterfly pattern. Histologically, the interstitium is relatively normal, the alveolar lining cells may be increased in number, and the alveoli and small airways are filled with a finely granular acidophilic material that is strongly PAS-positive. This material is a lipoprotein that is chemically similar to surfactant but has different physical properties.

The course is variable; some patients improve, while others die from respiratory failure or associated infection. Fungal infection, particularly with nocardia, is common. Bronchial lavage of each lung through a twin lumen Carlens tube with large amounts of normal saline containing heparin and acetyl cysteine has been reported to be an effective therapy.

Pneumoconiosis
Occupational exposure to certain irritant dusts produces a progressive but preventable form of diffuse alveolar damage. Dust particles are transported by macrophages to lymphoid tissue throughout the lungs. A spectrum of fibrogenic capacity ranging from the almost inert character of iron and soft coal particles to the intensely fibrotic character of silica is found.

Silicosis. Seen in hard coal and gold miners, grinders, granite cutters, workers in the abrasive industry, and foundry workers. Collagenous nodules form within the interstitium and coalesce as the disease progresses. Varying sized nodules, more marked in the upper lobes with calcification and cavitation, are seen on the chest radiograph. The eggshell calcifications of hilar lymph nodes are characteristic. Tuberculosis may complicate the clinical course; fibrosis appears to be progressive, even when the patient leaves the offending environment.

Coalworkers' pneumoconiosis. Inhalation of coal dust produces little fibrosis unless significant amounts of silica are present with the coal. However, peribronchial compression by the characteristic focal dust macule, if it is deposited in sufficient amounts, leads to the development of focal emphysema.

Pulmonary disease in American coal miners may be a varying mixture of the fibrogenic effect of silica inhalation and the obstructive effect of macrophages and granulomata laden with tobacco smoke and carbon particles. It may present as centrilobular emphysema, as almost asymptomatic "black lung," or as progressive coalworkers' pneumoconiosis. The presence of silicotic nodules or associated tuberculosis may contribute to the progressive disease.

Asbestos. This substance is one of the most dangerous encountered in the workplace. There are two main types: chrysotile, which accounts for 90% of world production, and crocidolite or blue asbestos. The disease develops in workers engaged in the production of the material as well as those involved in its use, such as pipe fitters, insulation workers, and demolition workers. Recently, exposure of individuals not ordinarily involved with these activities has been emphasized. Asbestos fibers remain within the lung for the life of the individual and produce disease only after a latent period of 10-15 years.

There are three distinct problems associated with this material. (1) *Asbestosis* or white lung is a form of progressive pulmonary fibrosis indistinguishable from the other forms described above. (2) *Bronchogenic carcinoma* is ten times more common in cigarette smoking asbestos workers, but in nonsmoking asbestos workers it is as rare as in other nonsmokers. *Calcified pleural plaques* are characteristic but present no problem, while (3) *pleural and peritoneal mesothelioma* are invariably fatal. Mesothelioma was a rare disease until the widespread use of asbestos; at present, more than 80% of mesotheliomas are believed to be asbestos-related.

Pulmonary Involvement in Collagen Vascular Disease
Rheumatoid Arthritis. Five types of pulmonary manifestations, which may coexist, have been described.

1. Pleuritis with or without effusion is found in 50% of patients at autopsy; 8% of men and 2% of women have pleural effusion on chest radiograph. This fluid is an exudate similar to that found in synovial fluid, with large numbers of both neutrophils and mononuclear cells; the protein and lactic dehydrogenase are high, while the glucose is low. Black granules within polymorphonuclear leukocytes release rheumatoid factor.
2. Necrobiotic nodules are morphologically similar to subcutaneous nodules and are usually asymptomatic unless they cavitate.

3. Caplan's syndrome is the presence of single or multiple well-defined parenchymal nodules, 0.5-5 cm in diameter, in coalworkers and others exposed to irritant inhalants. The joint manifestations frequently appear at the same time.

4. Diffuse alveolar disease is seen in a significant percentage of patients and ranges from abnormal pulmonary function studies with normal chest radiographs through interstitial pneumonitis to end stage fibrosis with honeycombing. Usually, there is a high titer of the rheumatoid factor. Up to 20% of patients with diffuse alveolar disease may have rheumatoid arthritis. The disease usually occurs following onset of arthritis but at times precedes it, making diagnosis difficult.

5. Pulmonary arteritis with hypertension is a rare association with rheumatoid arthritis.

The variable emergence of rheumatoid lung disease, the phenomenon of Caplan's syndrome, and the high frequency in men compared to women suggest that cigarette smoking and occupational inhalants in individuals with the rheumatoid diathesis may produce specific pulmonary abnormalities.

Systemic lupus erythematosus. Pleuritis and pleural effusion are seen in 50-75% of patients at some time during their course. The fluid is exudative, has low complement concentration and high protein as in rheumatoid arthritis. However, the cell counts tend to be lower, and glucose is not markedly depressed. Basal atelectasis, acute lupus pneumonitis, diffuse alveolar disease, and diaphragmatic dysfunction are also seen.

Progressive systemic sclerosis. Interstitial fibrosis is found at autopsy in almost all; pulmonary function studies reveal restrictive disease with impairment of diffusion. Increases in pulmonary vascular resistance are common, and many have evidence of right ventricular failure; pulmonary vascular lesions appear to be independent of parenchymal disease and may occur in its absence. Pleural effusion is rare. Association of bronchiolar carcinoma with pulmonary fibrosis has been confirmed.

Sjögren's syndrome. The dryness of the mouth, eyes, and other mucous membranes including the tracheobronchial tree are due to glandular atrophy with lymphocytic infiltration. Mucus plugging leads to airway obstruction and pneumonitis. Rarely, extraglandular lymphocytic infiltration leads to an interstitial pattern and, pathologically, a spectrum from benign to malignant lymphoproliferation is seen. When the sicca complex is accompanied by rheumatoid arthritis, pleural effusion and interstitial disease may occur.

Wegener's granulomatosis. Necrotic lesions of the upper respiratory tract with rhinorrhea, severe sinusitis, nasal ulcerations, and otitis media are frequent. The pulmonary manifestations include bilateral nodular infiltrates with cavitation that may be evanescent, disappearing and reappearing without therapy. Necrotizing granulomatous vasculitis is seen on biopsy. Calcification of parenchymal lesions and pleural effusions are uncommon. The agent of choice is cyclophosphamide and long-term remissions are common.

CHRONIC AIRFLOW OBSTRUCTION

Chronic airflow obstruction (CAO) is a common, underdiagnosed condition that presents as a complex of pulmonary symptoms or may complicate the course of other diseases such as acute myocardial infarction, pneumonia, or peptic ulcer. The term chronic obstructive lung disease (COLD) implies anatomic airway obstruction and embraces chronic bronchitis, emphysema, asthma, and bronchiectasis; the more limiting expression, chronic airflow obstruction, recognizes that reduced expiratory airflow may be due to either airway disease or loss of the recoil pressure of the lung, which is the driving force for expiratory airflow.

Three components of chronic airflow obstruction are recognized:

1. *Emphysema* is defined in anatomic terms and is an increase in size of air spaces distal to the terminal bronchiole, due to either dilatation or destruction of walls. *Panacinar or panlobular emphysema* describes uniform enlargement, *proximal acinar or centrilobular emphysema* predominantly involves the area of the respiratory bronchioles. While considerable variation exists and both types may occur in the same individual, the former is commonly associated with alpha-1 antitrypsin deficiency and the latter with cigarette smoking and inflammation. *Distal acinar or paraseptal emphysema* produces subpleural bullae and may be the major cause of spontaneous pneumothorax; *irregular emphysema* refers to the localized airspace dilatation produced by other pulmonary conditions that lead to scarring.

2. *Chronic bronchitis* is defined in clinical terms and is usually diagnosed when sputum production occurs on most days for at least three months in the year for at least two successive years. Reid showed that increases in the bronchial mucus-secreting glands and in specialized goblet cells located in both large and small airways are responsible for the cough and sputum production.

3. *Small airways disease*, a term coined by Hogg, Macklem and Thurlbeck, emphasizes that asymptomatic involvement of airways less than 2 mm in diameter may antedate symptomatic disease and may be recognized by measurement of maximal midexpiratory flow rates (MMFR).

An emphysema-like change occurs in many older individuals. Alveolar volume and surface area decrease, while alveolar duct volume increases; more than 50% of subjects over the age of 60 have this ductasia. These alterations result in a decrease in lung recoil, increase in residual volume, and a decrease in expiratory flow rates; Fletcher estimates that the $FEV_{1.0}$ decreases by 15 ml/year.

ETIOLOGY AND PREVALENCE

Consecutive autopsy studies showed that 70% of individuals over the age of 50, living in a large city (Saint Louis, Missouri) had evidence of emphysema; none of the nonsmokers but 19% of heavy smokers had severe emphysema, while mild or moderate disease was found in 36% of nonsmokers and 57% of heavy smokers. Fletcher, in a prospective clinical study, found that 12% of moderate smokers and 26% of those smoking more than 15 cigarettes each day developed evidence of airflow obstruction ($FEV_{1.0}$ below 2.5 liters). None of the nonsmokers developed CAO, and 25% of the smokers who did never exhibited sputum production, emphasizing the importance of routine spirometry in the evaluation of cigarette smokers.

Exposure to certain viruses such as influenza, high concentrations of air pollution, defective cilia as in Kartagener's syndrome, IgA deficiency, and alpha-1 antitrypsin deficiency may all be risk factors for pulmonary disease. Inheritance of the homozygous state (ZZ phenotype) reduces the alpha-1 antitrypsin concentration to 10% of normal and is associated with severe emphysema, usually of the panacinar type. Evidence of small airways malfunction has been found in MZ but not in MS heterozygotes; antitrypsin activity is 55-60% of normal in MZ, 80-85% in MS.

CLINICAL MANIFESTATIONS

Variable mixtures of small airway disease, mucous gland hyperplasia, mucus plugging, centriacinar and panacinar emphysema, and pulmonary vascular abnormalities lead to a wide spectrum of presentation with at least three clusters appearing as syndromes:

1. *Predominantly bronchitic* with productive cough, wheezing, and variable dyspnea.

2. *Pink puffer (type A)* with severe, relatively fixed dyspnea, variable cough, hyperinflation with increased total lung capacity, underweight, small heart on chest radiography, low cardiac output, close to normal oxygen, and carbon dioxide tensions.

3. *Blue bloater (type B)* with large poorly ventilated but perfused lung regions that lead to hypoxemia, hypercapnia, acidosis, corpulmonale, polycythemia, and CNS abnormalities including papilledema. Cardiac enlargement is present on chest radiographs, and the patients tend to be overweight.

Darnhorst coined the terms pink puffer and blue bloater in 1955. While earlier studies emphasized that the blue bloater frequently had considerable bronchitis with little emphysema, much overlap exists. Probably, the presence of centriacinar emphysema, small airway disease, and mucous gland hypertrophy leads to areas of poor ventilation while blood flow is maintained. In the pink puffer, panacinar involvement destroys blood vessels and vasoconstriction shunts blood away from poorly ventilated areas, reducing hypoxemia and hypercapnia.

Lindsay and Read characterized these patients as "responders" who protect themselves from hypoxemia by redirecting blood flow from poorly ventilated areas; oxygen, theophylline, or sympathomimetic amines may abolish this local constrictor response and produce hypoxemia. About one-third of patients appear to be "nonresponders" who could not redistribute blood flow. Of great importance is the intensification of ventilation-perfusion inequality by inactivity, sedation, oxygen administration, or respiratory infection, converting a pink puffer into a blue bloater.

PULMONARY FUNCTION TESTING

Simple spirometry separates obstructive from restrictive lung disease. A reduced vital capacity with a ratio of $FEV_{1.0}$ to FVC greater than 0.70 suggests restrictive disease; a normal or slightly reduced vital capacity with a $FEV_{1.0}/FEV$ less than 0.60 is diagnostic of chronic airflow obstruction.

Destruction of alveolar surface area leads to a decrease in diffusing capacity for carbon monoxide so that the DL_{C0} correlates well with the degree of emphysema. A decrease in expiratory flow rates may occur with either emphysema or bronchitis; decrease in lung recoil suggests the former, a decrease in airway conductance disproportionate to the decrease in recoil the latter.

Early small airway disease may be identified by the maximal midexpiratory flow rate (MMFR), by increased closing volume, or by measurement of flow-volume curves, breathing room air, and helium.

TREATMENT

Except for encouraging patients to stop smoking and removing them from dusty environments, the treatment for chronic airflow obstruction is largely symptomatic. Fletcher showed that the $FEV_{1.0}$ in smokers declined at a rate of about 100 ml per year; following discontinuation of smoking, the decline was about 40 ml per year. Since Burrows and Earle have shown that survival is related to $FEV_{1.0}$, the importance of this is obvious. (See Table 2-5.)

The presence of resting tachycardia, severe impairment of

TABLE 2-5—SURVIVAL IN CHRONIC AIRFLOW OBSTRUCTION

FEV_{1+0}	Five-Year Survival
Greater than 1.2 L	80%
0.8 to 1.2	60%
Less than 0.75	40%

diffusing capacity, or chronic hypercapnia reduces these figures by 25%.

GOALS OF SYMPTOMATIC THERAPY

Clearance of secretions. The patient needs education to aid him in the frequent removal of mucopurulent secretions by coughing, breathing humidified warmed air, and bronchodilator therapy. Sequence of bronchodilatation-hydration-ventilation-expectoration is more effective than pharmacologic expectorants.

Bronchodilator therapy. Most patients benefit, even though spirometry fails to document improvement. Mixtures of bronchodilators and sedatives are contraindicated. Both oral and nebulized bronchodilators are useful, the former for sustained bronchodilatation, the latter to assist in clearance of secretions (see bronchial asthma).

Antibiotics. Should not be used prophylactically, but should be taken whenever symptoms of bronchitis or dyspnea increase. Early treatment at the patient's discretion will produce quick improvement; delay before seeing a physician may result in exacerbation. Since the pneumococcus and *H. influenzae* are the usual organisms involved, penicillin G, ampicillin, or tetracycline are effective. *H. influenzae* is relatively insensitive to the cephalosporins, so they should not be used. Trimetheprim-sulfamethoxazole is also active against *H. influenzae*. Cultures should be taken where possible and therapy adjusted as indicated.

Breathing retraining and aids to everyday activity. Usually supervised by an experienced nurse, these are rewarding. Controlled exhalation prevents airway collapse, and synchronization of physical activity with exhalation increases exercise tolerance.

These techniques are probably more important than "diaphragmatic" breathing.

Oxygen enrichment without aggravation of hypercapnia. This can be accomplished by "low-flow" oxygen, delivered by a venturi mask calibrated to deliver 24-28% oxygen or by nasal cannula and an oxygen flow rate of 2-3 liters/minute. Intubation and mechanical ventilation are rarely indicated but must be considered if P_{CO_2} rises rapidly, P_{O_2} cannot be raised above 55, cardiac arrhythmias develop, or if the patient is somnolent or hypotensive. Nocturnal hypoxemia, caused by progressive airway closure and atelectasis, may require oxygen at night, even if the P_{O_2} during the daytime is above 55 mm Hg. Ear oximetry showed that nocturnal P_{O_2} fell below 40 mm Hg in 7 of 10 patients (below 30 in one) with severe obstuctive disease. Administration of oxygen,2 liters/minute, prevented these marked changes.

Other therapy. Diuretic therapy and digitalis are indicated if right or left ventricular failure is present. *Phlebotomy* is probably indicated when the hematocrit is above 55. Phlebotomy and replacement with equal volumes of dextran 40 has been shown to increase cardiac output during exercise. *Corticosteroids* may be used as a bronchodilator in patients with unstable cardiac rhythm where use of catecholamines is undesirable. *Carbonic anhydrase inhibitors* reduce bicarbonate concentration and may improve respiratory center sensitivity, but they increase acidosis and must be carefully used.

Intermittent positive pressure breathing. Probably, this is useful only in patients who are unable or unwilling to take deep breaths. It may be used together with humidification and bronchodilator instillation to foster clearance of secretions in individuals with wheezing, although it is difficult to demonstrate advantages of IPPB over compressors and hand-held nebulizers in clinical trials.

PULMONARY NEOPLASM
A circumscribed lung mass may be primary or secondary carcinoma, lymphoma, benign tumor, or granuloma. The solitary mass or coin lesion is a well circumscribed mass less than 6 cm in

diameter; the chances of malignancy increase with age, and thoracotomy is usually indicated if previous films are unavailable and the diagnosis cannot be otherwise made. In bronchogenic carcinoma, 5-year survivals approach 50%.

Larger or irregular masses are almost always carcinoma. The prevalence of lung cancer has been increasing dramatically since 1900 and is now the most common form of human cancer. A history of heavy smoking and bronchitis strongly favors the diagnosis of cancer when a lung mass is present. Asbestos and uranium workers have an increased incidence of bronchogenic carcinoma; synergism with tobacco is suggested, since the smoking asbestos worker has 90 times more lung cancer than a nonsmoker; the usual mortality ratio for lung cancer comparing smokers with nonsmokers varies between 9 and 12 and is dose-related.

Histologic classification is important for prognosis and therapy: 40% are undifferentiated, 35% are squamous cell, 20% adenocarcinoma, 5% bronchoalveolar. Small cell undifferentiated are termed oat-cell carcinomas.

Diagnosis. Hemoptysis, chest pain, recent onset of cough, and weight loss are common presenting symptoms. In one prospective study, 10% of patients with hemoptysis were found to have cancer. One study revealed that 79% of undifferentiated, 56% of adenocarcinomas, and 38% of squamous cell had extrathoracic metastases to brain, liver, adrenals, bone, and other sites. Intrathoracic spread may involve the recurrent laryngeal nerve and produce hoarseness, diaphragmatic paralysis due to phrenic nerve involvement, superior vena caval, obstruction, or Horner's syndrome due to invasion of the cervical sympathetic trunk.

A group of systemic syndromes, usually with oat cell carcinoma, demonstrate the ability of primitive cells to synthesize polypeptide hormones. These syndromes include:

1. Hormonal with hypercalcemia, inappropriate secretion of ADH, Cushing's syndrome, and gynecomastia.
2. Neuromuscular with profound myopathy, cortical cerebellar degeneration, and peripheral neuropathy.

3. Connective tissue and bone abnormalities such as clubbing, generalized hypertrophic osteoarthropathy, dermatomyositis and scleroderma and acanthosis nigicrans.

4. Vascular with migratory thrombophlebitis.

5. Hematologic with hemolytic anemia and thrombocytopenic purpura.

A variety of diagnostic procedures are available: bronchoscopy with biopsies for central lesions, brush biopsy, or percutaneous biopsy for peripheral lesions. Percutaneous techniques frequently show high yields but produce hemorrhage and pneumothorax in inexperienced hands.

Indications for mediastinoscopy vary but the statistics (Table 2-6) from Whitcomb provide some data.

Treatment. While overall results are discouraging, Weiss (Table 2-7) has shown that there is a subset of young individuals with squamous cell carcinoma who have 5-year survivals in excess of 20%. Operative mortality increases with age. Right pneumonectomy had greater mortality than left pneumonectomy.

Therapy of inoperable disease is controversial. Aggressive local radiotherapy with doses above 5500 rads appears to improve median survival, but radiation pneumonitis appears with levels above 4000 rads. Prophylactic cranial radiotherapy in patients with oat-cell carcinoma confined to the chest and supraclavicular area improves survival. Methotrexate in combination with other drugs may be useful in squamous cell carcinoma.

TABLE 2-6—FREQUENCY OF MEDIASTINAL LESIONS

All patients	38%
Undifferentiated	60%
Squamous	11%
Central	50%
Peripheral	20%
Visible on radiograph	56%

**TABLE 2-7—SURVIVAL IN 547 MEN WITH
BRONCHOGENIC CARCINOMA**

Age	Operative Death	Five-Year Survival
Under 50	11.4%	19.3%
50-59	9.5	18.4
60-69	13.9	13.4
Over 70	18.3	10.0
Overall	12.4%	15.7%

Cell Type	Operative Death	Five-Year Survival
Squamous	12.1%	21.1%
Undifferentiated*	14.3	8.4
Adenocarcinoma	11.4	12.7
Mixed	6.2	None
Overall	12.4	15.7

* Includes small and large cell undifferentiated.

Two recent studies emphasize problems in inoperable patients. Laing et al. reported that chemotherapy decreased median survival time substantially. Johnson et al. used combined therapy in small-cell carcinoma (doxorubicin, vincristine, cyclophosphamide, and radiotherapy, 3,000 rad to thorax and 2,000-3,000 rad to whole brain) and observed a complete clinical remission in 20 of 21 patients. Greco et al. used a similar program and observed a 1-year survival of 75% in 32 patients with disease clinically located to the chest.

BRONCHIAL ADENOMA
Up to 10% of surgically excised tumors are slowly growing, centrally located bronchial adenomas. They may present with hemoptysis or symptoms of obstruction and are somewhat more common in women. Many are carcinoid adenomas and may present with a typical carcinoid syndrome. Metastases are rare, and operative results are excellent.

Carcinoid adenomas could be called benign oat-cell tumors, since they arise from neural crest tissue like pancreatic alpha and beta cells, thyroid C cells, and enterochromaffin cells. These cells have been termed APUD cells (amine precursor uptake and amino acid decarboxylatation), and the resultant tumors, apudomas.

ASTHMA

Asthma is probably best defined as an increase in airway responsiveness to a variety of stimuli; enhanced responsiveness may be identified by measuring pulmonary function before and after administration of parasympathomimetic agents such as methacholine or carbachol.

Before diagnosing asthma, the following other causes of wheezing must be ruled out: chronic airflow obstruction, foreign body, bronchogenic carcinoma, bronchial adenoma, endobronchial granuloma, allergic bronchopulmonary aspergillosis, tracheal stenosis, pulmonary embolism, upper airway obstruction, left ventricular failure, polyarteritis nodosa, Wegener's granulomatosis, and the carcinoid syndrome.

Increased airway responsiveness is found in about 2% of the general population; symptoms appear before the age of 10 in 50%, and the male to female ratio is 2:1 in children but equalizes or even becomes reversed after puberty. Diagnosis is facilitated by dividing the responsive population into two groups, based on the major stimuli eliciting bronchospasm, allergic or idiosyncratic.

Allergic Asthma

Up to 50% of patients may have a seasonal variation, family history, association with rhinitis, positive wheal and flare skin reactions, airway constriction following challenge with aerosolized antigen, and increased concentrations of IgE in serum. Sensitivity to molds, animal dander, feathers, and materials found in the workplace such as toluene di-isocyanate (TDI) may produce nonseasonal asthma.

The reaginic antibody IgE is found in low concentrations in most individuals. In one study, means for three age groups were:

2 years, 10 IU (about 20 ng/ml); 10 years, 39 IU; and adults, 26 IU. Concentrations up to 50,000 IU are found in atopic individuals and in patients with helminthic infestations. Asthma in younger patients is more closely associated with elevated IgE than that in older individuals. About 13% of Caucasians appear to have genes associated with high IgE; the genetic control is related to both X and 6 chromosomes (HLA chromosome). Of interest in the relationship of heredity and environment is the observation that parasites can stimulate high IgE in those without genetic predisposition. A new analysis, radioallergosorbent test (RAST) measures antigen-specific IgE and rarely produces false-positives, except with house dust.

IgE and IgA producing B cells are located in the lamina propria of skin and of mucosal surfaces like the bronchial epithelium. Two IgE molecules attach to a mast cell and are bridged by an antigen, leading to the extrusion of mast cell granules and release of mediators including histamine, slow-reacting substance of anaphylaxis, platelet-activating factor, and eosinophil chemotactic factor of anaphylaxis. Histamine, probably the most important, produces increased capillary permeability, smooth muscle contraction, and stimulation of certain neural afferents, producing pruritis and vagal responses. Eosinophilia with asthma, parasitic infestations, hay fever, and certain drug reactions results from the eosinophilic chemotactic factor released by the type I reaction described above. Eosinophilia can also occur with type III and IV hypersensitivity responses.

Idiosyncratic Asthma

After eliminating the group of obstructive causes listed above, a large number of patients without obvious allergic proclivity are identified. Mecholyl provocation testing generally reveals increased bronchial reactivity. Several groups have been described: (1) following viral respiratory disease, (2) association with ingestion of aspirin and other nonsteroidal antiinflammatory agents, nasal polyposis, and sinusitis, and (3) following exposure to occupational or environmental pollutants. Frequently, etiologic factors cannot be identified, but systematic detective work is essential.

Nonsteroidal inflammatory agents may be factors in 2-10% of asthmatics. These agents inhibit prostaglandin synthetase and lead to a deficiency of Prostaglandin E_2 (PGE_2). It is postulated that in these individuals, PGE_2 rather than beta adrenergic tone may be the most important counterbalance to constrictor influences.

CLINICAL PRESENTATION

Cough and dyspnea are seen in most patients. Episodic presentation with nocturnal onset is common. Frequently, expectoration of stringy mucus (Curschmann's spirals) terminates the episode. Airway constriction is evidenced by increased airway resistance (measured by body plethysmography) and decreased $FEV_{1.0}$ and peak flow rates. Most patients present with mild respiratory alkalosis and hypoxemia. Increasing obstruction with reduction of $FEV_{1.0}$ to below 25% of predicted leads to hypoventilation with crossover of PCO_2 to normal levels and rapid increase leading to respiratory acidosis. Certain clinical and physiologic clues suggest severe disease that might result in sudden death:

1. Decrease in wheezing with loss of breath sounds.
2. Pulsus paradoxicus, right atrial and right ventricular hypertrophy, and atrial arrhythmias.
3. Rising carbon dioxide tension to "normal" levels.
4. Peak flow rates measured by a peak flow meter below 130 liters/minute. While 20% of asthmatics may present with hypercapnia, vigorous therapy frequently prevents the need for intubation.

The status between episodes influences treatment and prognosis. Persistent cough and evidence of small airway disease indicates chronic airway involvement.

TREATMENT

Management must be highly individualized. Identification of causal factors and specific treatment with hyposensitization, environmental control, antibiotics, and clearance of secretions where appropriate are important.

Acute exacerbations should be evaluated by sequential measurement of $FEV_{1.0}$ and by arterial blood gas analysis. Frequently, spirometry is simpler and more useful than repeated arterial puncture. Adrenergic agonists and theophylline are the cornerstones of bronchodilator therapy and act by directly increasing the cellular concentration of cyclic adenosine monophosphate. Since they do this by different mechanisms (adrenergic agonists increase production of cyclic AMP by stimulating adenylcyclase, while theophylline decreases its destruction by inhibiting phosphodiesterase), the two classes of agents are additive.

Most patients are treated in an emergency room or office; initial treatment is with either adrenergic agonists (subcutaneous epinephrine or terbutaline) or aminophylline, the soluble salt of theophylline. Dosage recommendations for both are shown in Table 2-8. It is important to achieve theophylline serum levels of 10-20 $\mu g/ml$; lower levels are generally ineffective, and higher levels may produce insomnia, anorexia, nausea, vomiting, sinus tachycardia, cardiac arrhythmias, or seizures. Knowledge of prior plasma levels and doses previously administered is helpful in understanding atypical responses. Cigarette smokers and individuals receiving barbiturates have increased clearance of theophylline; reduced clearances are seen in patients with liver disease or congestive heart failure.

A recent study involving the house staff from the Peter Bent Brigham Hospital demonstrated that subcutaneously administered epinephrine increased $FEV_{1.0}$ an average of 0.76 liter, nebulized isoproterenol 0.79 liter and aminophylline 0.23 liter, when given as initial therapy to patients arriving at an emergency room. Side effects for all agents and differences between the two beta agonists were not observed. These data suggest that short-acting sympathomimetic agents produce better and more rapid improvement in acutely ill asthmatics than intravenous theophylline and also emphasize the importance of $FEV_{1.0}$ measurements to monitor therapy. If objective improvement cannot be demonstrated, both sympathomimetic drugs and theophylline should be used, but hospitalization considered, since the combination substantially increases the likelihood of cardiovascular side effects.

While there is no clear-cut evidence that administration by intermittent positive pressure breathing is more effective than

TABLE 2-8—ADRENERGIC AGONISTS AND THEOPHYLLINE IN ASTHMA

Preparation	Dose	Route	Frequency
Epinephrine	0.003-0.005 mg/kg	S.C.	Every 20 minutes up to 3 doses
Terbutaline	0.25 mg	S.C.	Every 30 minutes up to 3 doses
	2.5-5 mg	p.o.	Every 6-8 hours
Theophylline	Load: 4-8 mg/kg	I.V.	Given over 15-30 minutes
	Maintenance: Continuous: 0.9 mg/ kg/hr*	I.V.	Continuous infusion
	Intermittent: 4-8 mg/kg	I.V. or p.o.	Every 6-8 hours
Metaproterenol	10-20 mg	p.o.	Every 6-8 hours

Nebulized bronchodilators		
Epinephrine	320 µg (2 inhalations)	Inhalation	Every 4-6 hours p.r.n.
Isoproterenol	250 µg (2 inhalations)		
Metaproterenol	130 µg (2 inhalations)		
Isoetharine	340 µg (1 inhalation)		
Nebulized steroids			
Beclomethasone	100 µg (2 inhalations)	Inhalation	Every 6-8 hours (may give up to a maximum of every 2 hours if needed, then taper back to maintenance)
Dexamethasone	250 µg (3 inhalations)		
Chromolyn sodium	20 mg	Inhalation	Every 6 hours (gradually taper to maintenance)

* 0.68 mg/kg/hr if over 50; 0.45 mg/kg/hr with liver disease or congestive failure.

that by metered inhalation, the delivery with large tidal volumes and concurrent nebulization of water may be valuable. In theory, the use of newer specific beta-2 agonists such as metaproterenol is desirable because of reduction of cardiovascular side effects and because of an extended length of activity. The longer action derives from the resistance of these compounds to inactivation by the enzyme, catecholomethyl transferase.

Corticosteroids are very useful in the treatment of acute exacerbations and of status asthmaticus. Initial doses of 40-60 mg or more of prednisone may be required; rapid reduction in dose is usually possible and should be based on clinical status and sequential spirometry.

Two relatively new agents have been effective in long-term control. Cromolyn prevents mast cell mediator release and is indicated in patients with allergic asthma. Nebulized beclomethasone apparently alters immune responses directly and allows for major reductions in oral corticosteroid dosage. Other studies have suggested that enhanced vagal activity may aggravate constriction of larger airways; parasympatholytic agents like atropine may be useful if these observations are confirmed.

The plethora of active pharmacologic agents complicates the selection of an appropriate therapeutic program. Turner-Warwick has provided a useful and pragmatic framework for long-term management:

1. *Brittle*—unpredictable decreases in airflow best treated by an aerosol bronchodilator.
2. *Morning dippers*—exaggeration of usual diurnal variation with predictable severe morning impairment treated by long-acting bronchodilators before retiring.
3. *Irreversible*—chronic reduction of airflow with empiric use of bronchodilators and steroids.
4. *Drifters*—showing little response to bronchodilators but almost complete improvement with corticosteroids.

PULMONARY EMBOLIZATION AND INFARCTION

The diagnosis of acute pulmonary embolization (APE) is difficult; 50-60% of patients with autopsy evidence of APE were not diagnosed during life. The incidence of APE at autopsy is 15-60%

depending on the patient population, and about 40% of individuals diagnosed as APE had other conditions such as bronchopneumonia, congestive heart failure, or viral pneumonitis. APE is usually multiple, more common in the lower than in the upper lung fields, and more than 80% arise from the leg veins. Infarction complicates embolization in 25% of instances but rises to 90% in cardiac patients.

A national cooperative study (Table 2-9), conducted between 1968 and 1970, randomized 160 patients to either heparin or urokinase. Mortality was 9% and 7% in the two groups, but a

TABLE 2-9—A NATIONAL STUDY OF 160 PATIENTS RANDOMIZED TO HEPARIN OR UROKINASE, 1968-1970.

CLINICAL OBSERVATIONS			
Dyspnea	81%	Rales	53%
Pleuritic pain	72	Increased pulmonary S_2	53
Apprehension	59	Tachycardia	43
Cough	54	S3 or S4	34
Hemoptysis	34	Diaphoresis	34
Temperature > 37.8°C	42	Phlebitis	33

ELECTROCARDIOGRAPHIC OBSERVATIONS	
Rhythm disturbances	11%
P pulmonale	4
QRS Abnormalities	65
Clockwise rotation (V4)	28
Clockwise rotation (V5)	8
$S_1 S_2 S_3$	9
$S_1 Q_3 T_3$	11
Pseudoinfarction*	11
ST-T wave abnormalities	64

RADIOGRAPHIC OBSERVATIONS	
Consolidation	41%
Atelectasis	20
Pleural effusion	28
Diaphragmatic elevation	41
Distension of proximal pulmonary arteries	23

* ST or T wave changes associated with prominent Q waves

National Cooperative Urokinase-Pulmonary Embolism Trial. Circulation (Suppl II) 47:1, 1973 number of measurements demonstrated more rapid resolution with urokinase. In both treatment groups combined, perfusion defects resolved in 55% at 14 days; 78% at 6 and 12 months; at 12 months, 16% had residual defects greater than 10% of total perfusion. Since all diagnoses were confirmed by angiocardiography, the following frequency of manifestations appears reliable.

Fifty percent had normal values for LDH, SGOT, and bilirubin; 16% had abnormalities of all three. LDH was elevated in 40%, bilirubin in 12%, and SGOT in 27%. Wacker's triad (elevated LDH and bilirubin with normal SGOT) was found in 4%; 54.2% had fibrinogen levels above 450 mg/dl; 22.7% had plasminogen levels below 1.75 units/ml. Right ventricular pressures averaged 44/9 mm Hg; right atrial pressure was 6. Twenty-four hours later, right ventricular pressures in patients given urokinase had fallen to an average of 33.7/6.5; there was no change in diastolic pressure in the heparin group, but right ventricular systolic fell to 41 mm Hg.

Arterial oxygen tension was below 80 mm Hg in 90% and below 70 mm Hg in 75% of patients.

TREATMENT

Heparin should be administered as soon as possible by either continuous or intermittent methods. Most believe the best technique is a loading dose of 75 IU per pound, followed by 10 IU/pound/hour by a constant infusion pump into a plastic catheter placed above the antecubital fossa. Subsequent dosage should be adjusted to maintain the partial thromboplastin time (PTT) at 1.5-2.5 times normal or the Lee-White clotting time (CT) to 2.0-2.5 times normal. If this is not possible, intermittent administration with 10,000 units every 4 hours for the first day, with subsequent dosages based on measurement of PTT or CT 1 hour before the next dose is scheduled. Bleeding may be controlled by the slow intravenous administration of protamine diluted in physiologic saline. One approach is to administer an amount equal to half of the last dose of heparin but not in excess of 100 mg; each 100 units of heparin represents 1 mg. Increasing heparin requirements suggest active thrombosis.

Heparin therapy should be continued for 7-10 days. Warfarin

should be initiated several days before discontinuation of heparin and continued for at least 6 weeks. The duration of warfarin therapy is controversial; some authorities recommend continuation for 3-6 months depending on the clinical situation.

The national urokinase study described above defined massive APE as one with obstructions or significant filling defects in two or more lobar pulmonary arteries or an equivalent amount of emboli in other vessels; submassive APE was obstruction or filling defect in at least one segmental pulmonary artery. A 12-hour urokinase infusion in addition to heparin therapy is probably indicated with massive APE, particularly if the patient is in shock.

Insertion of a vena caval umbrella (probably more desirable than other vena caval interruption techniques) is indicated if anticoagulants are contraindicated or if another massive APE occurs while the patient is on anticoagulant therapy. It is not indicated with a minor recurrence, since this may be related to the initial embolus.

PULMONARY HYPERTENSION: PULMONARY HEART DISEASE

Pulmonary hypertension should be considered whenever there is evidence of right ventricular systolic overload (right ventricular hypertrophy on EKG) or right ventricular failure (jugular venous distension, edema, hepatomegaly, ascites). Tricuspid valvular, right ventricular myocardial or pericardial disease, and myxoma or other tumor produce these manifestations but are not associated with significant elevations in pulmonary arterial pressure unless there is significant left ventricular impairment present.

Pulmonary hypertension is classified as follows:

A. Passive elevation secondary to left atrial hypertension
  1. Mitral stenosis
  2. Left ventricular failure
B. Increased pulmonary blood flow: hyperkinetic hypertension
  1. Atrial septal defect

C. Increased pulmonary vascular resistance
  1. Anatomic obliteration of vascular bed
  2. Vasoconstriction
D. Polycythemia: increased viscosity of the blood

Pulmonary hypertension when secondary to some other process is treated by treating the underlying disease. Oxygen and phlebotomy are important when chronic pulmonary disease is the cause; recent studies have shown significant decreases in pulmonary vascular resistance with either 12-hour or 24-hour continuous administration of oxygen. A recent multi-institutional study sponsored by the National Institutes of Health demonstrated that 24-hour administration was substantially more effective than 12-hour, particularly in patients with markedly reduced ventilatory function.

Primary pulmonary hypertension. This is relatively rare when unrelated to other disease conditions, more common in women than in men, and may be due to thromboembolism, intimal hyperplasia, or muscular hypertrophy. It is difficult to determine the precise morphologic changes clinically, but muscular hypertrophy is more susceptible to pharmacologic intervention. Patients present with exertional dyspnea but not orthopnea, syncope with effort, precordial pain, and weakness. Cyanosis may occasionally occur because of right-to-left shunting through a foramen ovale rendered incompetent by high right atrial pressures. It is difficult to separate such patients from patients with pulmonary hypertension due to intracardiac shunting. Prominent atrial contraction waves are seen in the jugular venous pulse, and a parasternal heave indicates right ventricular hypertrophy. The second heart sound is closely split, and the pulmonic component is accentuated. An ejection sound and atrial gallop are common; an early diastolic murmur of pulmonic insufficiency or a holosystolic murmur of tricuspid insufficiency may be present. The electrocardiogram exhibits very tall and peaked P waves, indicating right atrial enlargement and right ventricular hypertrophy with or without a "strain" pattern. Chest radiography reveals right ventricular enlargement, prominent main pulmonary artery, and underperfused peripheral arteries.
Treatment has been generally unsatisfactory, although acute

studies with beta adrenergic agonists or alpha adrenergic blocking agents (agents that apparently increase cyclic AMP) have shown a reduction in pulmonary vascular resistance. Two recent studies have shown that oral hydralazine, 200-300 mg daily in divided doses, or diazoxide, 300 mg/daily, improved symptomatology dramatically and reduced pulmonary vascular resistance substantially. Since improvement was sustained for 6 months, long-term therapy with either of these agents appears appropriate.

ACUTE RESPIRATORY FAILURE

A sudden reduction in arterial oxygen tension to below 50 mm Hg is termed *acute respiratory failure*. Since the physiology of oxygen uptake differs from that of carbon dioxide elimination, hypoxemic patients may have normal, elevated, or reduced carbon dioxide tensions. In general, an elevated carbon dioxide tension suggests respiratory failure associated with chronic airways obstruction; a normal or reduced tension suggests the adult respiratory distress syndrome.

Chronic Airways Obstruction

Hypoxemia is due to unequal distribution of ventilation to perfusion; as the ventilation-perfusion ratios fall, hypoxemia worsens. Carbon dioxide tensions above 60 mm Hg usually suggest an intercurrent respiratory infection or the injudicious use of either oxygen or sedation. A vicious circle ensues as alveolar hypoventilation leads to a rising carbon dioxide tension and a falling oxygen tension. Polycythemia increases blood viscosity, while acidosis and hypercapnia produce pulmonary arteriolar constriction. Together these factors lead to right ventricular failure with elevated jugular venous pressure, edema, hepatomegaly, and ascites. Drowsiness or coma is an important finding and indicates a rising carbon dioxide tension. Increased bicarbonate concentrations within the respiratory center limits the hydrogen ion response to rising carbon dioxide tension so that the center becomes insensitive. Respiration is driven by peripheral chemoreceptors, which respond to hypoxemia; administration of oxygen reduces the chemoreceptor drive and further reduces alveolar ventilation.

Therapy includes the administration of low-flow oxygen by either nasal cannula (flow rate, 1-2 liters/minute) or with a ventimask designed to deliver no more than 28-35% oxygen. Vigorous therapy with antibiotics, bronchodilators, humidification, cough techniques, acetozolamide (Diamox), phlebotomy, digitalis, and corticosteroids usually increases alveolar ventilation. Not all these agents are indicated for all patients. Usually, if a definite pneumonitis is not present, broad-spectrum antibiotics should be instituted following sputum and blood cultures. If pneumonitis is present, antibiotic therapy should be based on results of sputum examination.

The Adult Respiratory Distress Syndrome (Shock Lung)

The sudden onset of respiratory failure in a patient with relatively normal lungs is termed the adult respiratory distress syndrome. Hypoxemia is due to filling of alveolar units with fluid or infectious material, or to atelectasis. Hyperventilation is common, so that low carbon dioxide tensions are generally present.

Etiologic events include shock from any cause, sepsis, trauma, aspiration, drug overdose, pulmonary congestion, bacterial or viral pneumonitis, and other acute lung diseases. Decreased production of surfactant by type II granular pneumocytes and increased filtration of plasma contents into interstitial and alveolar spaces reduce pulmonary compliance and produce arterial hypoxemia. Certain units are completely unventilated but perfused, and produce a venoarterial shunt. In other units, interstitial edema may lead to a true diffusion block; in still other units, small airway closure occurs during expiration, leading to venoarterial shunting during part of the respiratory cycle. High concentrations of oxygen are necessary to overcome the effects of venoarterial shunting and raise arterial oxygen tensions to near normal values. A vexing paradox is that high concentrations of oxygen may further damage lung tissue.

Inappropriate activation of the immune system appears to increase capillary permeability. Sepsis, hypoxia, shock, and other factors appear to activate the complement cascade. Capillary injury activates the Hageman factor, producing intravascular coagulation, and also leads to platelet aggregation. The net effect is the release of mediators that increase pulmonary capillary permeability, dilate capillaries (bradykinin), and occlude capillaries with sticky leukocytes and platelets. Recent studies have shown that aggregating platelets release thromboxane A_2, a potent vasoconstrictor; treatment with specific thromboxane inhibitors substantially decreases mortality from endotoxin shock in experimental animals.

The most important treatment technique is early intubation with positive pressure ventilation; positive end-expiratory pressure (PEEP) increases functional residual volume and decreases venoarterial shunting. Positive end-expiratory pressure should be instituted early in all patients. The use of intermittent mandatory ventilation with PEEP, instead of controlled ventilation, improves oxygenation and maintains venous return and cardiac output. Recent studies have suggested that continuous positive airway pressure, delivered by mask without intubation, may be effective in certain individuals with normal alveolar ventilation. While patients must be closely monitored, the following approach is useful: end-expiratory pressure for hypoxemia, artificial ventilation for augmenting alveolar ventilation.

The second treatment principle is the maintenance of vascular volume. Corticosteroids in high doses (methyl prednisolone, 30 mg/kg administered once or twice) reduce mortality in septic shock and reverse immunologic abnormalities. Until specific antimediator agents are available, high-dose steroids appear relatively safe and probably decrease capillary permeability in the acute respiratory distress syndrome. One study has shown that PGE_1 reduces permeability in experimental animals previously treated with endotoxin.

Central venous and pulmonary wedge pressures should be maintained at close to normal levels by administration of crystalloid or colloid solutions such as albumin. Crystalloids should be infused initially and followed by colloid if atrial pressures do not increase to desired levels. Furosemide reduces total body water but also appears to shift fluids from the interstitium to the vascular space. Sympathomimetic vasopressor agents must be avoided.

Empyema is active infection or pus in the pleural fluid, usually resulting from an adjacent bacterial pneumonia or rupture from lung, or subdiaphragmatic abscess. Common bacterial agents include *S. aureus, Pseudomonas, Klebsiella, Pneumococcus* and anerobic organisms. Empyema fluid in its early stages may be a thin serous exudate; bacteria may be identified by gram stain and the pH is usually below 7. Closed chest tube draining or a limited thoracotomy may be necessary.

Pneumothorax may occur following trauma or in association with lung necrosis and a resultant broncho-pleural fistula; a *tension pneumothorax* occurs if the pathway to the pleural space is one-way. *Spontaneous pneumothorax* occurs in young adults, aged 18 to 45, and results from rupture of small subpleural blebs, usually at the apex. Sudden pleuritic chest pain with dyspnea is common. Differentiation from the hyperventilation syndrome is facilitated by obtaining radiographs in maximum expiration. Small pneumothoraxes may be observed, larger ones should be treated by aspiration or closed thoracostomy-tube drainage. Recurrence is noted in 50% of patients.

REFERENCES

Pulmonary Infections

Jacobs MR, Koornhof HJ, Robins-Browne RM, Stevenson CM, Vermaak ZA, Freiman I, Miller GB, Witcomb MA, Isaacson M, Ward JI, Austrian R: Emergence of multiply resistant pneumococci. N Engl J Med 299:735, 1978.

Levin DC, Schwarz MI, Matthay RA, LaForce FM: Bacteremic *Hemophilus influenzae* pneumonia in adults: report of 24 cases and review of the literature. Am J Med 62:219, 1977.

Toung TJK, Bordos D, Benson DW, Carter D, Zuidema GD, Permutt S, Cameron JL: Aspiration pneumonia: experimental evaluation of albumin and steroid therapy. Ann Surg 183:179, 1976.

Hamman L, Rich AR: Acute diffuse interstitial fibrosis of the lungs. Bull Johns Hopkins Hosp 74:177, 1944.

Heitzman ER: The Lung: Radiologic-Pathologic Correlations. St. Louis, Mosby, 1973.

Fraser DW, Tsai TR, Orenstein W, Parkin WE, Beecham HJ, Sharrar RG, Harris J, Mallison GF, Martin SM, McDade JE, Sheppard CC,

Brachman PS, et al.: Legionnaires' disease. I. Description of an epidemic of pneumonia. N Engl J Med 297:1189, 1977.

Cabot R, Scully RE, Galdabini JJ, McNeely BU: Case records of Massachusetts General Hospital. Case 979. N Engl J Med 300:301, 1979.

Scully RE, Galdabini JJ, McNeely BU: Case records of Massachusetts General Hospital. Case 32-1978. N Engl J Med 299:347, 1978.

Little JW, Hall WJ, Douglas RG Jr, Hyde RW, Speers DM: Amantadine effect on peripheral airways abnormalities in influenza: study in 15 students with natural influenza A infection. Ann Intern Med 85:177, 1976.

Whitely RJ, Soong SJ, Dolin R, Galasso GJ, Ch'ien LT, Alford CA, et al: Adenine arabinoside therapy of biopsy-proved herpes simplex encephalitis: National Institute of Allergy and Infectious Diseases Collaborative Antiviral Study. N Engl J Med 297:289, 1977.

Singer C, Armstrong D, Rosen PP, Walzer PD, Yu B: Diffuse pulmonary infiltrates in immunosuppressed patients. Am J Med 66:110, 1979.

Greenman RL, Goodall PT, King D: Lung biopsy in immunocompromised hosts. Am J Med 59:488, 1975.

Lauver GL, Hasan FM, Morgan RB, Campbell SC: The usefulness of fiberoptic bronchoscopy in evaluating new pulmonary lesions in the compromised host. Am J Med 66:580, 1979.

Winston DJ, Lau WK, Gale RP, Young LS: Trimethoprim-sulfamethoxazole for the treatment of *Pneumocystis carinii* pneumonia. Ann Intern Med 92:762, 1980.

International Symposium on Legionnaires' Disease. Ann Intern Med 90:489, 1979.

Wynne JW, Modell JH: Respiratory aspiration of stomach contents. Ann Intern Med 87:466, 1977.

Bynum LJ, Pierce AK: Pulmonary aspiration of gastric contents. Am Rev Respir Dis 114:1129, 1976.

Lau WK, Young LS: Trimethoprim-sulfamethoxazole treatment of *Pneumocystis carinii* pneumonia in adults. N Engl J Med 295:716, 1976.

Pleural Effusion and Tuberculosis

Light RW, MacGregor MI, Luchsinger PC, Ball WC Jr.: Pleural effusions: the diagnostic separation of transudates and exudates. Ann Intern Med 77:507, 1972.

Funahashi A, Sakar TK, Kory RC: Measurements of respiratory gases and pH of pleural fluid. Am Rev Respir Dis 108:1266, 1973.

Long MW, Snider DE Jr, Farer LS: U.S. Public Health Service cooperative trial of three rifampin-isoniazid regimens in treatment of pulmonary tuberculosis. Am Rev Respir Dis 119:879, 1979.

Byrd RB, Horn BR, Solomon DA, et al.: Treatment of tuberculosis by the nonpulmonary physician. Ann Intern Med 86:799, 1977.

Falk A, Fuchs GF: Prophylaxis with isoniazid in inactive tuberculosis. Chest 73:44, 1978.

Johnston RF, Wildrick KH: The impact of chemotherapy on the care of patients with tuberculosis. Am Rev Respir Dis 109:636, 1974.

Diffuse Alveolar Disease

Scadding JG: Fibrosing alveolitis. Br Med J 2:686, 1964.

Crystal RG, Fulmer JD, Roberts WC, et al.: Idiopathic pulmonary fibrosis: clinical, histologic, radiologic, physiologic, scintigraphic, cytologic, and biochemical aspects. Ann Intern Med 85:769, 1976.

Gadek JE, Kelman JA, Fells G, Weinberger SE, Horwitz AL, Reynolds HY, Fulmer JD, Crystal RG: Collagenase in the lower respiratory tract of patients with idiopathic pulmonary fibrosis. N Engl J Med 301:737, 1979.

Carrington CB, Gaensler EA, Coutu RE, FitzGerald MX, Gupta RG: Natural history and treated course of usual and desquamative interstitial pneumonia. N Engl J Med 298:801, 1978.

Liebow A: Definition and classification of interstitial pneumonias in human pathology. Prog Resp Res 8:1, 1975.

Dreisin RB, Schwarz MI, Theofilopoulos AN, Stanford RE: Circulating immune complexes in the idiopathic interstitial pneumonias. N Engl J Med 298:353, 1978.

Daniele RP, Dauber JH, Rossman MD: Immunologic abnormalities in sarcoidosis. Ann Intern Med 92:406, 1980.

Johns CJ, Zachary JB, Ball WC Jr: Ten-year study of corticosteroid treatment of pulmonary sarcoidosis. Johns Hopkins Med J 134:271, 1974.

Schatz M, Patterson R, Fink J: Immunologic lung disease. N Engl J Med 300:1310, 1979.

Schlueter DP: Response of the lung to inhaled antigens. Am J Med 57:476, 1974.

Israel HL, Patchefsky AS: Treatment of Wegener's granulomatosis of lung. Am J Med 58:671, 1975.

Chronic Airways Obstruction

Hogg JC, Maclem PT, Thurlbeck WM: Site and nature of airway obstruction in chronic obstructive lung disease. N Engl J Med 278:1355, 1968.

Laraya-Cuasay LR, DeForest A, Huff D, Lischner H, Huang NN: Chronic pulmonary complications of early influenza virus infection in children. Am Rev Respir Dis 116:617, 1977.

Eliasson R, Mossberg B, Camner P, Afzelius BA: Immotile cilia syndrome: congenital ciliary abnormality as etiologic factor in chronic airway infections and male sterility. N Engl J Med 297:1, 1977.

Hall WJ, Hyde RW, Schwartz RH, Mudholkar GS, Webb DR, Chaubey YP, Townes PL: Pulmonary abnormalities in intermediate alpha-1-antitrypsin deficiency. J Clin Invest 58:1069, 1976.

Fletcher C, Peto R, Tinker C, Spiezer F: The natural history of chronic bronchitis and emphysema. New York, Oxford University Press, 1976.

Burrows B, Earle RH: Course and prognosis of chronic obstructive lung disease. N Engl J Med 280:397, 1969.

Flick MR, Block AJ: Continuous in-vivo monitoring of arterial oxygenation in chronic obstructive lung disease. Ann Intern Med 86:725, 1977.

Gump DW, Phillips CA, Forsyth BR, McIntosh K, Lamborn KR, Stouch WH: Role of infection in chronic bronchitis. Am Rev Respir Dis 113:465, 1976.

Harrison BDW, Davis J, Madgwick RG, Evans M: Effects of therapeutic decrease in packed cell volume on responses to exercise of patients with polycythemia secondary to lung disease. Clin Sci 45:833, 1973.

Cherniack RM, Svanhill E: Long-term use of intermittent positive-pressure breathing (IPPB) in chronic obstructive pulmonary disease. Am Rev Respir Dis 113:721, 1976.

Lindsay DH, Read J: Pulmonary vascular responsiveness in the prognosis of chronic obstructive lung disease. Am Rev Respir Dis 105:242, 1972.

Dornhorst AG: Respiratory insufficiency (Frederick W. Price Memorial Lecture). Lancet 1:1185, 1955.

Lagerson J: Nursing care of patients with chronic pulmonary insufficiency. Nurs Clin North Am 9:165, 1974.

Cancer

Knowles JH, Smith LH Jr.: Extrapulmonary manifestations of bronchogenic carcinoma. N Engl J Med 262:505, 1960.

Weiss W: Operative mortality and 5-year survival rates in men with bronchogenic carcinoma. Chest 66:483, 1974.

Whitcomb ME, Barham E, Goldman AL, Green DC: Indications for mediastinoscopy in bronchogenic carcinoma. Am Rev Respir Dis 113:189, 1976.

Acosta JL, Manfredi F: Selective mediastinoscopy. Chest 71:150, 1977.

Johnson RE, Brereton HD, Kent CH: Small cell carcinoma of the lung:

attempt to remedy causes of past therapeutic failures. Lancet 2:289, 1976.

Laing AH, Berry RJ, Newman CR, Peto J: Treatment of inoperable carcinoma of bronchus. Lancet 2:1161, 1975.

Phillips TL, Miller RJ: Should asymptomatic patients with nonoperable bronchogenic carcinoma receive immediate radiotherapy? Yes. Am Rev Respir Dis 117:405, 1978.

Greco FA, Richardson RL, Snell JD, Stroup SL, Oldham RK: Small cell lung cancer. Complete remission and improved survival. Am J Med 66:625, 1979.

McNeil BJ, Weichselbaum R, Pauker SG: Fallacy of the five-year survival in lung cancer. N Engl J Med 299:1397, 1978.

Lawson RM, Ramanathan L, Hurley G, Hinson KW, Lennox SC: Bronchial adenoma: review of 18-year experience at Brompton Hospital. Thorax 31:245, 1976.

Asthma and Pulmonary Hypertension

Rossing TH, Fanta CH, Goldstein DH, Snapper JR, McFadden ER Jr, et al.: Emergency therapy of asthma: comparison of the acute effects of parenteral and inhaled sympathomimetics and infused aminophylline[1-3]. Am Rev Respir Dis 122:365, 1980.

Ruskin JN, Hutter AM Jr: Primary pulmonary hypertension treated with oral phentolamine. Ann Intern Med 90:772, 1979.

Klinke WP, Gilbert JAL: Diazoxide in primary pulmonary hypertension. N Engl J Med 302:91, 1980.

Rubin LJ, Peter RH: Oral hydralazine therapy for primary pulmonary hypertension. N Engl J Med 302:69, 1980.

Acute Respiratory Failure

Bone RC: Treatment of adult respiratory distress syndrome with diuretics, dialysis, and positive end-expiratory pressure. Crit Care Med 6:136, 1978.

Springer RR, Stevens PM: The influence of PEEP on survival of patients in respiratory failure. Am J Med 66:196, 1979.

Douglas ME, Downs JB: Pulmonary function following severe acute respiratory failure and high levels of positive end-expiratory pressure. Chest 71:18, 1977.

3

Digestive System

CONTROL OF DIGESTIVE SECRETIONS

Many important conditions arise from the leakage of corrosive gastric secretions backward into the esophagus, forward into the small intestine, or through the mucosal barrier into cells lining the stomach. The importance of vagal control of alimentary motility and gastric secretion has been known for years; the identification of a group of humoral substances provides additional insight into the sequential steps that allow release of gastric juice into the stomach, prevent reflux into the esophagus, alkalinize gastric contents as it passes into the duodenum, and turn off gastric secretion when no longer necessary.

At least 35 physiologically active peptides have been identified as products of the diffuse endocrine system (see page 319); many of these are found in the stomach, intestine, and pancreas as well as the central nervous system (CNS). Although commonly called gastrointestinal hormones, they are part of a generalized regulatory system modifying the behavior of many effector cells. Those active in the gastrointestinal system fall into two families with similar amino acid sequences. The gastrin group (big gastrin with 34 amino acids, small gastrin with 17 and cholecystokinin) is generally stimulatory; the secretin group (secretin, glucagon, vasoactive intestinal polypeptide, and gastric inhibitory polypeptide) is generally inhibitory. Cholecystokinin illustrates the diffuse roles for a single messenger; it is produced in the gut but is also found in high concentration in the cerebral cortex, where it may well influence behavior.

The polypeptides produced in the gastrointestinal tract, vagal activity mediated through the release of acetylcholine, histamine, and other factors stimulate and inhibit the sequential steps of digestion. Histamine is found in high concentrations in the gastric mucosa and is presumed to be a primary regulator of acid secretion, potentiating the action of the vagus and gastrin. H_2 inhibitors decrease acid production in response to either vagal or gastrin stimulation.

The cephalic phase of digestion begins with vagal activity that arises from hypothalamic activation. Gastric distension also increases vagal activity; antral distension leads to the release of gastrin from specific cells in the pyloric region. Combined neural and humoral stimulation leads to secretion of active digestive juice as the parietal cells secrete hydrochloric acid and the chief cells secrete pepsin. Positive feedback or enhancement occurs as vagal stimulation increases gastrin release. At some point, hydrochloric acid inhibits gastrin secretion by a direct effect on the pyloric mucosa, signaling the end of the *gastric phase* and the beginning of the *intestinal phase* of digestion. Acid reaching the duodenum stimulates the release of secretin from S cells in the duodenal mucosa; secretin acts to neutralize the acid chyme by stimulating the release of alkaline pancreatic and hepatic secretions. Fat in the duodenum releases gastrointestinal inhibitory polypeptide and cholecystokinin, both of which inhibit acid secretion; the latter also stimulates pancreatic secretions and gallbladder contraction.

Peptic Esophagitis and Heartburn

Widespread radiography of the alimentary canal has revealed the high frequency of hiatus hernia, gallstones, and diverticula, forcing clinicians to decide their relationship to a variety of symptoms. Both reflux esophagitis and sliding hiatal hernias occur in large numbers of individuals over the age of 40, suggesting their causal relationship and encouraging surgical procedures to replace the wayward gastric segment below the diaphragm. More recent observations suggest this belief to be erroneous and emphasize that reflux is related mainly to the competency of the lower esophageal sphincter, the corrosive nature of the gastric contents, and the sensitivity of the esophageal mucosa.

Separation of symptoms due to reflux from those related to coronary artery disease becomes a major clinical problem. Heartburn typically occurs after large meals, particularly when the person is recumbent, and is aggravated by positional changes enhancing reflux. It may be epigastric or retrosternal, is commonly described as burning or aching, and may radiate to the same distribution as anginal pain. It is occasionally relieved by sublingual nitroglycerine, but relief usually requires more time than the 2-3 minutes needed for disappearance of angina.

Radiographic and endoscopic changes are late; reflux may be visualized radiographically but occurs without symptoms in 25% of individuals. Biopsy will reveal inflammatory changes consistent with reflux. Confirmation that chest pain is due to reflux may require the instillation of 300 ml of 0.1N hydrochloric acid into the stomach, with measurement of pH above and below the lower esophageal sphincter, or at two levels of the esophagus. Intraesophageal pH above 5 suggests sphincter competence.

Simple treatment is the ingestion of small meals and the avoidance of recumbency for 2-3 hours after eating. Avoiding specific foods known to produce symptomatology and elevation of the head of the bed are also important. Anticholinergic drugs are not useful because they decrease the alkalinity of the esophagus, peristaltic activity, and sphincter tone. A cholinergic agent, bethanechol (Urecholine, 25 mg before meals and at bedtime), increases sphincter tone and may be used in the unresponsive patient. Antacids and cimetidine reduce the irritant nature of gastric fluid but have inconsistent effects on symptomatology.

Chronic reflux of acid juices is believed to transform the squamous esophageal epithelium into columnar (Barrett) epithelium. This epithelium is premalignant; adenocarcinoma develops in 5% of patients. Surgical antireflux techniques may lead to regression of columnar epithelium and could prevent the development of carcinoma.

Peptic Ulcer Disease

Loss of surface epithelium with extension below the muscularis mucosa is termed ulceration; surface lesions without muscular extension are termed erosions. Ulceration in areas bathed by gastric juices are called peptic ulcers and include esophageal, gastric, duodenal or jejunal ulcers.

Duodenal ulcer. Four times as common as gastric ulcer, it occurs about two to three times per 1000 men each year. The incidence appears to be declining; at one time, certain occupational groups such as taxicab drivers had a prevalence approaching 10%. Most ulcers are found within 3 cm of the pylorus. They may be erosions or true ulcers, may produce fibrosis with gastric obstruction, may perforate into the peritoneal cavity or into adjacent organs such as the pancreas, and may produce massive upper gastrointestinal bleeding by eroding a major arterial branch.

Duodenal ulcers do not occur in the absence of acid and are more common in hypersecretors. More than 50% of patients are hypersecretors, as evidenced by increases in basal and maximal acid output. A variety of physiologic abnormalities predisposing to increased acid secretion have been identified: more parietal cells, increased sensitivity to pentagastrin, and faulty autoregulation of gastric secretion. These abnormalities may be genetic since peptic ulcer is three times more common in the relatives of ulcer patients than in the general population. Patients have a higher frequency of blood group O, are more likely to be nonsecretors of AB(H) antigens into gastric juice, and have an increased frequency of HLA-B5 and genes leading to an increased serum concentration of pepsinogen I. Duodenal ulcer is also associated with cigarette smoking, hyperparathyroidism, cirrhosis, chronic pancreatitis, cystic fibrosis, pulmonary emphysema, and rheumatoid arthritis.

The diagnosis of duodenal ulcer is suggested by classic food-pain relationships, with pain or discomfort beginning several hours after eating, when gastric acid secretion increases following the suppression associated with duodenal activity. It may awaken the patient in the early hours of the morning and frequently occurs when individuals skip meals. Constant pain, nausea, vomiting, anorexia, or weight loss indicate perforation, obstruction, or an associated gastric ulcer. Radiographic evaluation may be negative with duodenal erosion or may show bulbar scarring with chronic ulcer disease. Endoscopy is somewhat more accurate, since inflammatory changes or bleeding may permit correlation of structure with clinical presentation.

NATURAL HISTORY AND THERAPY

The cyclic nature of duodenal ulcer disease makes evaluation of therapy difficult. More than 25-40% heal with placebo treatment, and there is a 95% chance of recurrence. Clinical studies are notoriously unreliable, since there is little correlation between the presence of symptoms, endoscopic evidence of healing, and subsequent recurrence.

High doses of antacid (120 mEq, 1 and 3 hours after meals and before retiring) have been shown to increase ulcer healing by elevating the gastric pH to above 5. The choice must be individualized for each patient. Calcium carbonate preparations are contraindicated if there is evidence of renal calculi, dehydration, electrolyte imbalance, constipation, or fecal impaction. Aluminum hydroxide may be constipating, lower serum phosphate, and have high sodium concentrations. Magnesium salts have laxative effects and may be absorbed, producing hypermagnesemia, particularly in patients with abnormal renal function. Several useful antacids are listed in Table 3-1.

Palatability and side effects differ widely. Improved compliance and chance for healing require trial selection of several different antacids with high neutralizing capacity. Potency published in package inserts is frequently expressed in varying units. Clinical studies have shown that placebo and antacid have similar effects on symptomatology but that high-dose antacids increase healing. In one study with 144 mEq given as suggested above, healing was noted in 78% compared to 45% with placebo. Anticholinergic agents also decrease acid secretion substantially and should be

TABLE 3-1—Comparison of Commonly Used Antacids

Brand Name	Active Components	mEq H+ Neutralized per 1.0 ml	Capacity *
Mylanta II	Equal amounts of Mg and Al Hydroxide	4.1	124
Maalox	Almost equal Mg and Al Hydroxide	2.6	78
Gelusil	Equal amounts	1.3	40
Amphogel	Aluminum hydroxide	1.9	58

* Capacity in mEq/30ml to raise pH of 0.1 N HCL to pH3 for 2 hr.

used in difficult situations; they have not been shown to improve healing rates over those of placebo, however.

An important adjunct to antacid therapy is cimetidine, an H_2-receptor antagonist which blocks acid secretion from the parietal cell. It appears to be the first effective, acceptable, and palatable agent generally available for the treatment of peptic ulcer. One comparative study with 300 mg four times daily (with meals and before retiring) for 3-4 weeks showed healing in 70% compared to 37% with placebo and 55-60% with antacids given in high dose. Recurrence rate within 1 year on maintenance cimetidine is 20% compared to 60-70% with placebo; its important role in high-level acid secretors is shown by the observation that most individuals with the Zollinger-Ellison syndrome respond. The obvious advantage of cimetidine over antacid is better patient acceptance and compliance. Side effects are infrequent but include dizziness, headache, rash, changes in gastrointestinal motility, mental changes, bradycardia, alterations in renal function (creatinine elevated in 10%), elevation in transaminase or alkaline phosphatase to twice normal in 3-5%, rare hepatitis, gynecomastia in up to 4%, reduction in sperm count within normal levels, rare impotence or loss of libido, and potentiation of the anticoagulant effect of warfarin. For these reasons, the prudent physician should limit long-term use to resistant patients—at least for the present.

Surgical treatment is indicated for (1) perforation, (2) organic obstruction, (3) intractable hemorrhage, or (4) refractoriness to medical therapy. Like medical therapy, the goal is the reduction of hydrochloric acid and pepsin secretion. Some form of vagotomy and resection to include the gastrin-producing cells of the antrum will reduce parietal cell activity.

Gastric Ulcers (GU)

Less frequent than duodenal ulcers, gastric ulcers are three to four times as common in men as in women. They tend to occur between 45 and 55 but have been seen at any age, and are found most often in the antrum or at the junction of the antrum and fundus, usually single and on the lesser curvature or in the prepyloric area.

The exact cause of gastric ulceration is unknown. Decrease in gastric emptying could stimulate gastrin release by producing antral distension, or bile refluxing through the pylorus could damage the gastric mucosal barrier. The clinical manifestations are not as clear-cut as in duodenal ulcer disease. Pain or discomfort may be vague, less localized, more diffuse, and unpredictably related to meals. Nausea, vomiting, anorexia, and weight loss are common and occur even in the absence of obstruction. Unlike duodenal ulcers, 10% of gastric ulcers are malignant.

Radiography will differentiate between benign and malignant lesions in 90% of patients. Endoscopy will identify the remaining ulcers. Endoscopy with biopsy and cytology has an accuracy of more than 90% in the differentiation of benign from malignant lesions. Errors are usually in the direction of false-negatives. Histamine-fast achlorhydria increases the likelihood of carcinoma, and endoscopic or surgical biopsy is indicated.

A strict controlled course of medical therapy is appropriate in a patient who produces acid and has radiographic features of a benign ulcer or whose endoscopy with biopsy and cytology is benign. The medical regimen consists of antacid (q2h), cimetidine, 300 mg q6h, and bed rest. Anticholinergic drugs are contraindicated because they delay gastric emptying. Carbenoxalone, not yet available in the U.S., is slightly less effective than cimetidine. Radiography is repeated in 3 weeks; endoscopy with biopsy and cytology should be performed if the ulcer has not been reduced to half its original size and if it had not been performed initially; if an initial biopsy was benign, operation should be considered. If healing is evident, the regimen should be continued for another 3 weeks and radiographic evaluation repeated again. Because a carcinoma is frequently associated with ulceration which will partially respond to treatment, surgery is indicated unless healing is complete. Cimetidine produces a 70-80% response rate in 6-8 weeks; extending the therapy to 3 months may improve the response rate to nearly 100%.

Stress-Induced and Drug-Induced Ulcers

These agents produce acute, superficial, and multiple erosions confined to the body and fundus of the stomach, often asymptomatic. Bleeding is the most frequent clinical manifestation. Stress ulcers occur with burns (Curling's ulcer), severe sepsis, or injury. Ischemia is probably the most important factor in their development and not hypersecretion of gastric juice or elevated endogenous corticosteroids.

The precise causative pathways of drug-induced ulcerations or erosions are unknown. The most common offenders are alcohol and acetylsalicylic acid, which injure the mucosal epithelial barrier and allow the back-diffusion of hydrogen ion and pepsin. Corticosteroids, nonsteroidal antiinflammatory agents (phenylbutazone, indomethacin), and colchicine are also associated with peptic ulceration.

Cushing's Ulcers

Cushing's ulcers occur in neurosurgical patients with recent intracranial surgery or brain injury. These are full thickness ulcers involving stomach, duodenum, or esophagus, and they produce bleeding. Cushing's ulcers have high acid output and hypergastrinemia. These ulcers are managed with antacid therapy, cimetidine, and nasogastric suction to remove acid.

Stomal and Gastrojejunal Ulceration

A recurrent ulcer may occur in the duodenum, on the jejunal side of a gastrojejunal anastomosis (marginal or anastomotic ulcer), but only rarely in the stomach. The symptoms are vague; the major complaint is pain, which is poorly localized and may not be relieved by food or antacid. The patient may frequently present with a complication (bleeding, obstruction, or perforation). A rare but well-known complication is gastrojejunocolic fistula with pain, weight loss, diarrhea, and steatorrhea; the latter results from colonic contamination and bacterial overgrowth.

Recurrent ulcer is established by either radiography or endoscopy. Once established, Zollinger-Ellison syndrome, retained antrum, and incomplete vagotomy must be excluded before any further surgery is performed. Recurrent ulcers should be managed surgically; vagotomy, distal gastric resection, or transthoracic vagotomy (if the original vagotomy is functionally incomplete) may be necessary.

The Zollinger-Ellison Syndrome (ZE)

Benign or malignant gastrin-producing tumors or diffuse islet cell hyperplasia may stimulate hypersecretion and produce peptic ulcer disease. Most of these tumors are pancreatic, but 10% are found in other locations, such as the duodenum. Although 50-60% are malignant, the malignancy is of low order, and patients may survive 8 to 10 years even with hepatic metastases. Multiple endocrine adenomas, especially in the parathyroid, pituitary, adrenal, and thyroid glands, occur in 10-20% of the patients and a common familial incidence is found. (See chapter 6, Multiple Endocrine Neoplasia (MEN) Syndromes.) The ZE syndrome without other endocrine tumors is generally regarded as a forme fruste of MEN I.

Patients with the Zollinger-Ellison syndrome may present with usual duodenal ulcer symptomatology but most often have fulminant ulceration with complications. The diagnosis is suggested if ulcers occur in unusual sites (jejunum or the postbulbar duodenum) and are multiple or recurrent.

The clinical manifestations of this syndrome are mainly due to increased acid secretion. The gastrin-secreting cells are always quite active so that basal secretion approaches maximum secretion. Basal rates of 10-30 mEq per hour are present. Further stimulation by histamine produces a small increment (if any) in acid production, since the stomach is maximally stimulated. A ratio of basal to maximally stimulated secretion of 0.6 or more is suggestive but not diagnostic. Diarrhea and malabsorption may be found in up to 50% of patients.

The ulceration is quite resistant to medical therapy. Cimetidine, in doses of 300-600 mg q6h, will control symptoms in many patients; however, the underlying tumor is unaffected and may continue to grow and metastasize. Therefore, use of cimetidine should generally be restricted to preoperative control or management of the high-operative-risk patient. Because these lesions are multiple and often metastatic, total gastrectomy is recommended despite a 10-15% mortality rate. In cases without total gastrectomy, the total mortality rate is 90%. Postoperative gastrin levels should be obtained to assess operative success and local or metastatic recurrence.

Acute Gastritis

Acute gastritis is a general term applied to acute ulceration, diffuse erosion, or hemorrhage of the mucosal surface. Although descriptive endoscopic labels are frequently applied (hemorrhagic gastritis, stress ulceration, erosive gastritis, etc.), they all appear related to loss of the normal protective barrier which prevents back-diffusion of hydrogen ion into the gastric mucosa. When the proximal duodenum is also involved, the term acute gastroduodenal ulceration is used.

The generalized stress response or agents such as alcohol, salicylates, bile salts, urea, and others disrupt the barrier. Prevention may be possible by the use of antacids, cimetidine, or gastric drainage. The efficacy of these attempts is generally not clear. Initial treatment uses the same measures. If unsuccessful, infusion of vasopressin (Pitressin) through a catheter placed in the left gastric artery is frequently effective. If bleeding persists, total gastrectomy may be necessary but is associated with a high mortality. Depending upon the underlying disease state, mortality from acute gastritis may reach 60%.

DISEASES OF THE SMALL INTESTINE

Diseases of the small intestine may produce lower abdominal cramping pain, intestinal obstruction, change in bowel habits, passage of either tarry or bloody stools, or evidence of malabsorption. The latter syndrome is relatively common and frequently difficult to diagnose and treat.

Diseases Causing Malabsorption

Physiology of Absorption. The 22 ft of small intestine are lined by a specialized columnar epithelium, thrown into a myriad of villi that markedly increase surface area. Evaluation of small intestinal histology by Rubin tube or Crosby capsule has provided much basic and clinical information about intestinal absorption and its malfunction. *Fat* is hydrolyzed to fatty acids and monoglycerides by pancreatic lipase; bile salts enter the small intestine, change the properties of lipase so that it is active in the duodenum, and also act as detergents to form small aggregates (micelles) that help to solubilize intestinal contents. Four separate mucosal steps then lead to fat absorption: (1) free fatty acids and monoglycerides bind with proteins in mucosal cells; (2) they are re-esterified to form triglycerides; (3) apoproteins are added to form lipoproteins; and (4) the lipoprotein is secreted into lymph.

Carbohydrates are split into small hexose units by salivary and pancreatic amylase; disaccharides are difficult to absorb as such but are split into simple sugars by lactase, sucrase, and maltase located in the brush border of intestinal mucosal cells.

Proteins are digested to polypeptides by pepsin and the pancreatic enzymes (trypsin, chymotrypsin, and carboxypeptidase); different amino acids appear to be absorbed by specific transport systems. A variety of other mechanisms account for the adsorption of *cholesterol* and the fat-soluble *vitamins A, D, E, and K,* of *calcium,* and of *iron. Folate* is absorbed as a monoglutamate; *bile salts* and vitamin B_{12} are absorbed by the terminal ileum.

Manifestations of Malabsorption. Malabsorption of fat leads to increased stool bulk. Diarrhea occurs if mucosal inflammation leads to increased secretion or if unabsorbed bile salts and long-chain fatty acids prevent water absorption by an osmotic effect. Changes in vascular and mucosal permeability produce transudation of plasma proteins into the intestinal lumen (exudative enteropathy). Both serosal and mucosal surfaces must be involved and the loss of albumin leads to dependent edema, while the plasma concentrations of immunoglobulins, lipoproteins, and fibrinogen are also reduced. Malabsorption of specific substrates produces osteomalacia, anemia, and bleeding diatheses.

Laboratory Studies. Malabsorption of fat is evidenced by the finding of excess fat and visible oil droplets by stool examination. Undigested meat fibers may also be seen; unabsorbed meat and fat suggest pancreatic disease. *Carbohydrate absorption* is evaluated by the oral administration of 25 gms of D-xylose; normally, 4 or more gms are excreted in the urine within 5 hrs. Renal insufficiency or gastric retention will produce false positive. B_{12} absorption can be evaluated by a three-stage Schilling test and malabsorption of other metabolites by analysis of plasma concentrations.

A careful clinical evaluation including radiography of the small intestine to identify pancreatic calcification or evidence of small bowel disease can usually separate maldigestion (hepatic or pancreatic) from malabsorption. Table 3-2 presents a useful classification of factors causing malabsorption. Histological study can separate diffuse mucosal disease such as sprue from abnormalities in DNA synthesis, infiltration by specific disease processes, or parasitic infestations.

Biochemical Defects of the Surface Absorptive Cells

Celiac sprue. Also called gluten-sensitive enteropathy, celiac disease, adult celiac disease, idiopathic steatorrhea, and nontropical sprue, this produces either general malabsorption or malab-

TABLE 3-2—CAUSES OF MALABSORPTION

1. Biochemical defects of the surface absorptive cells
2. Structural defects of epithelium due to abnormal DNA synthesis
3. Structural defects of intestine due to specific diseases
4. Hypoglobulinemia
5. Short bowel syndromes
6. Bacterial overgrowth syndromes
7. Infections

sorption limited to specific nutrients. Characteristic pathologic findings of a mucosal biopsy near the ligament of Treitz include flat mucosal surface, subtotal villous atrophy, hypertrophied crypts with increased mitotic figures, cuboidal or flattened epithelial cells, decreased brush border, and increased plasma cells, lymphocytes, or polynuclear leukocytes in the lamina propria. There is clinical improvement upon removing gluten-containing cereal grains (wheat, rye, barley, and oats) from the diet. Celiac sprue usually begins within the first 3 years of life. However, cases often appear in adults who have had no apparent childhood manifestation of the disease. The condition appears to predispose to development of lymphomas, and patients with dermatitis herpetiformis usually have the intestinal lesion of celiac sprue.

Steatorrhea, abnormal D-xylose test, abnormal small-bowel x-rays, anemia, weight loss, and increased secretion of fluids, electrolytes, and protein are present. Treatment consists of a gluten-free diet, substituting rice, soybeans, and corn. Corticosteroids have been used in patients with resistant disease.

Tropical sprue. The symptoms of malabsorption were first observed in tropical settings, presumably due to some infectious agent. When it was found in other climates it was called nontropical sprue. Tropical sprue remains an important entity that involves residents of tropical areas; visitors to such areas may also develop symptoms suggesting an infectious cause. Recently,

tetracycline and folic acid have been shown effective in these
patients.

Disaccharide deficiencies. Deficiency of brush border enzymes
may cause isolated instances of carbohydrate malabsorption.
Lactase deficiency with symptoms following milk ingestion is the
most important of these syndromes and presents with gastrointestinal discomfort. Congenital lactase deficiency in infants becomes symptomatic after the introduction of milk products into
their diet. Primary lactase deficiency in adults occurs most
commonly in Orientals and blacks.

Abetalipoproteinemia. This is a rare, inherited condition due to
abnormality of two of the fat re-synthesizing steps discussed
above. Chylomicra are not secreted into the lymphatic system.
Biopsy shows fat droplets in mucosal cells but not in the
lymphatics. Associated manifestations include hypolipidemia,
cerebellar ataxia, retinitis pigmentosa, and acanthocytosis.

Structural Defects of Epithelium Due to Abnormal DNA Synthesis

Abnormalities in DNA synthesis are seen in pernicious anemia
and nutritional folate deficiency. On biopsy, shortening of villi
and reduction in mitotic activity together with cystic crypt
epithelium is observed. True villous atrophy may be found in
kwashiorkor and after treatment with antimetalbolites that impair DNA synthesis (methotrexate and 5-fluorouracil). Irradiation for abdominal and pelvic malignancies may produce radiation enteritis with decreased mitosis, shortened walls, and
fibrosis. Malabsorption and chronic diarrhea may result.

Structural Defects of Intestine Due to Specific Diseases

Infiltrative diseases of the lamina propria and submucosa include
Whipple's disease, intestinal lymphoma, intestinal lymphangiectasia, eosinophilic gastroenteritis, amyloidosis, mast cell disease,
tuberculosis, carcinomatosis and regional enteritis.

Whipple's disease. The classic features are fever, arthritis, lymphadenopathy, and steatorrhea. Malabsorption of fat is severe, and proteins leak into the intestinal lumen; absorption of vitamin B_{12} and xylose is not impaired. Diagnosis is established by intestinal biopsy, and the findings include infiltration of the lamina propria with foamy macrophages that stain positively with PAS. Treatment is with penicillin or tetracycline.

Intestinal lymphoma. In the small intestine, this may be isolated or generalized. It may be localized or diffuse; diffuse intestinal lymphoma is the most common malignancy, causing malabsorption and leading to a severe protein-losing enteropathy. Diagnosis is made by peroral or surgical biopsy. Surgical resection is the treatment of localized disease, radiotherapy and chemotherapy of more diffuse disease.

Intestinal lymphangiectasia. Dilatation of the intestinal lymphatics may be congenital or acquired. In acquired disease, it is usually the result of mesenteric lymphatic obstruction from a primary retroperitoneal disease. In both diseases, protein-losing enteropathy is prominent but malabsorption minimal. Biopsy is necessary for diagnosis, and treatment is directed toward the underlying disease in acquired cases.

Eosinophilic gastroenteritis. A hypersensitivity syndrome, this disease is characterized by nausea, vomiting, diarrhea, and abdominal cramps; peripheral eosinophilia is recognized by finding eosinophils in the lamina propria. There is moderate to severe malabsorption of D-xylose and fat and a significant loss of protein. Upper GI with small bowel follow-through studies shows an infiltrative pattern. Treatment consists of eliminating the offending food or giving steroids.

Hypoglobulinemia

Absence of plasma cells in the lamina propria is evidence of immunoglobulin deficiency. Diarrhea is common in patients with congenital agammaglobulinemia or hypoglobulinemia. Malabsorption and diarrhea are seen in the dysgammaglobulinemias. Deficiency of IgA and IgM favors intestinal infection; some patients, for example, have giardiasis which responds to treatment.

Short Bowel Syndrome

Ileal resection produces malabsorption of fat and fat-soluble vitamins. Failure of bile salt absorption produces steatorrhea, and unabsorbed bile salts provoke salt and water secretion, producing a severe watery diarrhea known as choleric enteropathy. The prototype of the short bowel syndrome is the extensive resection performed therapeutically in patients with morbid obesity. Jejunal resection is much better tolerated, since the ileum takes over much of the absorptive function.

Cholestyramine reduces intestinal water secretion; substitution of medium-chained triglycerides for usual dietary fat reduces steatorrhea. There is increased oxalate absorption and formation of urinary oxalate stones in patients with ileal resection, so that ingestion of high oxalate foods must be reduced; parenteral B_{12} administration is indicated.

In patients with a Billroth II anastomosis (gastrectomy and gastrojejunostomy), the duodenum is bypassed and steatorrhea and mild malabsorption may result. Pancreatic enzyme replacement or conversion of the gastrojejunostomy to a gastroduodenostomy may be necessary.

Bacterial Overgrowth Syndromes

In intestinal stasis syndromes, which may be the result of surgically created loops, interluminal fistulas, multiple diverticula, or chronic intestinal obstruction, there is bacterial overgrowth in the proximal small intestine. The bacteria are usually anaerobic and similar to colonic flora; B_{12} malabsorption and bile salt deconjugation are noted. Antibiotic therapy will usually eliminate both malabsorption of vitamin B_{12} and steatorrhea. Surgery is indicated for the treatment of gastrojejunocolic fistula with continual colonic contamination of the small intestine, since antibiotics are of little value. Stasis syndromes also occur, with primary impairment of intestinal motility such as scleroderma involving the bowel wall or visceral neuropathy secondary to diabetes mellitus.

Infections

Giardia lamblia. This flagellated protozoan parasite is found in the United States, South America, and most countries and proliferates in the proximal intestine, producing acute or chronic diarrhea and steatorrhea. *Giardia* is found more frequently in the stools of children than adults and may occur with hypogamma-globulinemia and nodular lymphoid hyperplasia. Diagnosis requires the identification of the protozoas in stool, duodenal drainage, mucous smears, or mucosal biopsies. Treatment is with either metronidazole or quinacrine hydrochloride.

Strongyloides stercoralis. This is a roundworm found in warm, rural areas of the United States and in tropical and subtropical areas. Identification of the larvae in duodenal secretions or stool confirms the diagnosis. Infestation may cause nonspecific abdominal symptoms, diarrhea, and steatorrhea. Occasionally, the organism will migrate and cause fever and acute pulmonary and hepatic symptoms.

Infections with the hookworm Necator may cause anemia as a result of chronic blood loss, diarrhea, and weight loss.

TUMORS OF THE GASTROINTESTINAL TRACT

Frequently asymptomatic until inoperable, malignant tumors of the alimentary canal may be diagnosed by radiographic and endoscopic examination; an early sign may be occult bleeding. The 5-year survival is generally low, so that considerable energy should be expended in identifying premalignant lesions and removing them. Therapy is ordinarily a combination of surgical and radiotherapeutic techniques, with chemotherapy used for both early and late disseminated disease. Regional chemotherapy has been of value in some situations.

Esophageal Carcinoma

Carcinoma of the esphagus occurs mainly in older men and is associated with smoking, alcohol, achalasia, and reflux esopha-gitis. Half of the tumors are in the midesophagus; tumors of the proximal two-thirds are derived from the squamous epithelium, while many of those in the distal third are adenocarcinomas developing from gastric tissue or from Barrett columnar epithelium. Dysphagia for solids and ultimately liquids is the presenting manifestation. The 5-year survival is 5-10%.

Gastric Carcinoma

The prevalence of carcinoma of the stomach has declined in the United States over the past several decades, but the disease remains common in Japan, South America, and Eastern Europe. There appears to be an increased prevalence in Hispanics in the United States because of an irritant diet containing hot peppers and other spices. It is twice as common in men and two to four times more common in relatives. Risk factors include atrophic gastric mucosa, partial gastrectomy, and gastroenterostomy for peptic ulcer disease. More than 5% of patients with pernicious anemia develop carcinoma of the stomach. The tumor, an adenocarcinoma, is found in both the antrum and body of the stomach; the lesser curvature is more commonly involved than the greater curvature.

Upper abdominal discomfort, postprandial pain, iron deficiency anemia, and weight loss are common presenting symptoms. The tumor is locally invasive and may spread to esophagus, duodenum, pancreas, colon, or liver. Lymph node metastases are common, and involvement of the thoracic duct produces enlargement of left supraclavicular or Virchow nodes. The tumor may metastasize to peritoneum, rectum (Blumer shelf), umbilicus, peritoneum, liver, ovaries, lung, or brain. Presenting symptoms are frequently due to metastatic disease.

Radiographic abnormalities are found in 90%, but biopsy is necessary for precise diagnosis. If multiple biopsies are obtained, the accuracy exceeds 98%. The prognosis varies with the extent of disease. Five-year survivals are as high as 80% with disease localized to the mucosa or submucosa, 10-20% when the serosa is involved. Surgical cure rates vary widely, however, and 50% survivals for 5 years have been reported, particularly with smaller tumors and without lymph node involvement.

Primary gastric lymphomas and leiomyosarcoma comprise 5% and 1-3% of all gastric tumors respectively. *Primary lymphoma of the stomach*, usually histiocytic or lymphocytic, has a substantially better prognosis, especially if the serosa and adjacent lymph nodes are not involved; up to 50% may survive 5 years. Hodgkin's disease of the stomach is uncommon, but a significant number of histiocytic lymphomas and lymphosarcomas ultimately involve the stomach. *Leiomyosarcomas* occur in somewhat older patients, are large, usually confined to the upper part, and tend to ulcerate so that bleeding is found in one-third of patients. Peritoneal and liver metastases are relatively common; a palpable mass is observed in half of patients.

Benign and Premalignant Growths of Stomach and Intestine

A number of polypoid growths biopsied at endoscopy may be benign or pre-malignant; precise histologic diagnosis is obviously critical. Hyperplastic lesions imply increased numbers of almost normal cells, while neoplastic lesions appear abnormal with unusual architecture, active mitoses, or absence of sufficient underlying stroma. Invasion of a polypoid stalk or other misplaced mucosal cells suggests malignancy.

A papillary gastric lesion may be malignant, a benign epithelial polyp, or a papillary adenoma. Eighty to 90% of noncarcinomatous polypoid masses are hyperplastic nonneoplastic epithelial polyps, measuring less than 2 cm in diameter. The remainder are papillary adenomas composed of neoplastic epithelium, usually larger than 2 cm and prone to malignant degeneration. Both of these benign growths occur more frequently in individuals with achlorhydria or pernicious anemia, or in those over 50 years of age. Occult bleeding is a common presenting manifestation; the diagnosis is established by biopsy.

Diffuse gastric polyposis is a rare condition in which the gastric mucosa is covered with numerous sessile or pedunculated epithelial polyps, of which 20-30% become malignant. Leiomyomas are of little clinical significance unless they are large (greater than 3 cm), in which case they can cause a massive bleed.

Treatment is local excision for small tumors and a partial gastrectomy for larger tumors. Other rare benign gastric tumors include lipomas, schwannomas, leiomyoblastomas, hemangiomas, lymphangiomas, and fibromas.

Four inheritable syndromes of intestinal polyposis have been described. *Familial multiple colonic polyposis.* This consists of adenomatous polyps located throughout the colon. Transmitted by an autosomal dominant gene, the polyps uniformly become malignant. The polyps often present in childhood or adolescence with rectal bleeding and diarrhea; the treatment is colectomy, and the entire family should be screened once the diagnosis is established.

Gardner's syndrome. Adenomatous polyps are combined with associated benign lesions such as lipomas, fibromas, sebaceous cysts, and osteomas of the jaw and skull bones. The polyps uniformly become malignant by the age of 40.

Peutz-Jeghers syndrome. Multiple hamartomas of the entire alimentary track and melanotic spots on the lips, buccal mucosa, and skin are characteristic. Most of the polyps occur in the small intestine. The polyps are generally not considered premalignant, although malignant degeneration has been reported in several instances. In contrast, 10% of gastric and duodenal hamartomas become malignant.

Juvenile polyposis. A syndrome of multiple inflammatory polyps involving small and large intestines. It may be isolated or in association with alopecia. Hyperpigmentation and nail dystrophy constitute the Cronkhite-Canada syndrome. These polyps are benign and do not become malignant, but they may be confused with the premalignant polyps of familial polyposis.

MALIGNANT TUMORS
Adenocarcinoma. Adenocarcinoma of the small intestine is a rare tumor accounting for less then 1% of GI cancers. Adenocarcinomas may arise from villous adenomas or adenomatous polyps. Located in the duodenum or proximal jejunum, the tumors are found more frequently in men over 50, who present with pain, bleeding, or obstruction. Cramping abdominal pain, anorexia, and weight loss are common symptoms. Distal or local metas-

tases are found in 50% of these patients at the time of diagnosis. The surgical cure rate is 15-20%.

Lymphoma. This occurs in young patients and is usually located in the distal small intestine. Abdominal pain, bleeding, or palpation of an abdominal mass are the principal features of leiomyosarcomas, which occur in older men and are found anywhere in the intestine. Treatment is by surgical resection, and the cure rate approaches 50%.

Carcinoid Syndrome

Carcinoid tumors, representing less than 1% of all GI tumors, are the most frequent benign tumor of the small bowel. However, they account for approximately 20% of all malignant tumors of the small intestine. These tumors are derived from enterochro-maffin cells (of the peripheral division of the diffuse endocrine system), which secrete a group of humoral substances, principally 5-hydroxyindoles including serotonin and 5-hydroxytryptophan as well as histamine, bradykinin, and on occasion polypeptide hormones. They are diagnosed usually because of bleeding or obstruction with resultant surgical exploration and resection. The majority of carcinoid tumors do not produce the carcinoid syndrome.

The clinical picture of carcinoid syndrome, which occurs in 20-30% of patients with malignant carcinoid tumor, varies with the site of the tumor—midgut, foregut, or associated with teratomas of ovary or testes. The classical carcinoid syndrome is produced by a tumor of the terminal ileum. The ileal tumors may occur in the appendix and fail to metastasize. Tumors of the terminal ileum secrete principally serotonin, which is largely inactivated by the liver until significant hepatic metastases allow escape into the systemic circulation with production of symptomatology. Serotonin produces gastrointestinal hypermotility, diarrhea, and malabsorption. It produces endocardial fibrosis, resulting in right heart and to a lesser extent left heart abnormalities. Typically tricuspid incompetence with pulmonary stenosis is seen. Tumors of foregut origin, stomach, and bronchus lack the decarboxylase necessary for the conversion of 5-hydroxytryptophan (5-HTP) to

5-hydroxytryptamine (serotonin), but secrete polypeptide hormones including insulin, gastrin, glucagon, and ACTH and are associated with multiple endocrine neoplasia syndrome (MEN). Eating frequently provokes symptoms, with histamine-secreting carcinoid of the stomach. The metastastic behavior of these tumors also varies with site of origin. Tumors of the ileum metastasize principally to the liver, whereas tumors of foregut origin tend to metastasize to bone and lung. Attacks of the syndrome can be provoked by anxiety or by eating. Besides cutaneous flushing, patients experience tachycardia and hypotension. Bradykinin, a potent vasodilator, is released when kallikreins from the tumor activate plasma kininogen. In some patients, a deficiency of nicotinamide develops when large quantities of tryptophan are diverted to serotonin production.

Diagnosis can be confirmed by measurements of 5-HIAA (hydroxyindole acetic acid) in a 24-hour urine specimen. (Levels may be falsely elevated due to excessive ingestion of bananas, walnuts, and cough syrups.)

Management includes local surgery, removal of hepatic metastases, and pharmacologic management. Where the tumor produces excessive histamine, the combined use of H_1 blockers such as diphenhydramine and H_2 blockers such as cimetidine are indicated. The serotonin antagonist methysergide is useful in combatting the diarrhea but may produce retroperitoneal fibrosis. In patients with tumors of foregut origin, the flushing may sometimes be prevented with steroids or phenothiazines.

Carcinoma of the Colon

There are 100,000 new diagnoses of colorectal carcinoma in the United States each year; the 5-year survival of 41% has been unchanged for the past 25 years. The second most prevalent malignancy in men, colorectal cancer has also become the second most common in women because of the decline in uterine malignancy, although the rapid increase in carcinoma of the lung will soon make that more prevalent than bowel cancer in women. Colonic carcinoma is more common in women, rectal cancer more common in men. Fifteen percent are found in the caecum and ascending colon, 10% in the transverse colon, and 75% in the descending colon. More than 60% are within reach of the sigmoidoscope, but a recent study has emphasized that the flexible scope can detect many more than the rigid instrument. Winnan et al. detected colorectal disease in 4.1% with rigid sigmoidoscopy; the figure increased to 16.1% with flexible instruments. Fifty-one polypoid lesions were identified with the flexible scope, and 82% of these were beyond the average colonic length of 20 cm visualized by the rigid scope. They recommend that physicians be trained in flexible sigmoidoscopy, since the morbidity of the examination is minimal.

Changes in bowel habits and bleeding are common with left-sided lesions, lower abdominal pain and iron deficiency anemia with right-sided lesions. Since benign and malignant lesions present with identical symptomatology, identification of premalignant lesions is of great importance.

Four types of polyps may be identified by biopsy: neoplastic (adenomatous polyps and villous adenomas), hyperplastic, hamartomas, and inflammatory polyps. The latter three types offer little or no potential for malignant degeneration in the colon. *Adenomatous polyps* are the most common neoplastic lesion of the colon. Eighty percent are located in the rectum and sigmoid colon; their frequency rises sharply after the age of 50, with a slight male predominance and a peak in the 70s. Sessile or pedunculated, they are premalignant, especially when located in sigmoid colon or rectum. The rate of malignant degeneration in multiple congenital adenomatous polyposis is 100%. *Villous adenomas* are similar but are frequently larger, sessile, soft, friable, and prone to bleeding. They are also premalignant. Carcinoma of the colon may be prevented by removal of these lesions and close observation of patients with documented risk factors such as a family history of juvenile polyposis, Peutz-Jeghers syndrome, or ulcerative colitis.

Treatment is surgical resection in the absence of distal metastases. The resectability of colonic tumors is 95%, and the operative mortality is 4%. The 5-year survival rate in patients with cancer limited to the bowel wall is 70% and less than 35% in patients with disseminated disease. Following surgical resection,

18% of patients are discovered to have recurrent tumor in the suture line. In patients with documented metastases, chemotherapy with 5-FU (fluorouracil) is palliative.

INFLAMMATORY BOWEL DISEASE

The response of infectious inflammatory bowel diseases such as salmonellosis and shigellosis to antibiotics unmasked at least two "new" disorders that did not appear directly related to an infectious agent: ulcerative colitis and regional enteritis (Crohn's disease). The etiology of both is unknown, and there is considerable overlap in about 20% of patients so that precise separation is impossible. Several pathologic features permit separation in most patients, however. Crypt abscesses are characteristic of ulcerative colitis but may be found in Crohn's disease, ischemic colitis, and infectious bowel disease. Granulomas are rare in ulcerative colitis, and loss of goblet cells with decrease in mucus is very rare in Crohn's disease.

At present, it appears likely that both disorders represent the interaction of certain infectious agents and an abnormal immune response (both nature and nurture). Viruses, L or inactive forms of certain bacteria, and at least one specific agent *(Yersinia)* have been suggested as etiologic agents. Both diseases have been associated with extraintestinal manifestations that suggest autoimmunity such as erythema nodosum, arthritis, uveitis, and hemolytic anemia. Patients with inflammatory bowel disease and ankylosing spondylitis have a high frequency of HLA-B27 histocompatibility genes. Lymphocytotoxic antibodies are found in 40% of patients; others contain an antibody to colon epithelial tissue. Peripheral lymphocytes are frequently cytotoxic for colonic epithelium, and killer T cells have been found in mesenteric lymph nodes. Such discoveries have added some rationale to the use of antimicrobial and inflammatory agents in the treatment of these disorders.

Ulcerative Colitis

Ulcerative colitis or proctocolitis is an inflammatory bowel disease that affects the mucosa of the distal colon and rectum but may involve the entire colon. The disease commonly begins between ages 25 and 45, and is more common in whites and among females. Although ulcerative colitis is uncommon in Israel, it is two to four times more prevalent among American Jews than non-Jews. The disease is uncommon in the elderly, but attacks in persons over 65 are associated with high morbidity and mortality.

The rectum is always involved in disease; rectal disease is called proctitis. From the rectum, the disease progresses proximally in the colon. The microscopic and pathologic features—hemorrhage, ulceration, and crypt abscesses—are nonspecific and limited to the mucosa and submucosa. Patients present with constipation and passage of blood or mucus with the stools. Patients often have urgency to defecate followed with only small amounts of blood and mucus. Diarrhea and other constitutional symptoms follow these initial symptoms in months to years. There then will be 10 to 30 bowel movements daily, with associated tenesmus. The disease can be described further as mild, moderate, or severe.

In *mild colitis* (60% of cases), the disease is confined to the distal colon and rectum. In only 15% does it progress to the remainder of the colon. Patients with mild colitis have three to five stools per day and do not have extracolonic or systemic manifestations. Physical and laboratory examinations are usually normal. Treatment consists of Lomotil tablets 1-2 q.i.d. or deodorized tincture of opium 10-20 drops in water q.i.d.; sulfasalazine (Azulfidine) 4-6 gm/day, and corticosteroid enemas. Mortality from acute attacks in patients with mild colitis is 0.4%.

Patients with *moderately severe colitis* (25% of total) usually have five bloody mucus stools each day, with cramping pain and rectal urgency. Systemic symptoms and findings include low-grade fever, anorexia, weight loss, and fatigue. Physical examination reveals tenderness over the distal colon. Laboratory tests may show an anemia and an elevated alkaline phosphatase in 25%. In these patients, prednisone 40-80 mg/day is added. If there is no response in 2 weeks, a trial of 40-80 u ACTH I.M./day is indicated. Mortality from an acute attack is 2%.

In *severe colitis*, patients usually require hospitalization, because the mortality rate from an acute attack ranges from 10-

25%. These patients have profuse or constant loose bloody stools, temperatures of 38-40°C, anorexia, weight loss, and a distended tympanitic abdomen. If severe, intravenous fluids with electrolyte replacement are indicated as well as nasogastric suction. Prednisone 100 mg I.V./day or ACTH 40-80 u/day in a slow continuous drip may be given. If toxic megacolon is present, ampicillin 4-8 gm/day I.V. is necessary. Proctocolectomy may be necessary.

Diagnosis of ulcerative colitis consists of sigmoidoscopy, rectal biopsy, barium studies, and if indicated, colonoscopy. On sigmoidoscopy, there will usually be a coarse granular mucosal surface and friable mucosa; the latter is always present in active disease. Characteristic findings in ulcerative colitis with rectal biopsy are atrophy of the mucosal glands and polymorphonuclear leukocytes in the crypts of Lieberkühn (crypt abscesses). Characteristic barium study findings in ulcerative colitis are loss of haustral markings, foreshortened colon, loss of redundancy in the rectosigmoid region, and a mottled appearance of barium and roughening at the barium-mucosa interface. Colonoscopy is indicated in patients with disease beyond the sigmoidoscope or when there is a possibility of malignant change.

Other conditions to be considered in the differential diagnosis of bloody diarrhea include trauma secondary to foreign objects, bacterial colitis, ischemic colitis, diverticulitis, Crohn's disease, and irritable colon syndrome.

Complications associated with ulcerative colitis include toxic megacolon (1-3%), perforation (3%), stricture (10%), hemorrhage (4%), and carcinoma (2.5-5%). Toxic megacolon is a medical emergency, and if the patient does not respond to medical management, a total proctocolectomy is recommended. Even with drug and supportive therapy, the mortality rate of toxic megacolon is 15-50%. One-third of all patients who die of ulcerative colitis have a colonic perforation. High-dose steroid therapy may mask signs of abdominal peritonitis.

The risk of developing cancer of the colon with ulcerative colitis is related to duration of the disease (2.5-5% after 10 years, 15% after 20 years, and 20-25% after 25 years), involvement of the entire colon, frequent exacerbations, and severity of the initial attack. Stricture in the rectosigmoid area will develop in approximately 10% of patients with ulcerative colitis. Surgery is required because the stricture must be distinguished from scirrhous carcinoma.

Extracolonic complications of ulcerative colitis include skin lesions (erythema nodosum and pyoderm gangrenosum, 3.5%), aphthous mouth ulcer (10%), iritis and severe bilateral episcleritis (5-10%), migratory arthritis (5-10%), and liver disease (fatty infiltration, 40%; pericholangitis, 30-50%; postnecrotic cirrhosis, 3%; sclerosing cholangitis, 0.5%; and bile duct carcinoma, 0.5%).

Crohn's Disease: Granulomatous Ileitis, Colitis, and Ileocolitis

Granulomatous involvement of the terminal ileum (classic Crohn's disease) is characterized by chronic inflammation of all layers of the bowel. The etiology of Crohn's disease is unknown, but females predominate and the disease develops between ages 20 and 40, with a peak incidence at 30.

Gastroenterologists generally accept that classic regional ileitis (the original Crohn's disease) and granulomatous colitis constitute variations of the same disease—"granulomatous ileocolitis," now called Crohn's disease. Approximately 50% of patients have both ileal and colon involvement, while the remaining one-half are divided equally between patients with Crohn's disease restricted to the small intestine and with disease only in the colon.

Analysis of 569 patients randomized by the National Cooperative Crohn's Disease Study shows that the average interval from the onset of symptoms to diagnosis was 35 months; it was less for colitis than for those with isolated small bowel disease. The small bowel was involved in 89%; disease was limited to the small bowel in 39%. The colon was involved in 69%, and disease was limited to it in 11%. More than 90% complained of diarrhea and abdominal pain. Weight loss occurred in 85%, fever in 56%, lower GI bleeding in 41%, anal fissure, abscess, or fistula in 36%, arthritis or spondylitis in 19%, internal fistulae in 16%, enterocolitis fistula in 5%, iritis in 4%, hepatitis or pericholangitis in 4%, and erythema nodosum or pyoderma gangrenosum in 5%.

Laboratory findings in Crohn's disease are anemia due both to iron and folate deficiency, mild leukocytosis, and hypoalbuminemia. Radiography reveals segmental involvement of two or more areas, most commonly in the ascending colon, with intervening normal "skip" areas. Transmural bowel involvement produces an eccentric convex defect, protruding into the lumen and producing "thumbprinting" on one side only.

The differential diagnosis includes amebic colitis, diverticulitis, ischemic colitis, and intestinal tuberculosis.

Sigmoidoscopy reveals gross ulcerations (0.5-1 cm in diameter), which may be stellate in shape. Friability is minimal compared to ulcerative colitis. Biopsy reveals linear ulcers which extend into the submucosa, granulomas, and evidence of chronic inflammation with mononuclear cell infiltration.

Natural history in the cooperative study demonstrated that 32% of placebo patients experienced spontaneous remission in 17 weeks and that 53% of these remained in remission for 24 months. Surgical removal of disease, absence of perianal disease, and mild nature made remission more likely. Patients receiving steroids before randomization to placebo worsened more than those who had not previously been on steroids. Neither steroids nor azathioprine appeared superior to placebo.

A more recent study by Present et al. evaluated the 2-year effect of 6-mercaptopurine (6-MP) administered for 6 months and compared to placebo. Cross-over data demonstrated a 67% beneficial response to 6-MP compared to an 8% response with placebo. Steroids could be reduced or discontinued in 75% of the 6-MP group and 36% of the placebo. Only 7 of 68 patients had major side effects, all of which were reversible. These data suggest that immunosuppressive agents be tried after an initial trial with sulfasalazine (or tetracycline as suggested by one study) and steroids.

Fifty-five to 60% of patients require surgical therapy within 5 years because of failure of medical therapy or from complications of the disease, such as intraabdominal fistulas or strictures. Despite the high recurrence rate and poor results with medical therapy, the overall mortality rate is 5% per year.

DISEASES OF THE LARGE INTESTINE
Diverticulosis

Colonic diverticula are saccular outpouchings at points of vascular entry that lack a muscular coat and consist of a mucosal layer covered by serosa. Approximately 95% of diverticula are sigmoidal. Diverticulosis is rare in persons under 30 years of age, and approximately 50% are over 60 years of age. Males and females are affected equally. Although the exact etiology is unknown, it has been suggested that low-residue, high carbohydrate diets common in affluent countries, along with the use of purgatives, may be responsible. The disease is rare in rural black Africans, Koreans, Japanese, and Russians, all of whom consume a high-fiber diet. The most common cause of extensive lower gastrointestinal bleeding is diverticulosis. In contrast, patients with diverticulitis ooze but rarely bleed massively. In diverticulosis, bleeding is the result of ulceration of the mucosa and may be massive because of the concentration of intraluminal vessels in the area of the diverticulum. Approximately 75% of patients bleed from a diverticulum in the right colon. Diagnosis is made by the history of passage of red blood per rectum, negative gastric aspirate, angiographic evidence of bleeding, negative sigmoidoscopy, and identification of diverticula by barium enema. In most patients, bleeding subsides spontaneously. If bleeding persists, blood replacement, vasopressin infusion, or surgery may be necessary.

Diverticulitis

Ten to 12% of patients with diverticulosis have the inflammatory pathologic changes of diverticulitis. The etiology of diverticulitis is thought to be a microperforation of the involved diverticulum with varying degrees of peritonitis. These perforations may result in inflammation of the serosa, pericolic fat, intestinal wall, or peritoneum. Diverticulitis may be either acute or chronic.

Clinical features include pain in the left lower quadrant and a change in bowel habits (frequent loose movements, constipation, or diarrhea followed by severe constipation). Physical examination may reveal left lower quadrant tenderness, peritoneal rebound, palpable mass in 25-50% of patients, distension, and tympany. Fever, tachycardia, and leukocytosis are common features.

Carcinoma of the colon and the irritable bowel syndrome are important in the differential diagnoses of a patient presenting with the above complaints and findings. Complications of diverticulitis include obstruction, perforation, and fistula, the most common being colovesical found in 6-28% of patients.

Acute, uncomplicated diverticulitis is best treated medically with bed rest, soft or liquid diet, stool softener, and antibiotics, usually ampicillin. Emergency surgery is indicated in patients with generalized peritonitis, persistent intestinal obstruction, or evidence of abscess. If possible, surgery should be delayed since the mortality rate is 15-23% with emergency surgery, 1.5% when elective.

Intestinal Obstruction

Intestinal obstruction may be complete or incomplete, acute or chronic, intermittent or continuous. It is important to determine whether there is also interference with the blood supply (strangulation), since gangrene, perforation, or peritonitis may result.

Mechanical obstruction may be intramural, mural, or extramural. Polyps, bezoars, gallstones, foreign bodies, congenital diaphragms, meconium, or fecal impaction are important intramural causes. Diverticulitis, hematoma, strictures due to malignancy, irradiation, or inflammatory bowel disease are mural causes. Extramural etiologies include adhesions, nonstrangulated hernias, and annular pancreas. Mechanical obstruction that interferes with the vascular supply to the intestine may be caused by intussusception, volvulus, strangulated hernia, or closed loop obstruction due to adhesions; hernias or adhesions account for approximately 70% of the cases of mechanical obstruction. In general, mechanical obstruction will require surgical relief and paralytic obstruction will respond to conservative measures.

Irritable Colon Syndrome

This syndrome, also known as mucus colitis or spastic colitis, is characterized by abdominal pain, believed to be of colonic origin, constipation, diarrhea, and often the passage of mucus. Actually there is no inflammation, and the term colitis is technically incorrect.

Several etiologic factors have been suggested: emotional or psychologic causes (80% of the patients), infectious diarrhea (25% of patients), and laxative abuse (30% of patients).

Clinically, women are afflicted more commonly than men (2:1). Onset is between the ages of 20 and 50 years. The pain of irritable colon is variable and may be colicky, gripping, or constant and felt most often in the left lower quadrant or hypogastrium. The symptom is called the splenic flexure syndrome if the pain is in the left upper quadrant with radiation to the shoulder and left arm. Bowel habits vary, with constipation the usual problem but often alternating with diarrhea. Passage of mucus, anxiety, headache, insomnia, and weakness are common features of the syndrome. Tenderness is elicited with palpation, especially over the left lower quadrant, and the sigmoid is often palpable. Laboratory evaluation is usually normal, although sigmoidoscopy may occasionally reveal hyperemia of the mucosa or excessive mucus.

Reassurance is an important aspect of therapy. Irritant laxatives must be eliminated in patients with constipation, and good bowel habits established. The patient should be instructed to eat a high-fiber diet consisting of fruit, vegetables, and bran. Anticholinergics and hydrophilic colloids are often useful.

Megacolon

Megacolon can be divided into two categories: congenital (Hirschsprung disease or aganglionic megacolon) and acquired megacolon, both of which are characterized by dilatation of the colon and obstinate constipation.

Hirschsprung's disease. Absence of the myenteric nerve plexus in the wall of the pelvic colon and upper rectum. Males are affected more often than females, and symptoms of constipation, abdominal distention, and vomiting date from birth. Barium enema reveals a small rectum, a narrowed segment above the rectum, and then a wide dilatation of the colon full of retained feces. A rectal biopsy showing absence of the nerve plexus confirms the diagnosis. Treatment consists of surgical resection of the abnormal segment of colon.

Acquired megacolon. This may be associated with endocrine disorders (cretinism) or the abuse of drugs such as chlorpromazine. Psychologic factors are also important. The barium examination usually shows no narrowed segment, and the dilatation extends down to the anus. The rectum is full of feces. Most cases of acquired megacolon can be managed conservatively by treating the cause if known, high-residue diets, and the judicious use of laxatives.

DISEASES OF THE PANCREAS

The pancreas produces both endocrine and exocrine secretions. The exocrine secretions, produced by tubuloacinar glands of serous cells, account for almost the entire mass of the pancreas and are concerned with the digestion of protein and fat. These secretions, the pancreatic juice, are delivered to the duodenum via the pancreatic duct. There are two principal endocrine hormones: insulin, produced by the beta cells, and glucagon, produced by the alpha cells, which are concerned with carbohydrate metabolism. Pancreatic juice is alkaline and contains carbonate, potassium, and sodium and three enzymes: amylase (diastase), lipase, and trypsin. The alkaline medium is necessary for enzyme function.

Serum amylase is the most useful diagnostic test, although it may be elevated in pseudocyst, abscess, neoplasm, pancreatic trauma, parotitis, renal failure, intestinal obstruction, perforation or infarction, ruptured ectopic pregnancy, diabetic ketoacidosis, burns, pregnancy, and other neoplasms such as lung, ovary, or esophagus. Lipase elevations may distinguish between pancreatic and other sources; isoenzyme identification can separate pancreatic and salivary amylase. Urinary amylase should be markedly elevated in acute pancreatitis because renal clearance is increased, perhaps due to a specific and transient renal tubular abnormality. The ratio of amylase to creatinine clearance is calculated in the following manner:

$$\text{Ratio} = \frac{U_{amyl}}{P_{amyl}} \div \frac{U_{creat}}{P_{creat}}$$

A ratio of greater than 6% suggests pancreatitis. Amylase clearance is low in renal failure and macroamylasemia.

Pancreatic study has been revolutionized by computed tomography and ultrasonography. Plain films may demonstrate pancreatic calcification or localized gas in hepatic flexure of jejunum—the "sentinel" loop. Barium radiography may show distorted duodenal mucosal folds or displacement of the stomach.

Minimal elevation of bilirubin or moderate biliary obstruction limit the usefulness of oral or intravenous cholangiography. Percutaneous cholangiography, valuable in over 95% of cases, may reveal biliary obstruction or a pancreatic mass. Jaundice does not preclude the usefulness of this test.

Fiberoptic endoscopy permits direct visualization of the ampulla of Vater and retrograde cannulation of the papilla with injection of contrast material to visualize the biliary and pancreatic ducts. In experienced hands, the success rate is 70-80%.

Acute Pancreatitis

Acute pancreatitis is most commonly associated with alcoholism and biliary tract disease. It arises from enzymatic autodigestion of the pancreas and may proceed to hemorrhagic necrosis with the formation of a local or generalized peritonitis.

Biliary tract disease. This disease is found in 30-60% of patients with pancreatitis. A gallstone may obstruct the ampulla of Vater, with resultant reflux of fluid from the common bile duct into the pancreatic duct. More frequently, however, obstruction cannot be demonstrated, and it is thought that the composition of bile is altered and reflux of the juice leads to pancreatitis. Although the exact mechanism is unknown, *alcohol* accounts for 20-60% of all cases of pancreatitis. Alcohol may directly damage acinar tissue, resulting in secondary obstruction of pancreatic ducts. Other causes are *direct injury* (penetrating peptic ulcer or surgical injury), *metabolic and systemic disorders* (hyperparathyroidism, hyperlipidemia, hereditary pancreatitis with aminoaciduria), *pregnancy*, *drugs* (thiazides, isonazid, sulfonamides, indomethacin, and steroids), *ascariasis,* and *mumps.*

The clinical features of acute pancreatitis include severe upper abdominal pain, which may radiate to the back. Bending forward or flexing the knees may relieve the pain. The majority of patients have nausea and vomiting. Alcoholic pancreatitis occurs most frequently in men, and pancreatitis associated with biliary tract disease is more common in women.

Physical examination usually reveals a tachycardia and a low-grade temperature (100-102°F). Signs of dehydration may be present. The abdomen is usually slightly tender, nonrigid, and painful with palpation. Ascites may be present if pancreatic fluid has escaped into the peritoneal cavity. Alcoholic pancreatitis should be suspected if stigmata of liver disease are present. Band keratopathy supports the diagnosis of pancreatitis secondary to hypercalcemia. Skin xanthoma suggest hyperlipemic pancreatitis.

There are no specific tests for acute pancreatitis, but an elevated serum amylase within the first 12-48 hours and increased renal clearance of amylase are supportive. Serum lipase may be high; WBC usually exceeds 10,000-18,000. Serum alkaline phosphatase and bilirubin may be elevated. Pancreatic swelling causes common duct obstruction.

The differential diagnosis includes perforated peptic ulcer, acute cholecystitis, dissecting or expanding abdominal aneurysm, lead poisoning, acute intermittent porphyria, sickle cell crisis, familial Mediterranean fever, Henoch-Schönlein's purpura, and tabetic crisis. Acute myocardial infarction should always be suspected in patients with severe midepigastric pain.

Complications are shock, pneumonia, atelectasis, and pleural effusions. Approximately 10-25% develop transient hyperglycemia and glycosuria; others have hypocalcemia with tetany and positive Chvostek and Trousseau signs. Pancreatic pseudocysts and abscess may occur later.

Treatment. Aimed at decreasing pancreatic activity and correcting fluid and electrolyte abnormalities. Intestinal secretions stimulate pancreatic secretion and must be removed; gastric suction is traditional, but duodenal drainage may be necessary for optimal results because of intestinal stasis. Glucagon administration reduces gastric and pancreatic secretion and may be useful but apparently has not reduced mortality. Pain should be controlled but morphine avoided, because it produces sphincter of Oddi spasm. Antibiotics are indicated if biliary tract infection is present. Surgical drainage is necessary for biliary tract sepsis, pancreatic abscess, and bleeding or expanding cyst.

Chronic Pancreatitis

Chronic pancreatitis produces abdominal pain, weight loss, and pancreatic insufficiency. Complications include pseudocyst and abscess, pancreatic calcification, and diabetes mellitus. When pain is minimal, differentiation from carcinoma is difficult.

Diabetes develops in 15-20% of patients with noncalcific pancreatitis and 70-75% of those with pancreatic calcifications. If 80% of pancreatic function is lost, steatorrhea will develop.

Diabetes mellitus should be treated by a restriction of carbohydrate intake and insulin. Viokase is useful in the treatment of steatorrhea as well as the use of medium chain triglycerides. Antacids should be administered with exogenous pancreatic enzymes to protect them from inactivation by gastric acidity (keep pH above 4.5). Weight gain and improvement of general nutritional status are the principal goals of enzyme replacement therapy.

Carcinoma of the Pancreas

Pancreatic carcinoma is the fourth most common cause of neoplastic death in the United States; risk factors include alcohol, cigarette smoking, and food additives, and perhaps coffee drinking. The major features are pain, weight loss, and a rapid course leading to death, usually within a year.

Courvoisier's sign, a dilated, nontender gallbladder in a jaundiced patient, is characteristic in carcinoma of the head of the pancreas. Patients with pancreatic carcinoma usually develop mild diabetes. Metastases to liver, bones, peritoneum, and thoracic organs are common features.

A recent evaluation of seven diagnostic procedures showed that abnormal pancreatic secretory function and ultrasonography were the most useful. Computed tomography may be even better, since it allows a more general evaluation of the abdomen, retroperitoneum, and biliary ducts. Percutaneous fine-needle biopsy may obviate surgery in certain situations.

The tumor mass with involvement of adjacent structures may be outlined radiologically. Carcinoembryonic antigen (CEA) is positive in a high proportion of cases, but it is also positive in chronic benign pancreatitis. In a patient who appears with obstructive jaundice, carcinoma of the head of the pancreas must be differentiated from choledocholithiasis and tumors of the ampulla of Vater, two conditions that are readily accessible to surgery. Ampullar tumors usually obstruct both pancreatic and common bile ducts and tend to bleed. Characteristic signs of ampullar carcinoma include the passage of silvery slate-gray stools, which are the result of biliary and pancreatic insufficiency. These stools are acholic and contain excess fat.

Resection of tumors of the pancreatic head include total pancreatectomy, or Whipple's procedure, which includes resection of antrum, duodenum, and common bile duct along with gastrojejunostomy and biliary-enteric fistula. These procedures are largely palliative to relieve jaundice and itching. Five-year cures are rare.

DISEASES OF THE LIVER

The liver plays a prominent role in the metabolism of many substrates and is responsible for the synthesis of albumin and several coagulation factors as well as drug detoxification and inactivation of steroid and nonsteroid hormones. The liver forms bilirubin, is responsible for the secretion of bile, and stores vitamins and minerals. The hepatic mononuclear macrophages (Kupffer's cells) are an important body defense mechanism.

Approximately 250-350 mg of bilirubin is formed daily, primarily from the heme of senescent red blood cells. Heme is converted to biliverdin in the spleen, kidney, and liver by the microsomal enzyme, heme oxygenase. Biliverdin is reduced to bilirubin by biliverdin reductase. Bilirubin is then delivered to the hepatocyte surface, where it is bound to two soluble cytoplasmic proteins, Y and Z. It is then solubilized intracellularly by the microsomal enzyme bilirubin glucuronyl transferase, which conjugates it to a glucuronide. Phenobarbital stimulates the activity of this enzyme. The conjugated pigment is secreted into the bile and delivered to the small intestine, where it is reduced by bacterial enzymes to urobilinogen. Most of the urobilinogen is excreted in the feces, but a small amount is reabsorbed and re-excreted by the liver into the bile (enterohepatic circulation). Trace amounts of urobilinogen appear in the urine.

The serum of normal adults contains approximately 0.5-1.0 mg of bilirubin per 100 ml. Two pigment fractions are present in the serum, a conjugated water-soluble fraction (primarily bilirubin diglucuronide, which gives a direct Ehrlich diazo reaction) and an unconjugated fraction. The direct fraction is 0.25 mg/100 ml or less in healthy adults.

Disorders of Bilirubin Metabolism

Both conjugated and unconjugated bilirubin are found in patients with jaundice, but the dominance of one over the other provides valuable diagnostic information.

Unconjugated hyperbilirubinemia. Found with increased production due to hemolysis or ineffective erythropoiesis, congestive heart failure, previous right ventricular failure, or certain drugs such as rifampin.

Gilbert's syndrome. A common, autosomal dominant disorder with impairment of both hepatic uptake and conjugation. The evaluation is otherwise unrevealing, and treatment is unnecessary. The **Crigler-Najjar syndromes** are severe variants, commonly seen in children and associated with high bilirubin concentrations and kernicterus.

Predominantly conjugated hyperbilirubinemia. Found with hepatocellular abnormalities producing intrahepatic cholestasis or extrahepatic biliary obstruction; bile is found in the urine, and the sclerae may be deeply stained. The **Dubin-Johnson syndrome** is an autosomal recessive disorder of conjugated bilirubin secretion; a dark pigment is found in the liver, and the bromosulphalein (BSP) level is higher at 90 than 45 minutes, implying regurgitation of conjugated BSP. The oral cholecystogram shows absent or delayed visualization. In the **Rotor syndrome,** the dark pigment is absent and the oral cholecystogram negative.

The relationship of serum transaminase to hyperbilirubinemia is a useful diagnostic consideration. Levels greater than 500 units in a jaundiced patient support hepatocellular disease, particularly hepatitis; levels greater than 1000 units are almost diagnostic of hepatitis or shock with centrilobular necrosis, provided production by skeletal muscle has been excluded. Loss of parenchymal function is indicated by a decrease in albumin and prothrombin concentrations.

Complete obstruction. This is suggested by an absence of urinary urobilinogen. Differentiation is essential and is assisted by ultrasonography to identify calculi within the gallbladder or dilated intrahepatic or extrahepatic ducts. Percutaneous thin-needle transhepatic cholangiography or endoscopic retrograde evaluation may indicate the level of obstruction.

Acute Parenchymal Disease

Infectious causes are: (1) viral (Ebstein-Barr, hepatitis, cytomegalic, coxsackie, and herpes); (2) parasitic (amebiasis and toxoplasmosis); (3) spirochetal (leptospirosis and syphilis); and (4) septicemic. *Gram-negative bacteremia* may produce jaundice by a direct inflammatory effect and by decreasing cardiac output and splanchnic blood flow. Toxic substances producing acute disease are carbon tetrachloride, ethylene glycol, methylchloride, chloroform, halothane, dinitrophenol, arsenic and antimony compounds, ferrous salts, poisonous fungi *(Amanita phalloides)*, sulfonamides, isoniazid, phenylbutazone, thiouracil, phenothiazine, and alcohol. The liver pathology is either acute zonal necrosis (the most common being the central zone) or acute massive necrosis involving the entire hepatic lobule.

Viral Hepatitis

Three common and similar clinical disorders, hepatitis A, B, and non-A non-B, have been defined. Hepatitis A is caused by an RNA enterovirus that produces an antibody which peaks 2-3 months after infection and persists. The viral antigen circulates in low concentration and is rapidly cleared in the stool. There appears not to be a carrier state; the antibody confers immunity. Antibody identification is accomplished by immune-adherence, complement-fixation, or radioimmunoassay techniques. Hepatitis B is due to a double-stranded DNA virus; 3 viral particles are found in the serum of patients—small spherical and tubular forms representing surface antigen (HBsAg) and larger Dane particles which appear to be the complete virion and contain an inner core antigen (HBcAg) and an outer shell of HBsAg. The core may be the infective particle. HBsAg appears in the serum early in the course of hepatitis, often before a rise in SGOT; it is absent in 15-25% of patients. As HBsAg disappears, its antibody develops and appears to confer permanent immunity. In some patients, however, HBsAg persists and may lead to a carrier state. An additional antigen—the e antigen—that is somehow associated with lactic dehydrogenase and is distinct from HBsAg and HBcAg has been found in patients with persistent HBsAg states. HBeAg correlates with activity and infectivity and is found in 40-60% of individuals with chronic active hepatitis. Antibody to HBcAg and HBeAg is found in HBsAg carriers; antibody to c-antigen suggests recent or active infection, antibody to e antigen suggests limited disease activity and low-grade infectivity.

Hepatitis A is spread by fecal-oral contamination and has an incubation period of 14-42 days. Hepatitis B has an incubation period of 50-180 days and is common among narcotic addicts and in patients on hemodialysis or following organ transplantation. It has followed local dental anesthesia and accidental needle sticks among medical personnel. The virus is found in saliva, urine, semen, breast milk, and other body fluids; sexual partners frequently contract the disease. Fever, chills, headache, anorexia, malaise, nausea, vomiting, diarrhea, right upper quadrant discomfort, and distaste for cigarettes are common prodromal symptoms in all three varieties. Bilirubinuria, light stools, and jaundice occur 2-14 days later. Hepatic enlargement and tenderness, splenomegaly, lymphadenopathy, jaundice, and laboratory evidence of hepatocellular disease are found during clinical study.

Eighty percent of patients with hepatitis A recover fully in 4 months, the remainder in 6 months, although 2-5% relapse with recurrence of jaundice and elevation of transaminase; mortality is 1%. Mortality with hepatitis B may be as high as 30%. Immune globulin is an accepted preventive measure for contacts of individuals with hepatitits A; hyperimmune globulin may be used in intimate contacts and accidental needle-sticks associated with hepatitis B. A vaccine for hepatitis B is now available.

CHOLESTATIC HEPATITIS
Patients with viral hepatitis may present with a clinical picture of intrahepatic cholestasis, which resembles extrahepatic bile obstruction. Hyperbilirubinemia, increased serum alkaline phosphatase levels, and elevated transaminase levels are present. Bile stasis, hepatocyte necrosis, and portal inflammation are found on liver biopsy. Severe pruritus and jaundice are present.

SUBACUTE HEPATIC NECROSIS
Subacute hepatic necrosis, a variant of viral hepatitis, is found more often in hepatitis B than type A. The disease may present like classical viral hepatitis, but the clinical course is variable, including fluctuating bilirubin and transaminase levels and significant hypoalbuminemia and hyperglobulinemia. Physical findings include hepatosplenomegaly, spider angiomas, and edema or anasarca. Liver biopsy findings reveal confluent, intralobular hepatic necrosis bridging adjacent portal tracts. Approximately 30% of the patients go on to develop postnecrotic cirrhosis. Death may result from liver failure, hemorrhage, or infection.

ACUTE HEPATIC NECROSIS

This condition, also called fulinant hepatitis or acute yellow atrophy, is rare, more common in women, and characterized by the acute onset of massive cell necrosis, diminution of liver size, jaundice, mental confusion, aminoaciduria, coma, and in 60-90% of patients, death within a few weeks. The prothrombin time is prolonged, and bleeding is common. Liver biopsy reveals massive interlobular necrosis of most lobules.

Treatment is aimed at maintaining vital functions and correction of fluid and electrolyte abnormalities. Dietary protein should be restricted, and lactulose or neomycin should be administered to reduce bacterial colonization.

CHRONIC HEPATITIS

Hepatitis B or non-A, non-B may last more than 3-6 months and is then considered chronic. The term *chronic persistent hepatitis* implies a mild process with few symptoms but laboratory abnormalities; *chronic active hepatitis* produces significant symptomatology with necrosis and fibrosis on biopsy.

Chronic active hepatitis may be due to persistent infection or to immunologic response. Hepatitis B is a classic example of immune complex disease. In some patients, a serum sickness-like syndrome occurs acutely with arthralgias and rash; complexes containing antigen, antibody, and complement have been found in skin, synovial membranes, and glomeruli. The presence of LE cells and ANA antibodies in young women with liver disease initially was thought to represent a collagen disease of some sort and was dubbed "lupoid hepatitis." The finding of antibodies to smooth muscle in 80%, hemolytic anemia, thyroiditis, and other auto-immune phenomena suggests this to be an unusual immune response to hepatitis B antigen. Corticosteroids and immunosuppressive drugs appear to be useful.

Other patients with chronic active hepatitis have persistent HBsAg titers; persistence beyond 13 weeks has been shown to be a poor prognostic sign. Liver biopsy demonstrates necrosis that bridges portal triads and extends into adjacent lobules. One-quarter of these patients die and an additional one-third develop cirrhosis. There is also evidence that regenerative nodules may lead to hepatoma.

Toxic Liver Disease

Many toxic substances cause liver disease. Agents such as carbon tetrachloride, yellow phosphorus, the peptides of poisonous mushrooms, and others produce a dose-related or direct toxic effect. A large group of other substances, many used for therapeutic purposes, produce hepatic damage in certain individuals, suggesting a hypersensitivity response. These agents may produce either a parenchymal response or a cholestatic pattern that may be confused with extra-hepatic biliary obstruction. INH produces a mild increase in serum transaminase levels in 10% and a hepatitis-like pattern in 1% of individuals. The incidence increases with age. Other common drugs producing a similar illness include halothane, phenytoin, and methyldopa. Chlorpromazine produces intrahepatic cholestasis with jaundice in 1-2% of patients. Clinical features include fever, rash, joint pain, nausea, vomiting, and abdominal pain, pruritis, and jaundice. Peripheral eosinophilia is common, and bile stasis is found on liver biopsy. Discontinuation of the drug relieves the pruritis and jaundice, although the latter may persist for months to years. Erythromycin estolate, methimazole, para-aminosalicylic acid, and chlorpropamide may produce similar cholestatic drug reactions. Anabolic steroids, 17-alpha-alkyl-substituted testosterone derivatives, and oral contraceptives produce dose-related cholestasis without hepatocellular damage or inflammation.

Secondary Liver Involvement

Hepatosplenomegaly may be the first evidence of many systemic diseases. Jaundice is unusual, but substantial elevation in alkaline phosphatase is characteristic so that its disproportionate elevation relative to serum bilirubin may be a useful clue. Computed tomography or radionuclide scanning may suggest tumor, but a liver biopsy is usually necessary for precise diagnosis.

Cells not usually found in the liver infiltrate the parenchyma in leukemia, Hodgkin's disease, extramedullary hematopoiesis, and amyloidosis. Triglycerides accumulate in galactosemia, abetalipoproteinemia, and diabetes. Cholesterol esters are found in increased amounts in Tangier disease and cholesterol ester storage disease, while excessive hepatic phospholipids are found in Gaucher's disease, Niemann-Pick's disease, Wolman's disease, and Fabry's disease. Glycogen is increased in diabetes, and hepatic glycogen storage disorders and mucopolysaccharides accumulate in Hurler's syndrome. In both primary and secondary amyloidosis, hepatic amyloid deposition is a feature. Sarcoidosis, berylliosis, and certain drugs produce hepatic granulomas and may lead to hepatosplenomegaly, mimicking portal hypertension and postnecrotic cirrhosis. Infectious disease-producing hepatic granulomas include infectious mononucleosis, Q fever, syphilis, brucellosis, schistosomiasis, histoplasmosis, and tuberculosis.

The Porphyrias
Defects in any of the biosynthetic steps that lead to the production of heme, shown in Fig. 7-1 lead to an accumulation of heme precursors. The resultant symptoms are dependent on the enzymatic defect and its localization to bone marrow, liver, or both. The precursors excreted for each defect are shown within the brackets in Fig. 7-1. All except porphobilinogen fluoresce and produce sensitivity to sunlight.

ACUTE INTERMITTENT PORPHYRIA
A 50-60% reduction in the hepatic concentration of uroporphyrinogen 1 synthetase activity (inherited as an autosomal dominant) produces a syndrome with severe abdominal pain, nausea, vomiting, mental changes and peripheral neuropathy with flaccid paralysis. Unexplained abdominal pain together with excretion of urine that turns red on standing alerts the internist to an important diagnosis.

Both porphobilinogen and aminolevulinic acid are found in the urine; the former because it is proximal to the enzymatic block, the latter, because a decrease in heme synthesis increases the activity of ALA synthesis. Barbiturates, sulfonamides, and estrogens also induce ALA synthetase and may precipitate attacks.

The treatment of an acute attack includes chlorpromazine to suppress pain and either the oral or parenteral administration of glucose or propranolol to inhibit the induction of ALA synthesis.

Other porphyrias include the rare autosomal recessive disorder, erythropoietic porphyria; variegate porphyria (mixed hepatic porphyria) and hereditary coproporphyria, both autosomal dominant diseases; and erythrohepatic protoporphyria, an autosomal dominant disorder of childhood.

Hepatic Vein Occlusion (Budd-Chiari Syndrome)

An uncommon lesion, hepatic vein occlusion, may occur in the following situations: hematologic disorders that lead to increased viscosity; intra-abdominal malignancies such as hepatoma, hypernephroma, and metastatic liver disease; lesions of the inferior vena cava or hepatic veins; intra-abdominal sepsis; pregnancy; oral contraceptives; trauma; systemic venous hypertension due to right ventricular failure.

In 50% of patients, the obstruction is in the inferior vena cava at or near the entrance of the hepatic veins. Ascites, hepatomegaly with tenderness, and abdominal pain are the characteristic presenting features of hepatic vein occlusion. Hematemesis, shock, signs of an acute abdomen distention of superficial abdominal veins, leg edema, and mild jaundice are also seen. Serum bilirubin is mildly increased; serum alkaline phosphatase is moderately elevated, and during the acute phase, serum transaminase levels may be increased. The serum albumin level is decreased, and the prothrombin time is normal or mildly prolonged. In 60-70% of patients, the ascitic fluid protein is high (greater than 2.5 gm/100 ml).

Diagnosis is made by liver biopsy, which reveals centrilobular congestion with dilated sinusoids filled with red blood cells and moderate centrilobular necrosis. Central fibrosis is observed late in the course. Hepatic venous and inferior vena caval catheterization is usually required to establish the site of occlusion. The presence of esophageal varices may be demonstrated by superior or mesenteric arteriography, which also provides information about portal vein patency if surgical decompression of portal hypertension is being considered.

The prognosis is poor for patients with total occlusion of the hepatic veins, although venous recanalization can occur. Hepatic coma, variceal hemorrhage, intercurrent sepsis, or portal mesenteric thrombosis with intestinal infarction are the causes of death.

Chronic Liver Disease
CIRRHOSIS
Cirrhosis, a major health problem in the United States, is one of the ten leading causes of death. Cirrhosis may be described in morphologic or etiologic terms. Alcohol produces *portal or micronodular cirrhosis.* Multiple small nodules of regenerating liver tissue are separated from each other and normal parenchyma by thin bands of connective tissue. Severe hepatitis, hemochromatosis, Wilson's disease, and biliary cirrhosis produce *macronodular* or *post-necrotic cirrhosis;* larger irregular-sized regenerating nodules and coarse scars are scattered throughout. There is considerable blending of these two morphologic types; portal and post-nephrotic changes may be found in the same patient and transition from portal to post-necrotic cirrhosis has been observed in alcoholics.

ALCOHOLIC LIVER DISEASE
Excessive ingestion of alcohol produces a variety of liver problems as well as absorptive defects, peripheral neuropathy, and central nervous system disturbances (see chapter 10). While mixed lesions are common, alcoholic fatty liver, alcoholic hepatitis, and alcoholic cirrhosis are frequently diagnosed. Alcoholic hepatitis is characterized by hepatic cell degeneration, necrosis, inflammatory infiltrates, enlarged hepatocytes, and Mallory bodies (irregular or globular hyaline deposits within hepatocytes).

Mallory bodies may also be found in Wilson's disease, primary biliary cirrhosis, certain hepatomas, and other liver conditions. For some reason, cirrhosis more frequently follows alcoholic hepatitis than fatty liver.

Hematologic abnormalities in patients with alcoholic liver disease may result from direct bone marrow suppression, associated dietary deficiencies, malabsorption, blood loss from gastritis or varices, and hypersplenism. Anemia, leukocytosis, leukemoid reactions, and thrombocytopenia are particularly common. Leukopenia may result from marrow suppression or from hypersplenism. Megaloblastic anemias occur with folate deficiency and sideroblastic anemia from an impaired conversion of pyridoxine to pyridoxal phosphate. Occasionally, a bizarre bone marrow picture may suggest a myeloproliferate disorder but may improve with a nutritious diet and abstinence from alcohol.

Drug administration in patients with alcoholic liver disease is difficult because the drugs can have either an exaggerated or a decreased action, depending on the patient's hepatic drug-metabolizing ability. This activity is usually decreased.

Portal cirrhosis (alcoholic cirrhosis, Laennec's cirrhosis). May develop after 10 or more years of continued alcohol ingestion. Men outnumber women by two to one. Clinical features include nausea and vomiting, weakness, anorexia, fatigue, and weight loss. Jaundice persists in a variable fashion. Patients with portal hypertension often develop ascites.

Physical findings include hepatomegaly, spider angiomas, gynecomastia and testicular atrophy, cachexia, muscle wasting, splenomegaly, and abdominal varices. Less common findings include palmar erythema, parotid gland enlargement, clubbing, and Dupuytren's contractures. Frequently, a low-grade fever is found.

Progressive fibrosis produces portal hypertension and hepatic encephalopathy. Hepatic coma is frequently preceded by bleeding esophageal varices, renal failure, or sepsis. Death may occur with any of these or from hepatoma.

Liver function tests are an index to the severity of the process. Hyperbilirubinemia, moderate elevations of serum alkaline phosphatase, and mild to moderate rises in serum transaminase levels are usually seen. The prothrombin time is usually prolonged, and the serum albumin level is depressed. Mild elevations of the serum globulin and the gammaglobulin fractions are usually found. Hyponatremia, hypokalemia, hyperglycemia, and low blood urea nitrogen levels are characteristic. Renal tubular acidosis or renal failure (hepatorenal syndrome) often complicate cirrhosis.

A common feature of cirrhosis is respiratory alkalosis, which is secondary to CNS-mediated hyperventilation. Hypoxemia is common and may be aggravated by cardiomyopathy, pneumonia, and recurrent pulmonary infections. Ascites may elevate the diaphragm and reduce lung volume. Pleural effusion develops in 10-15% of patients with cirrhosis.

Although the diagnosis can be made clinically, liver biopsy is necessary to confirm it. Prognosis depends on the stage of the liver disease as well as continued alcohol consumption. Five-year survival rates of 50-60% are observed, especially in patients who abstain from alcohol. In patients who develop ascites, the rate is 15-30% and averages 10-20% in patients who develop esophageal variceal bleeding.

Aside from the complete abstention from alcohol, there is no definitive treatment of cirrhosis. Supportive care includes a high-carbohydrate, low-protein diet, vitamin supplementation, bed rest, and salt restriction, especially in patients with cirrhosis. Paracentesis is rarely indicated except for respiratory distress, because it may cause hypovolemia and renal insufficiency. The major concern is treatment of complications.

Postnecrotic cirrhosis. Affects women as often as men, and the patients are usually younger than those with alcoholic cirrhosis.

The only sign may be splenomegaly; the liver may be small. Persistent jaundice is an early sign; ascites is late. Pruritis is present in 10-15% of patients. Abdominal pain is a common complaint. While the patient with alcoholic cirrhosis presents with hepatocellular insufficiency, the patient with postnecrotic cirrhosis often presents with complications of portal hypertension.

If present in postnecrotic cirrhosis, anemia is due to either hypersplenism or iron deficiency anemia secondary to variceal hemorrhage. Splenic sequestration accounts for leukopenia with or without anemia. Liver function tests resemble those found in alcoholic cirrhosis. However, the hyperglobulinemia may be more marked and the hyperbilirubinemia more persistent.

The diagnosis of postnecrotic cirrhosis should be considered in nonalcoholic patients presenting with features of portal hypertension. A liver biopsy is necessary for definitive diagnosis. There is a poor prognosis in patients with persistent jaundice or recurrent variceal bleeding. They often die in hepatic coma, from primary liver cell cancer or exsanguination. Treatment of postnecrotic cirrhosis is the same as that of alcoholic cirrhosis.

Primary Biliary Cirrhosis

While secondary biliary cirrhosis is due to long-standing extra-hepatic biliary obstruction, the etiology of a characteristic disorder called primary biliary cirrhosis remains unclear. The syndrome suggests chronic intrahepatic cholestasis associated with drugs, although evidence for this etiology is missing. Hypersensitivity to phenothiazines or viral destruction following cholestatic hepatitis have been suggested. Several immunologic abnormalities have been described. More than 95% of patients have an IgG antibody to mitochondria, an antibody seen but rarely in other liver diseases. Elevated IgM levels are found in 80%; cryoproteins in 90-95%. These cryoproteins are immune complexes that fix complement. Abnormal lymphocyte transformation has also been observed, suggesting an abnormal immune response to some agent.

The primary feature of the disease at this stage is distortion, degeneration, necrosis, or hyperplasia of the interlobular bile duct epitheliun. Another characteristic feature is a paucity of interlobular bile ducts, with proliferation of atypical ductules, expansion of portal tracts, and portal fibrous deposition in a later stage. Postnecrotic cirrhosis and cholestasis is the histologic feature of end-stage disease. The disease has an insidious onset and usually affects women between the ages of 35 and 65.

However, 10-15% of patients are men. The major feature is a progressive pruritis, which is due to an increased concentration of bile salts in the skin. Jaundice may appear in several months to years. Steatorrhea and osteomalacia are common features. Splenomegaly is found in 50-60% of patients and increased skin pigmentation, with or without xanthelasma, in 30-40%. Hepatomegaly is found in the majority. Complications of advanced postnecrotic cirrhosis and portal hypertension are the hallmark of advanced phases. Cutaneous calcinosis, Raynaud's phenomenon, sclerodactyly, and telangiectasis (CRST syndrome) may develop in a small number of cases.

The major differential diagnostic problem is between primary biliary cirrhosis and cirrhosis secondary to prolonged extrahepatic obstruction (sclerosing cholangitis, carcinoma, or stricture of the bile ducts or gallstones). Diagnosis may be made by laparotomy, with operative cholangiography, liver biopsy, and percutaneous or retrograde cholangiogram.

Pruritis is relieved by the use of oral cholestyramine, but it should be remembered that this agent may increase steatorrhea. Phenobarbital may also control the pruritis. To prevent deficiency of the fat-soluble vitamins A, D, E, and K, parenteral doses may be given. Corticosteroids and immunosuppressive agents have no proven clinical efficacy.

DISEASES OF THE GALLBLADDER AND BILE DUCTS

Gallstone formation and inflammatory biliary tract disease occurs in 10% of males and 20% of females between the ages of 55 and 65 years. Approximately 2% of the 15 million people in the United States with gallstones have a cholecystectomy yearly. Thirty percent of patients with Crohn's disease have gallstones.

Bile is composed of cholesterol (5%), bile salts (65-90%) and phospholipid (5-25%). Biliary secretions help dispose of bilirubin and solubilize dietary fat, which is absorbed from the intestinal lumen. Bile salts are the principal constituent of bile and solubilize cholesterol. Bile salts have both hydrophilic (water-soluble) and hydrophobic (fat-soluble) properties, which are necessary for micelle formation. Phospholipids in the form of lecithin help solubilize cholesterol in the formation of micelles. The micelle with both phospholipid and bile salts maintains cholesterol in solution.

There are two major types of stones that form in the gallbladder and biliary tract. Approximately 80% are composed of cholesterol, and the other major type contains calcium bilirubinate (50-70% bilirubin) around a cholesterol nucleus. Cholesterol stones form because of a reduction in the pool of bile salts. With decreased bile salts, cholesterol becomes supersaturated and cholesterol microcrystals precipitate. The microcrystals aggregate and form radiolucent gallstones, measuring from a few millimeters to greater than a centimeter in size. Cholesterol stones are more common in the United States and Europe and bilirubinate stones are more common in the Orient (associated with biliary stasis and *E. coli* and *Ascaris lumbricoides* infection). Bilirubinate stones are radiopaque and can be seen on a plain abdominal x-ray film.

Cholelithiasis

Cholelithiasis develops in middle age and produces symptoms in approximately 30%. Elective cholecystectomy is the treatment of choice for patients under 50 years of age with asymptomatic cholelithiasis. Patients 50-60 years old who are in good health should also have cholecystectomy for asymptomatic stones. Patients over 60 should be followed closely. The overall mortality rate for cholecystectomy is 4% for patients greater than 60 years of age and 0.4% for patients less than 60.

Cholesterol supersaturation present in a patient's bile with cholesterol gallstones can be cleared in 85-90% of patients with the bile salt chenodeoxycholic acid (10-15 mg/kg/day). As long as the gallbladder is functioning, treatment with this salt lowers biliary cholesterol concentration. Although the mechanism is unknown, it has been shown that small radiolucent stones (4 mm or less) are cleared partially or completely in a year, and larger stones (5-10 mm or more in diameter) can be cleared in approximately 2-4 years. Approximately 20% of patients will have recurrent stones.

Chenodeoxycholic acid should be an excellent technique for preventing acute and chronic cholecystitis and will probably be approved for general use early in 1981.

ACUTE CHOLECYSTITIS

Acute inflammation of the gallbladder is almost always caused by a gallstone obstructing the cystic duct (90-95% of cases). If there is no demonstrable stone, bacterial infection or prior surgery of the biliary tract may be responsible. Patients present with acute abdominal pain. Pain due to biliary obstruction is steady, midepigastric with radiation to the right upper quadrant, around to the back or up between the scapulae. It is abrupt, severe, constant, and lasts 15-60 minutes, finally subsiding gradually. The pain varies in nature from a cramp to a pain described as excruciating, and the person relieves pain by assuming different positions. Anorexia, nausea, and fever (38-39°C) accompany the attack.

The gallbladder is palpable in 25-30% of patients. There is also subcostal tenderness in the right upper quadrant, pain with inspiration (Murphy's sign), and rebound. If there is diffuse abdominal tenderness after several days, perforation is a consideration. Secondary pancreatitis and abscess are considerations if localized tenderness exists in a patient who has been ill for several days. Scleral icterus is a sign that a stone has lodged in the common bile duct. The WBC ranges from 12,000-15,000/cu mm; serum amylase is elevated in 30-50%. Alkaline phosphatase and bilirubin are also high. Plain abdominal films will show calcifications in 12-15% of patients with gallstones. Failure to reveal opacification after a double oral dose of contrast material is indicative of obstruction of the cystic duct. Intravenous cholangiography to identify a common bile duct stone is indicated in three clinical situations: (1) history of colic, (2) elevated serum phosphatase three times normal, and (3) mild jaundice, i.e., bilirubin level of 3 mg/100 ml or more. Ultrasonography is nearly as reliable as an oral cholecystogram in demonstrating cholelithiasis or a distended gallbladder.

Differential diagnosis includes acute appendicitis with right upper quadrant pain (especially when the appendix is retrocecal or the cecum is in the subhepatic area) and an acute right pyelonephritis. Acute pancreatitis is often especially difficult to distinguish from acute cholecystitis, since both produce right upper abdominal tenderness or rebound pain, elevated serum amylase, and poorly visualized gallbladder on cholecystography.

Pneumonia, infarction of the right lung, myocardial infarction, and acute viral hepatitis or alcoholic hepatitis may present with right upper quadrant pain.

Emphysematous cholecystitis (three times more common in males than females) is caused by gas-forming bacteria such as *Clostridium perfringens*, anaerobic streptococci, or *E. coli*, and may present with sharp epigastric pain and elevation of liver function tests. An abdominal flat plate shows gas within the gallbladder.

Patients with acute cholecystitis should be hospitalized, given intravenous fluids, and have nasogastric suction. Morphine should be avoided because it causes spasm of the common bile and cystic ducts, but meperidine (Demerol) may be necessary to relieve pain (100 mg I.M. q3h). Antibiotics are not indicated unless the patient becomes toxic or develops peritonitis. Suggested antibiotics are penicillin (20 million units q24h or ampicillin (1 gm q4h I.V.) along with gentamycin (2-4 mg/kg q24h in divided doses).

Once stabilized, cholecystectomy should be performed in patients who are 60 years of age or less. Conservative medical therapy and antibiotic usage may be preferable in patients over 60 years of age or who are at high risk. In other patients, a simple cholecystectomy and stone extraction may be indicated. The status of the biliary tract should be evaluated by cholangiography through the drainage tube. In elderly patients who are at risk but with functioning gallbladders and who have cholesterol stones, an attempt to dissolve the gallstones with chenodeoxycholic acid is warranted.

Major complications are gallbladder necrosis and perforation.

Approximately 2% of patients with cholecystitis will perforate, but this is associated with a 25-30% mortality rate. Fistula formation between the colon or duodenum and gallbladder (cholecystoenteric fistula) occurs near the hepatic flexure. Surgical treatment consists of cholecystectomy, common bile duct exploration, and closure of the fistula. A gallstone passing through a cholecystoenteric fistula may produce an ileus, especially if the stones produce an obstruction at the ileocecal valve. The gallstone must usually be larger than 2.5 cm in diameter. Surgical extraction is the treatment of choice.

Chronic Cholelithiasis and Cholecystitis
CLINICAL MANIFESTATIONS

Many patients who have gallstones and suffer recurrent attacks of acute cholecystitis develop chronic cholecystitis. These patients develop a fibrotic gallbladder. The organs are incapable of secreting bile, and many develop transient jaundice with recurrent attacks.

On physical examination, there may be guarding or right upper quadrant tenderness. Because the gallbladder is scarred with fibrosis, it will not be enlarged and will therefore not be palpable.

Laboratory examination may reveal an elevated alkaline phosphatase or bilirubin, which may suggest chronic cholangitis or a common bile duct stone. Other laboratory tests are usually normal.

A diagnosis of chronic cholangitis may be made in 85-90% of cases in which there is failure to visualize the gallbladder after administration of a double dose of contrast material. This failure to opacify may be due to chronic fibrotic gallbladder disease or cystic duct obstruction. Ultrasonography has been helpful, especially in identifying cholesterol stones.

Because 3-5% of patients with acute or chronic cholecystitis have a normal cholecystogram, duodenal drainage may be useful, especially in patients with normal liver function tests and a normal oral cholecystogram but who are suspected of having gallbladder disease. Patients swallow a polyvinyl nasogastric tube, which is allowed to move to the distal duodenum. Then 75 ml of 33% magnesium sulfate is passed through the tube in order to stimulate emptying of the gallbladder. The duodenal contents are removed and examined for the presence of cholesterol crystals and bilirubinate granules. Presence of either of these crystals in the drainage implies supersaturation of one of the components of bile in the sediment.

Choledocholithiasis

Choledocholithias, the passage of a stone to the common bile duct from the gallbladder via the cystic duct, occurs in 12-15% of patients with chronic cholelithiasis. The stones usually lodge in the ampulla of Vater (point of insertion of the common duct into the second segment of the duodenum). Patients often present with shaking chills, jaundice, and severe right upper quadrant pain, which is colicky with a rapid onset and lasts up to an hour with associated nausea and vomiting. Large stones may obstruct the common bile duct, while smaller ones pass through the common bile duct into the duodenum. Patients usually have right upper quadrant or midepigastric guarding. There is no rebound tenderness unless there is common bile duct or gallbladder perforation.

On laboratory examination, there is an abrupt rise of both serum bilirubin and alkaline phosphatase, with a moderate rise in serum aminotransferase. Values for serum bilirubin are 5-10 mg/100 ml, and the alkaline phosphatase will be two and one-half to three times normal. Both of the elevations occur within 48-96 hours of the attack. An elevated serum 5'-nucleotidase or leucine aminopeptidase will verify the hepatic origin of the elevated serum alkaline phosphatase.

To differentiate between extrahepatic and intrahepatic causes of cholestasis and discover the site of obstruction, it may be necessary to perform intravenous cholangiography or transhepatic cholangiography. An oral cholecystogram will usually fail to opacify the gallbladder because of chronic cholecystitis associated with common bile duct obstruction with a stone. An intravenous cholangiogram reveals in a majority of cases an opacified dilated duct and a radiolucent filling defect in the distal duct.

Ultrasonography, a noninvasive procedure, may be useful in delineating disease in a patient with common bile duct obstruction who has an elevated bilirubin. Two other procedures include percutaneous transhepatic cholangiography and endoscopic retrograde cholangiopancreatography (ERCP). Percutaneous transhepatic cholangiography is indicated if obstruction of an intrahepatic biliary duct is suspected. Use of a small-bore needle carries little risk of bile peritonitis. ERCP is a direct catheterization of the common bile duct for the introduction of contrast material, allowing visualization of contrast material and study of the biliary tree. Carcinoma will usually have irregular margins, while an impacted stone will have a smooth-appearing defect.

Right upper quadrant and midepigastric pain can be confusing in establishing a differential diagnosis. A temporary obstruction of the common bile duct may be produced by an acute inflammation of the head of the pancreas. Acute pancreatitis can be differentiated by an upper GI series, which will show edematous, angulated folds in the descending portion of the duodenum with acute inflammation of the pancreatic head. If the diagnosis is still uncertain, the patient may be treated with nasogastric suction, which allows pancreatic edema to subside. An intravenous cholangiogram will then show a normal common bile duct in acute pancreatitis and a stone in choledocholithiasis.

Liver function tests will differentiate between acute biliary obstruction by a stone and ureterolithiasis, both of which may present in clinically similar ways. Acute intermittent porphyria can be differentiated by failure to produce strikingly elevated levels of alkaline phosphatase or bilirubin. A radioisotope scan or ultrasonography will help identify an obstruction of the major bile ducts caused by a large hepatic or amebic abscess. Clinically, the abscesses will not be acute in onset but will present as a chronic vague upper quadrant pain.

Pancreatic carcinoma must also be considered in the differential. Midepigastric pain is often severe, but liver function tests may be normal. Irregular margins of the tumor invading the duct will be seen by intravenous cholangiography and in patients with jaundice, transhepatic cholangiography, and/or ERCP. Narrowing and irregularity of either the small or large ducts caused by sclerosing cholangitis, a chronic process often associated with ulcerative colitis, can be distinguished by dilatation or presence of stones caused by choledocholithiasis by transhepatic or retrograde cholangiography.

The treatment of choice for choledocholithiasis is common bile duct exploration and removal of stones. A T-tube is left in the common bile duct and a cholangiogram is done 7-10 days postoperatively to determine whether any stones were left. If stones remain, instrumental extraction at 4-6 weeks may be attempted via the T-tube tract (the tube is left in place so that a rigid wall develops). From 10-15% of patients pass stones spontaneously. For remaining stones, a forceps equipped with a basket is introduced into the tract under fluroscopic control, and an attempt is made to crush and remove the stones.

Chemical dissolution of stones with a solution of 200 mM sodium cholate and 0.15 mM sodium chloride buffered to pH 7.5 may be attempted if instrumental extraction is unsuccessful. The solution is administered at 30 ml/hour. Cholestyramine 4 mg p.o. q.i.d. is also given to prevent cholic acid-induced diarrhea. Approximately 60% of patients will have reduction in stone size in 2 weeks.

Even after cholecystectomy and surgical reexploration, 2-5% of patients develop recurrent stones in the biliary tree with recurrent symptoms and hepatic dysfunction.

Chronic Cholangitis

Chronic cholangitis, a chronic inflammation in the hepatic biliary tract, will develop in a small number of patients with chronic cholecystitis. These patients present with fatigue, anorexia, weight loss, and intermittent chills and fever. Physical examination reveals moderate right upper quadrant tenderness and skin excoriations secondary to pruritis. Significant laboratory findings include a chronic elevation of serum alkaline phosphatase to two or three times normal. There is also an associated increase in serum leucine aminopeptidase and 5'-nucleotidase. Transient jaundice and a further elevation of alkaline phosphatase may occur with episodes of fever and chills.

Conditions leading to chronic cholangitis include common bile duct stricture, intrahepatic cholestasis, recurrent cholelithiasis, congenital hepatic fibrosis, biliary cirrhosis, and cholangiocarcinoma.

Patients with chronic cholangitis secondary to common bile duct stricture and who develop stones may require a choledochoduodenostomy to allow the stones to pass from the biliary tree. Intrahepatic cholestasis related to either viral or toxic hepatitis and appearing clinically like chronic cholangitis may also be caused by certain drugs, the most notable example being chlorpromazine.

Characterized by marked dilation of intrahepatic ducts, congenital hepatitis with fibrosis often presents with hepatosplenomegaly and associated cholangitis in early middle age. If severe portal hypertension develops, there may be bleeding varices. Fifty-five to 60% of these patients will also have cystic lesions in the kidneys and many of the patients will have stones in the gallbladder and common bile duct. Liver biopsy shows fibrosis of the liver, and the definitive diagnosis is made by transhepatic cholangiography, which will reveal gross sacculation of the intrahepatic ducts.

Cholangiocarcinoma, which may cause moderate liver enlargement and elevation of alkaline phosphatase without jaundice, usually occurs in one of the major branches of the biliary tree. These patients usually have some underlying hepatic disease. Diagnosis is established by ERCP or transhepatic cholangiography. Marked elevation in serum alkaline phosphatase and cholesterol with late-appearing jaundice are the hallmarks of primary biliary cirrhosis, a progressive inflammatory disease of the biliary radicles. Pruritis is the most common presenting complaint. Liver biopsy shows characteristic pathologic findings (granulomas in portal areas and abnormal biliary duct epithelium with segmental neutrophils), but they are not diagnostic.

If the site of biliary tract obstruction can be defined by newer techniques (ultrasonic scanning, transhepatic cholangiography, and ERCP), many of the lesions can be treated surgically before damage to the biliary tree becomes irreversible and secondary biliary cirrhosis develops. Computed tomography should also be considered since it allows evaluation of other abdominal organs.

Hyperalimentation in the Hospitalized Patient

Protein-energy starvation has been found in 25-60% of patients in general medical wards at teaching hospitals. Poor intake of calories together with malabsorption and hypermetabolism lead to a major nutritional deficit. While central venous hyperalimentation may be necessary when severe malabsorption is present, enteral alimentation appears to be a more physiologic substitute. Feeding mixtures such as Vivonex or Flexical may be given on a 24-hour basis, using a mechanical pump and nasogastric tube. Complications include obstruction of tube, gastrointestinal reaction to enteric feeding, or inability to utilize nutrients because of cardiac, hepatic, or renal abnormalities. The technique appears preferable in most situations to transvenous hyperalimentation.

Hepatorenal Syndrome

The classic syndrome is the development of oliguric renal failure in a patient with otherwise normal kidneys and advanced liver disease. Common in individuals with severe cirrhosis, hypoalbuminemia, and ascites, the cause is probably hypovolemia in the presence of an expanded interstitial space. Peritoneal-atrial and peritoneal-jugular (LeVeen) shunts return ascitic fluid to the circulation and may improve renal blood flow and glomerular filtration. Blendis et al. showed that cardiac output, PAH (para-amino-hippuric) and creatinine clearances, urine volume, and sodium excretion increased dramatically after return of ascitic fluid. While demonstrating the importance of vascular volume, the technique may have practical limitations since disseminated intravascular coagulation and thrombosis of the prostheses were not infrequent complications.

A variant of the hepatorenal syndrome is found in the patient with shock and poor splanchnic and renal blood flow. In these individuals, jaundice and oliguric renal failure complicate the overall management of the shock syndrome.

Primary Hepatoma

Hepatomegaly, right upper quadrant pain, mass, friction rub, or bloody ascites together with anemia, leukocytosis and elevated alkaline phosphatase suggests hepatoma. Hepatitis B appears to be an important causal factor but any form of chronic liver disease seems to predispose to its development. Scintiscans may not distinguish among hepatoma, other tumor, or cirrhosis but gallium scanning and angiography has been useful. Alpha-feto-protein serum concentrations are markedly elevated in at least two thirds of patients.

Prognosis is poor; most die within six to ten months.

Infectious Diarrhea

These syndromes are produced by bacterial, viral, and protozoan agents. *Shigella* and *Salmonella* are invasive and produce severe diarrhea, often bloody, as well as abdominal pain, fever, myalgia and headache. Systemic symptoms are more severe with *Shigella* and antibiotics appear effective. Systemic symptoms are less severe with *Salmonella,* and antibiotics may prolong the excretion of bacteria. A noninvasive diarrheal syndrome with minimal systemic symptoms is produced by cholera and by enterotoxi-genic *E. coli.* There are no rapid means for identifying those *E. coli* that produce enterotoxin. Some strains of *E. coli,* rare in the U.S., also produce an invasive diarrheal syndrome.

REFERENCES

Esophageal Disorders

Behar J et al: Medical and surgical management of reflux esophagitis: a 38-month report on a prospective clinical trial. N Engl J Med 293:263, 1975.

Bernstein LM, Baker LS: A clinical test for esophagitis. Gastroenterology 34:760, 1958.

Nakayama K, Kinoshuta Y: Cancer of the gastrointestinal tract. II. Esophagus: treatment—localized and advanced: surgical treatment combined with preoperative concentrated irradiation. JAMA 227:175, 1974.

Peptic Ulcer Disease

Fleischer D, Samloff MI: Cimetidine therapy in a patient with metiamide-induced agranulocytosis (letter). N Engl J Med 296:342, 1977.

Peterson WL, et al: Healing of duodenal ulcer with an antacid regimen. N Engl J Med 297:341, 1977.

Grossman MI, Guth PH, Isenberg JI, Passaro EP Jr, Roth BE, Sturdevant RAL, Walsh JH: A new look a peptic ulcer. Ann Intern Med 84:57, 1976.

Brimblecombe RW, Duncan WAM, Durant GJ, et al.: Characterization and development of cimetidine as a histamine H_2-receptor antagonist. Gastroenterology 74:339, 1978.

Richardson CT: Effect of H_2-receptor antagonists on gastric acid secretion and serum gastrin concentrations. Gastroenterology 74:366, 1978.

Bender HJ, Cocco A, Crossley RJ, et al.: Cimetidine in the treatment of duodenal ulcer: a multicenter double-blind study. Gastroenterology 74:380, 1978.

Hetzel DJ, Hansy J, Shearman DJC, et al.: Cimetidine treatment of duodenal ulceration: short-term clinical trial and maintenance study. Gastroenterology 74:389, 1978.

Gray GR, Smith IS, Mackenzie I, et al.: Long-term cimetidine in the management of severe duodenal ulcer dyspepsia. Gastroenterology 74:397, 1978.

Ippoliti AF, Sturdevant RAL, Isenberg JI, et al: Cimetidine versus intensive antacid therapy for duodenal ulcer: a multicenter trial. Gatroenterology 74:393, 1978.

Henn RM, Isenberg JI, Maxwell V, Sturdevant RAL: Inhibition of gastric acid secretion by cimetidine in patients with duodenal ulcer. N Engl J Med 293:371, 1975.

Upper Gastrointestinal Hemorrhage

Sandlow LJ, et al.: A prospective randomized study of the management of upper gastrointestinal hemorrhage. Am J Gastroenterol 61:282, 1974.

Schiller KFR, Truelove SC, Williams DG: Haematemesis and melaena, with special reference to factors influencing the outcome. Br Med J 2:7, 1970.

Diarrhea

Dupont HL, Formal SB, Hornuk RB, et al.: Pathogenesis of *Escherichia coli* diarrhea. N Engl J Med (parts I and II) 285:831, 1971.

Fedesco FJ, Markham R, Gurwith M, et al.: Oral vancomycin for antibestic-associated pseudomembranous colitis. Lancet 2:226, 1978.

Fedesco FJ, Stanley RJ, Alpers DH: Diagnostic feature of clindamycin-associated pseudomembranous colitis. N Engl J Med 290:841, 1974.

Phillips SF: Diarrhea: a current view of the pathophysiology. Gastroenterology 63:495, 1972.

Wolfe MS: Giardiasis. JAMA 233:1362, 1975.

Diseases of the Small Intestine

Finley JM, Hogarth J, Wightman KJR: A clinical evaluation of the D-xylose tolerance test. Ann Intern Med 61:411, 1964.

Drummey GD, Benson JA Jr, Jones CM: Microscopical examination of the stool for steatorrhea. N Engl J Med 264:85, 1961.

Rubin CE, Dobbins WO III: Peroral biopsy of the small intestine: a review of its diagnostic usefulness. Gastroenterology 49:676, 1965.

Benson GD, Knowlessar OD, Sleisenger MH: Adult celiac disease with emphasis upon response to the gluten-free diet. Medicine (Baltimore) 43:1, 1964.

Bloomer WD, Hellman S: Normal tissue responses to radiation therapy. N Engl J Med 293:80, 1975.

Hermans PE, Diaz-Buxo JD: Idiopathic late-onset immunoglobulin deficiency: clinical observations in 50 patients. Am J Med 61:221, 1976.

Hoskins LC, Winawer JJ, Broitman SA, et al.: Clinical giardiasis and intestinal malabsorption. Gastroenterology 53:265, 1967.

Tumors of the GI Tract

Wooley PV, MacDonald JS, Schein PS: Chemotherapy of malignancies of the gastrointestinal tract. Progr Gastroenterol 3:671, 1977.

Moertel CG: Clinical management of advanced gastrointestinal cancer. Cancer 36 (Suppl):675, 1975.

Winnan G, Berci G, Panish J, Talbot TM, Overholt BF, McCallum RW: Superiority of the flexible to the rigid sigmoidoscope in routine proctosigmoidoscopy. N Engl J Med 302:1011, 1980.

Winawer SJ, Sherlock P, Schottenfeld D, Miller DG: Screening for colon cancer. Gastroenterology 70:783, 1976.

Inflammatory Bowel Disease

Almy TP. Sherlock P: Genetic aspects of ulcerative colitis and regional enteritis. Gastroenterology 51:757, 1966.

Norland CC, Kisner JB: Toxic dilatation of colon (toxic megacolon): etiology, treatment and prognosis in 42 patients. Medicine 48:229, 1969.

Famer RG, Hawk WA, Turnbull RB Jr: Clinical patterns in Crohn's disease: a statistical study of 615 cases. Gastroenterology 68:627, 1975.

Singleton JW: National Cooperative Crohn's Disease Study (NCCDS): results of drug treatment. A cooperative study (abstract). Gastroenterology 72A:110/1133, 1977.

Hermos JA, Cooper HL, Kramer P, et al.: Histological diagnosis by peroral biopsy of Crohn's disease of the proximal intestine. Gastroenterology 59:868, 1970.

Drossman DA, Powell DW, Sessions JT Jr: The irritable bowel syndrome. Gastroenterology 73:811, 1977.

Fawaz KA, Glotzer DJ, Goldman H, Dickersin GR, Gross W, Patterson JF: Ulcerative colitis and Crohn's disease of the colon—a comparison of the long-term postoperative courses. Gastroenterology 71:372, 1976.

Goodman MJ, Kirsner JB, Riddell RH: Usefulness of rectal biopsy in inflammatory bowel disease. Gastroenterology 72:952, 1977.

Greenstein AJ, Janowitz HD, Sachar DB: The extra-intestinal complications of Crohn's disease and ulcerative colitis: a study of 700 patients. Medicine 55:401, 1976.

Dobbins WO III: Current status of the precancer lesion in ulcerative colitis. Gastroenterology 73:1431, 1977.

Kirsner JB: Observations on the medical treatment of inflammatory bowel disease. JAMA 243:557, 1980.

Mekhjian HS, Switz DM, Melnyk CS, Rankin GB, Brooks RK: Clinical features and natural history of Crohn's disease. Gastroenterology 77(part 2):898, 1979.

Present DH, Korelitz BI, Wisch N, Glass JL, Sachar DB, Pasternack BS: Treatment of Crohn's disease with 6-Mercaptopurine. A long-term, randomized, double-blind study. N Engl J Med 302:981, 1980.

Diseases of the Large Intestine

Painter NS, Burkett DP: Diverticular disease of the colon, a 20th century problem. Clin Gastroenterol 4:3, 1975.

Bradriff AJ: Treatment of symptomatic diverticular disease with a high-fibre diet. Lancet 1:664, 1977.

Heald RJ, Ray JE: Bleeding in diverticular disease of the colon. Proc R Soc Med 65:779, 1972.

McGuire HH Jr, Haynes BW Jr: Massive hemorrhage from diverticulosis of the colon: guideline for therapy based on bleeding patterns observed in fifty cases. Ann Surg 175:847, 1972.

Adams JT: The barium enema as treatment for massive diverticular bleeding. Dis Colon Rectum 17:439, 1974.

Larson DM, Masters SS, Spiro HM: Medical and surgical therapy of diverticular disease: a comparative study. Gastroenterology 71:734, 1976.

Boley SJ, Sammartano R, Adams A, DiBiase A, Kleinhaus S, Sprayregen
   S: On the nature and etiology of vascular ectasias of the colon:
   degenerative lesions of aging. Gastroenterology 72:650, 1977.

Diseases of the Pancreas

Farmer RG, Winkelman EI, Brown HB, Lewis LA: Hyperlipoproteinemia and pancreatitis. Am J Med 54:161, 1973.

Warshaw AL, Fuller AF Jr: Specificity of increased renal clearance of
   amylase in diagnosis of acute pancreatitis. N Engl J Med 292:325,
   1975.

Johnson SG, Ellis CJ, Levitt MD: Mechanisms of increased renal
   clearance of amylase/creatinine in acute pancreatitis. N Engl J Med
   295:1212, 1976.

Salt WB II, Schenker S: Amylase—its clinical significance: a review of
   the literature. Medicine 55:269, 1976.

DiMagno EP, Malagelada JR, Taylor WF, Go VLW: A prospective
   comparison of current diagnostic tests for pancreatic cancer. N Engl J
   Med 297:737, 1977.

Regan PT: Medical treatment of acute pancreatitis. Mayo Clin Proc
   54:432, 1979.

Cubilla AL, Fitzgerald PJ: Classification of pancreatic cancer (nonendocrine). Mayo Clin Proc 54:449, 1979.

Malagelada JR: Pancreatic cancer: an overview of epidemiology, clinical
   presentation and diagnosis. Mayo Clin Proc 54:459, 1979.

DiMagno EP: Medical treatment of pancreatic insufficiency. Mayo Clin
   Proc 54:435, 1979.

Kelly TR: Gallstone pancreatitis: pathophysiology. Surgery 80:488, 1976.

Adson MA: Surgical treatment of pancreatitis: review of a series. Mayo
   Clin Proc 54:443, 1979.

DeTroyer A, Naeije R, Yernault JC, Englert M: Impairment of pulmonary function in acute pancreatitis. Chest 73:360, 1978.

Diseases of the Liver

Conrad ME, Schwartz FD, Young AA: Infectious hepatitis—a generalized disease: a study of renal, gastrointestinal and hematologic abnormalities. Am J Med 37:789, 1964.

Grady FG, Lee VA: Hepatitis B immune globulin—prevention of hepatitis from accidental exposure among medical personnel. N Engl J Med
   293:1067, 1975.

Seeff LB, et al.: A randomized, double-blind controlled trial of the
   efficacy of immune serum globulin for the prevention of post-transfu-
   sion hepatitis. Gastroenterology 72:111, 1977.

Villarejos VM, Visona KA, Guterrez AD, Rodriguez AA: Role of saliva, urine and feces in the transmission of type B hepatitis. N Engl J Med 291:1375, 1974.

Krugman SH, Friedman H, Lothmer C: Viral hepatitis, type A: identification by specific complement-fixation and immune adherence tests. N Engl J Med 295:755, 1976.

Purcell RH, Dienstag JL, Feinstone SM, et al.: Relationship of hepatitis A antigen to viral hepatitis. Am J Med Sci 270:61, 1975.

Robinson WS, Lutwick LI: The virus of hepatitis, type B. N Engl J Med 295:1168, 1976.

Hoofnagle JH, et al.: Transmission of non-A, non-B hepatitis. Ann Intern Med 87:14, 1977.

Szmaness W, et al.: Hepatitis type A and hemodialysis: a seroepidemiologic study in 15 U.S. centers. Ann Intern Med 87:8, 1977.

Corey L, Stamm WE, Feorino PM, et al.: HBsAg-negative hepatitis in a hemodialysis unit. Relation to Epstein-Barr virus. N Engl J Med 293:1273, 1975.

Redeker AG, Mosley JW, Gocke DJ, McKee AP, Pollack W: Hepatitis B immune globulin as a prophylactic measure for spouses exposed to acute type B hepatitis. N Engl J Med 293:1055, 1975.

Gregory PB, Knauer CM, Kempson RL, Miller R: Steroid therapy in severe viral hepatitis: a double-blind, randomized trial of methylprednisolone versus placebo. N Engl J Med 294:681, 1976.

Galambos JT: Alcoholic hepatitis: its therapy and prognosis. Prog Liver Diseases. Popper H, Scaffner F, eds., Grune & Stratton Inc, New York, 1972, p. 567.

Conn HO: A rational approach to the hepatorenal syndrome. Gastroenterology 65:321, 1973.

Schenker S, Breen KJ, Hoyumpa AM Jr: Hepatic encephalopathy: current status. Gastroenterology 66:121, 1974.

Long RG, Scheuer PJ, Sherlock S: Presentation and course of asymptomatic primary biliary cirrhosis. Gastroenterology 72:1204, 1977.

Boyer JL: Chronic hepatitis—a perspective on classification and determinants of prognosis. Gastroenterology 70:1161, 1976.

Sherlock S: Predicting progression of acute type-B hepatitis to chronicity. Lancet II:354, 1976.

Knodel RG, Conrad ME, Ishak KG: Development of chronic liver disease after acute non-A, non-B posttransfusion hepatitis: role of γ-globulin prophylaxis in its prevention (part I). Gastroenterology 72:902, 1977.

Mistilis SP: Active chronic hepatitis. In Schiff L (ed.): Diseases of the Liver. Philadelphia, Lippincott, 1975, p 645.

Berman M, Alter HJ, Ishak KG, Purcell RH, Jones EA: The chronic sequelae of non-A, non-B hepatitis. Ann Intern Med 91:1, 1979.

Czaja AJ, Summerskill WHJ: Chronic hepatitis: to treat or not to treat? Med Clin of North Am 62:71, 1978.

Surgenor DMN, et al.: Clinical trials of hepatitis B immune globulin: development of policies and materials for the 1972-1975 studies sponsored by the National Heart and Lung Institute. N Engl J Med 293:1060, 1975.

Prince AM, et al.: Hepatitis B "immune" globulin: effectiveness in prevention of dialysis-associated hepatitis. N Engl J Med 293:1063, 1975.

Levin DM, Baker AL, Riddell RH, Rochman H, Boyer JL: Nonalcoholic liver disease: overlooked causes of liver injury in patients with heavy alcohol consumption. Am J Med 66:429, 1979.

Favero MS, Maynard JE, Leger RT, Graham DR, Dixon RE: Guidelines for the care of patients hospitalized with viral hepatitis. Ann Intern Med 91:872, 1979.

Seefe LB, Hoofnagle JH: Immunoprophylaxis of viral hepatitis. Gastroenterology 77:161, 1977.

Hoofnagle JH, et al.: Passive-active immunity from hepatitis B immune globulin: reanalysis of a Veterans Administration cooperative study of needle-stick hepatitis. Ann Intern Med 91:813, 1979.

Seefe LB, et al.: Type B hepatitis after needle-stick exposure: prevention with hepatitis B immune globulin. Final Report of the Veterans Administration Cooperative Study. Ann Intern Med 88:285, 1978.

The Hepatitis Knowledge Base. A Prototype Information Transfer System. AIMEAS 93 (1, Suppl. Part II)165-222, 1980.

Blendis LM, Greig PD, Langer B, Baigrie, Russe J, Taylor BR: Renal and hemodynamic effects of the peritoneovenous shunt for intractable hepatic ascites. Gastroenterology 77:250, 1979.

Pladson TR, Parrish RM: Hepatorenal syndrome: recovery after peritoneovenous shunt. Arch Intern Med 137:1248, 1977.

Diseases of the Gallbladder and Bile Ducts

Friedman GD, Kannel WB, Dawber TR: The epidemiology of gallbladder disease: observations in the Framingham study. J Chronic Dis 19:273, 1966.

Wenckert A, Robertson B: The natural course of gallstone disease: eleven-year review of 781 nonoperated cases. Gastroenterology 50:376, 1966.

Thistle JL, Hoffmann AF: Efficacy and specificity of chenodeoxycholic acid therapy for dissolving gallstones. N Engl J Med 289:655, 1973.

Vicary FR: Progress report: ultrasound and gastroenterology. Gut 18:386, 1977.

Iser JH, Dowling RH, Mok HYI, Bell GD: Chenodeoxycholic acid treatment of gallstones. A follow-up report and analysis of factors influencing response to therapy. N Engl J Med 293:378, 1975.

Bartrum RJ Jr, Crow HC, Foote SR: Ultrasonic and radiographic cholecystography. N Engl J Med 296:538, 1977.

Hoffman AF: The medical treatment of cholesterol gallstones. A major advance in preventive gastroenterology. Am J Med 69:4, 1980.

Hyperalimentation in the Hospitalized Patient
Heymsfield SB, Bethel RA, Ansley JD, Nixon DW, Rudman D: Enteral hyperalimentation: alternative to central venous hyperalimentation. Ann Intern Med 90:63, 1979.

4

The Kidney

RENAL FAILURE

The terms azotemia, uremia, and renal failure all refer to diminished renal function. Acute renal failure is frequently reversible; chronic renal failure is not and must be treated by chronic hemodialysis or renal transplantation. While failure to excrete appropriate amounts of hydrogen ion or to conserve free water is a type of renal failure, the term is usually used to describe failure to excrete nitrogenous waste products.

TESTS OF RENAL FUNCTION

Plasma creatinine concentrations are a better measurement of renal function than urea nitrogen. The renal clearance of creatinine is closer to that of inulin than any other endogenous substance; about half of the filtered urea diffuses back into the blood from the renal tubules, making urea clearance dependent on urine flow and a less reliable indicator of glomerular filtration. In addition, increased dietary protein or excessive protein breakdown does not increase the creatinine load. Creatinine clearance may be measured by obtaining a 24-hour urine sample and a single sample of blood during this period. Normal values for men are 97-140 ml/minute and for women, 85-125 ml/minute. A 2-hr creatinine clearance has recently been shown to be as accurate as the 24-hr clearance.

The normal concentrating mechanism allows a dehydrated individual to concentrate urine to 750-1400 mOsm per liter in the presence of a plasma osmolality of about 300. This corresponds to a urine-specific gravity of 1.020-1.032; protein, glucose, and radiographic contrast material produce artificially high values. Although a 12-18 hour overnight period of fluid withdrawal will not always produce maximal reabsorption, a specific gravity greater than 1.022 following withdrawal or after injection of 5 units of vasopressin in oil I.M. suggests that the concentrating ability is intact.

Acid excretion may be evaluated by administering 0.1 gm ammonium chloride per kilogram body weight in nonenteric coated capsules. A normal hydrogen ion excretion rate is identified by a reduction in urine pH to 5.3 or below.

ACUTE RENAL FAILURE

A sudden reduction in urine output to below 450 ml/day or 15 ml/hour may be the result of prerenal, renal, or postrenal causes. *Prerenal azotemia* denotes renal failure due to inadequate perfusion of an anatomically normal kidney. It may be caused by dehydration or shock and is extremely common in the febrile diabetic or elderly individual. *Postrenal* obstructive renal failure, like prerenal failure, is potentially reversible and may be due to bladder neck obstruction, acute pyelonephritis, or ureteral obstruction caused by malignant disease, stricture (postsurgical or radiation), or nephrolithiasis.

Renal failure due to intrinsic renal disease. Causes are (1) ischemic, (2) toxic, or (3) secondary to parenchymal renal disease. *Ischemic failure* follows prolonged shock or dehydration; it may also occur with diffuse renal vascular disease. *Toxic failure* is commonly due to heavy metals, ethylene glycol, or injudicious use of certain antimicrobials. At present, the failure to carefully adjust the dose of aminoglycosides to preexisting renal function is one of the most common causes of acute renal failure in the hospitalized patient.

Since prerenal failure occurs with normal kidneys while acute ischemic renal failure (sometimes called acute tubular necrosis) results in a global loss of renal function, the following differential criteria are useful.

	Urine Sodium	Urine/Plasma Osmolality	BUN/Creatinine in Plasma
Prerenal	< 10 mEq/liter	> 1.5	> 20
Renal	> 10 mEq/liter	< 1.5	< 10

The acutely damaged kidney cannot conserve water, wastes salt, and has marked reduction in glomerular filtration evidenced by a high plasma creatinine concentration. Examination of the urinary sediment is also extremely useful:

Prerenal: proteinuria, moderate amounts of granular and hyaline casts.

Renal: Acute necrosis: epithelial cells and casts, coarse granular casts, hemoglobin or red cell casts; proteinuria minimal. Glomerular diseases: proteinuria, hematuria, red cell casts.

Postrenal: Minimal sediment, but may include occasional red cells, white cells, and hyaline or granular casts.

CLINICAL COURSE AND TREATMENT

The initial or oliguric phase is characterized by progressive azotemia, hyperkalemia, and acidosis. Fluid overload may produce hypertension, congestive failure, and pulmonary edema. After a variable period of days to several weeks, urine output begins to increase, signaling the onset of the diuretic phase. Creatinine levels may increase at first, but when urine output reaches 800-1000 ml, it begins to fall. The onset of the diuretic phase must be accurately noted, since the urine output may increase from less than 15 ml/hour to more than 1000 ml/hour in several hours, leading to marked hypovolemia. Within days or weeks, the diuresis begins to diminish and the patient achieves a plateau of renal function.

Fluid intake during the oliguric phase should be limited to the urine output, any extrarenal losses, and about 400 ml/day for insensible loss. Caloric requirements are met by administering 150-200 gm of carbohydrate either orally or intravenously. If the catabolic state is severe, additional calories may be provided in the form of lipids; protein sources should generally be avoided.

Hyperkalemia is a serious complication; peaked T waves usually appear when the potassium rises above 5-6 mEq/liter and are an important early sign. Treatment includes:

1. Calcium gluconate or chloride, 1 gm I.V. (10 ml of a 10 percent solution) over 10-15 minutes.

2. Correction of acidosis with sodium bicarbonate.

3. Glucose and insulin, 1 unit insulin for each 3-4 gm of glucose (300 ml of 20 percent glucose in water, or 100 ml of 50 percent glucose in water added to 150 ml of 5 percent glucose, with 15 units regular insulin added to either) administered over 30-60 minutes.

4. Sodium polystyrene sulfonate resin (Kayexalate), 25-75 gm orally or by retention enema.

5. Peritoneal or hemodialysis with perfusate containing low concentrations of potassium (1 mEq/liter for peritoneal after 6-8 potassium-free exchanges; 2 mEq/liter for hemodialysis). Flattening of T waves with appearance of prominent U waves indicates potassium concentration below 3 mEq/liter. Ventricular ectopic beats may occur with hyperkalemia or hypokalemia and are more common in the digitalized patient. Hemodialysis is much more effective than peritoneal dialysis and is indicated for severe hyperkalemia.

While certain patients may be managed conservatively, many require dialysis. Indications include progressive acidosis, evidence of persistent fluid overload, hyperkalemia, and complications of marked azotemia such as encephalopathy and uremic serositis. Elevation of creatinine itself is generally not considered an indication.

COMMON CAUSES OF DEATH
Mortality rates range from 30-60% (highest with trauma or the postoperative state, intermediate in a medical setting, and lowest in obstetric patients); death is usually due to infections, fluid and electrolyte problems, gastrointestinal hemorrhage, and uncontrolled progressions of the underlying disease.

Chronic Renal Failure

The causes of acute renal failure may also lead to gradual but progressive loss of renal tissue. When somewhat more than 50% of renal parenchyma is destroyed, plasma creatinine begins to rise; when glomerular filtration rate falls below 20 ml/minute, symptoms related to accumulation of nitrogenous wastes, electrolyte and fluid disturbances, and imbalance of certain essential substances occur.

As glomerulotubular units are destroyed, surviving units hypertrophy and accommodate an increased load of solute and water. Polyuria is an early symptom, since the hypertrophied units have difficulty in concentrating and excreting a salt-poor urine. When glomerular filtration falls below 10 ml/minute, urine output may be limited and hypervolemia, hypertension, edema, and pulmonary edema may occur.

Data from transplant and dialysis registries reveal the following causes for chronic renal failure: glomerular diseases, 50-60%; interstitial diseases, 20-30%; polycystic diseases, 5-10%; renal vascular disease, 5%; drug nephropathy, 3%; other congenital diseases, 3%. Diabetes and analgesic abuse account for many patients in the first two categories. Treatable causes of chronic renal failure include urethral or ureteral obstruction, heart failure, infection, hypovolemia, hypercalcemia, hyperuricemia, hypersensitivity nephritis, toxic nephropathy, and analgesic nephropathy.

Symptoms include: (1) fatigue and lassitude, (2) nausea and vomiting, (3) pruritis (probably due to secondary hyperparathyroidism), (4) epistaxis and mucous membrane bleeding (secondary to platelet dysfunction caused in particular by retention of guanidinosuccinic acid), (5) cramps at night, numbness, and paresthesias (reflecting uremic peripheral neuropathy), and (6) edema.

Physical signs include: (1) asterixis, (2) edema, (3) evidence of anemia, (4) pericardial friction rub (uremic serositis), (5) loss of lower-extremity deep tendon reflexes, vibratory sense, and pain sensation, and (6) brown arcs in the distal fingernails of 35% of patients (Terry nails). Terry nails are also seen in 2% of normal subjects.

The anemia observed is generally normochromic and normocytic. Bone marrow activity is diminished because of decreased renal production of erythropoietin. A minor hemolytic component is also observed; uremic red cells have a normal survival in normal patients, while normal red blood cells have a diminished survival in uremic patients.

Although the precise pathways are not clear, phosphorous retention leads to hypocalcemia and increased parathormone secretion. Calcium concentrations then increase because of increased phosphate excretion, mobilization of bone calcium (producing osteitis fibrosa cystica or osteomalacia), and increased intestinal absorption of calcium (parathormone also facilitates conversion of vitamin D to the active form, 1,25 dihydroxycholecalciferol). Phosphate levels may be normal for longer periods of time because of secondary hyperparathyroidism.

Potassium retention is generally absent until urine output falls. Tubular secretion of potassium is enhanced by a high-sodium diet, so that salt restriction may lead to hyperkalemia. The plasma magnesium level does not rise until glomerular filtration falls below 30 ml/minute. Unless magnesium salts have been administered as laxatives or antacids, symptomatic hypermagnesemia with urinary retention, muscle weakness, drowsiness, and coma does not occur.

Uric acid levels usually do not rise above 10 mg/100 ml because of increased uricolysis in the intestine. Elevated levels together with symptoms of gouty arthritis suggest either gouty nephropathy or a gouty proclivity unrelated to the renal failure.

Treatment

1. Establish diagnosis and rule out treatable causes.
2. Reduce protein intake to 40 gm/day when symptoms appear.
3. Estimate salt and water needs depending on extracellular fluid volume (ECV). Plasma sodium concentration is a poor estimate of ECV, but 24-hour urinary sodium together with knowledge of sodium intake (usually 90-120 mEq/day when the patient avoids salty food and does not add salt or more than 200 mEq when food is salted freely) permits a reasonable estimate.
4. Treat acidosis with sodium bicarbonate, realizing that added sodium may increase extracellular volume.

5. Treat congestive heart failure with fluid restriction and diuretics. Thiazide diuretics are effective until the GFR reaches 15 ml/minute, furosemide until GFR falls to 3 ml/minute. Digitalis is rarely indicated except for arrhythmias; if used, digoxin dosage should be reduced about one-third and guided by frequent serum levels.

6. Treat hypertension by fluid restriction and by alpha methyldopa, propranolol, or thiazide diuretics (for nondiuretic antihypertensive effects).

Chronic hemodialysis. The arteriovenous fistula, a direct communication that arterializes venous forearm blood, has replaced the prosthetic arteriovenous shunt. The disequilibrium syndrome is an early neurologic syndrome, probably due to the sudden reduction in urea concentration and osmolarity. Urea is slowly transported across the blood-brain barrier; water is osmotically shifted into the central nervous system, leading to increased intracranial pressure. Dialysis dementia is a clinical syndrome from aluminum toxicity due to leaching aluminum from tubing and from small quantities in water used to prepare dialysate. While many of the effects of chronic renal failure are reversed by chronic hemodialysis, anemia may persist, peripheral neuropathy may still occur, and skeletal demineralization due to persistent parathyroid activity continues.

Certain drugs usually require supplemental dosage after dialysis. These include aminoglycosides, cephalosporins, penicillins, sulfonamides, chloramphenicol, trimethoprim, aminophylline, methyldopa, procainamide, immunosuppressive agents, salicylates, and phenobarbital. The mortality in patients undergoing chronic renal dialysis is about 10% per year. Half of the patients die from cardiovascular complications such as acute myocardial infarction and stroke; 25% die from infection, and the remainder die from progression of underlying disease, complications of therapy, or voluntary withdrawal from dialysis.

DIAGNOSIS OF RENAL DISEASE
A careful history should include recent respiratory or skin infections, recurrent urinary tract infections, arthritis, skin rash, history of hypertension, and use of drugs. Detailed questioning is

sometimes necessary to elucidate the inappropriate use of analgesics. The presence of hepatosplenomegaly suggests amyloidosis, an enlarged prostate or a cystocele may indicate urinary
tract infection, and polycystic kidneys may be palpable.

A fresh urine sample should be examined by the physician and
a urine culture obtained; the spun sediment should be studied for
cells and casts; more than 1-2 WBCs per HPF with bacteria
suggests a urinary tract infection, and more than 25 is presump-
tively diagnostic. Uric acid, antinuclear antibodies, rheumatoid
factor, and plasma proteins should be evaluated. Complement
may be depressed in certain nephritides, particularly acute streptococcal nephritis, membranoproliferative nephritis, and lupus
nephritis (Table 4-1).

GLOMERULAR DISEASE

The glomerulus may be injured by immune processes directed
against the kidney itself (antiglomerular basement membrane
disease), by a variety of soluble immune complexes trapped
within the glomerulus, and by a group of diseases that inciden-

TABLE 4-1—CAUSES OF HEMATURIA

Glomerular disease (see Table 4-2)

Trauma

Pyelonephritis and cystitis

Tuberculosis

Neoplasm

Thrombocytopenia and other coagulopathies

Foreign body

Hemoglobinopathy
  Sickle cell trait and disease

Systemic diseases

tally involve the kidney. These immune responses initiate an inflammatory response with activation of either classic or alternate complement pathways, migration of leukocytes, and activation of both the intrinsic coagulation cascade and the vasodilator kinin system.

A variety of etiologic and pathologic factors produce a similar clinical response: hematuria, proteinuria, excretion of red cells or hyaline casts, decreased glomerular filtration, and retention of salt and water. These manifestations may present as persistent asymptomatic urinary abnormalities, the nephrotic syndrome, an acute nephritic syndrome, or chronic renal failure. Because a group of different pathologic processes may produce similar clinical manifestations, the most useful diagnostic approach at this time is a pathologic classification that attempts to deduce etiology where possible. Such an approach obviously places renal biopsy with comprehensive histologic evaluation at the center of the diagnostic process (Table 4-2).

An afferent arteriole terminates in the lobulated capillary tuft that lies within an evagination of the proximal convoluted tubule (Bowman capsule). Three separate layers, the capillary endothelium, the basement membrane, and the visceral epithelium function as an incomplete barrier between capillary blood and capsular urine; a central stalk, the mesangium, contains 35-40% of the glomerular cells and plays a supporting and phagocytic role. The pathologic classification of glomerular disease is based on the location of abnormalities within the glomerulus. Lesions may be generalized (more than 90% of glomeruli), focal (less than a majority of the glomeruli), segmental (involvement of one or two lobules within a glomerulus), or diffuse (involvement of the majority of lobules within a glomerulus).

Poststreptococcal Glomerulonephritis

This relatively common acute nephritic syndrome is probably mediated by the deposition of immune complexes containing antibody and some streptococcal antigen within the glomerulus. It is classified as an acute diffuse endocapillary proliferative glomerulonephritis, and there is proliferation of mesangial cells

TABLE 4-2—SUMMARY OF GLOMERULAR DISEASES

Pathologic Classification	Urinalysis
Glomerulonephritis, Proliferative, endocapillary	RBC, WBC, RBC and WBC casts, proteinuria
Proliferative, extracapillary (Goodpasture's syndrome)	RBC, RBC and granular casts, proteinuria
Membranoproliferative (Measangial or hypocomplementemic)	Either proteinuria or RBC with RBC casts
Focal glomerulonephritis (Berger's or IgG-IgA)	Gross hematuria, RBC between episodes
Membranous glomerulopathy	Proteinuria, gross hematuria rare
Minimal change or foot process disease	Proteinuria, hyaline granular or waxy casts; Maltese cross
Focal sclerosing glomerulopathy	Proteinuria; microscopic hematuria

McPhaul JJ, Mullins JD: JCI 57:351-361, 1976.
Frequency figures are approximate and based on several series of serial renal biopsy data; McPhaul and Mullins, for example, found anti-GBM disease in 11%.

Immune Deposits	Clinical Features	Frequency
Granular IgG, C3 in GBM	Poststreptococcal, hypertension, edema, excellent prognosis	40-50%
Linear IgG, C3 in GBM	Insidious, rapidly progressive. Gross hypertension, nephrotic syndrome rare	2-5%
Coarse IgG, C3 in GBM	Nephrotic (50%), nephritic (20%), mixed (30%)	2-5%
IgG, IgA, C3 in mesangium	Fluctuating complement; recurrent hematuria, frequently with viral illness; good prognosis	2-5%
Granular IgG, IgM, IgA, C3	Nephrotic syndrome, hypertension late, ten-year survival, 25-75%	15-20%
None	Nephrotic syndrome, prognosis good	5-10%
None	Nephrotic syndrome, hypertension and BUN may rise early	5-10%

with lesser degrees of endothelial and epithelial proliferation. Proliferation of epithelial cells in Bowman's capsule may lead to crescent formation. Immunohistologic study with fluorescein-labeled immunoglobulin reveals a granular ("lumpy-bumpy") deposition of IgG and the C3 component of complement within the capillary wall. Electron microscopy shows electron-dense humps in the subepithelial portion of the capillary basement membrane; these humps are characteristic of immune-complex deposition.

Acute nephritis develops in up to 25% of individuals infected with group A hemolytic streptococcal types 1, 4, 12 (majority), 41, 49 (Red Lake strain), and 57. Pharyngitis and otitis media are the most common antecedent infections, although skin infections are frequent with type 49. Typically, dark urine or frank hematuria, edema, malaise, and hypertension are seen within 1-3 weeks of an acute infection. Bilateral abdominal pain is common. Hypertension, when severe, may be associated with encephalopathy and retinopathy. The urinary sediment contains red cells, red cell casts, and hyaline casts. Protein excretion ranges from 1-4 gm/24 hours; 20% of patients may have a transient nephrotic syndrome with excretion of up to 15 gm of protein in a 24-hour period. The antistreptolysin-O titer is elevated and may remain elevated at 6 months. Evidence of immune complex generation is the marked reduction in the C3 and late components of complement, with C1, C4 and C2 generally remaining normal (suggesting activation of the alternate or properdin pathway). Elevation of blood urea nitrogen and creatinine are seen when the disease is severe.

While streptococcal infection is the most common cause of postinfectious immune complex nephritis, the disease is also seen following a variety of other infections including pneumococcal or enterococcal disease, staphylococcal bacteremia, secondary syphilis, typhoid fever, varicella, mumps, infectious mononucleosis, coxsackie viremia, falciparum malaria, toxoplasmosis, Guillain-Barré syndrome, and viral hepatitis (particularly type B).

Treatment is directed toward fluid retention and hypertension. Diuretics are useful, but cardiac glycosides play little role since edema is related to hypervolemia rather than to any problem with myocardial contractility. Hypertension is due to a decrease in glomerular filtration and also to activation of the renin-angiotensin system. Control of fluid retention usually controls hypertension in most patients, but parenteral hypotensive agents may be necessary if there is evidence of encephalopathy. Probably more than 90% of children heal completely, but recent studies suggest that about 30% of adult patients may develop evidence of chronic renal disease.

Rapidly Progressive Glomerulonephritis

Diffuse crescent formation, leading to the term acute diffuse extracapillary glomerulonephritis, is seen in association with an acute nephritic syndrome that may produce chronic renal failure in 3-9 months. While frequently the cause is not known, it may be seen in association with poststreptococcal nephritis, Henoch-Schonlein purpura, systemic lupus, Wegener's granulomatosis, and periarteritis nodosa. In the idiopathic variety, initial symptoms are nonspecific, and the disease progresses insidiously. Hypertension, gross hematuria, and the nephrotic syndrome are rare; urinalysis reveals the signs of glomerular damage already described.

The most striking histologic finding is diffuse, extracapillary, parietal proliferation of epithelial cells leading to crescent formation in more than 50% of glomeruli. Necrosis, a prominent polymorphonulear leukocyte exudate, and fibrin deposition within Bowman's capsule are also common. One-third of patients demonstrate a linear staining (smooth-linear) for an anti-glomerular basement membrane IgG antibody, and circulating antibodies to basement membrane may also be identified. Another one-third demonstrate granular staining with immunofluorescence microscopy suggestive of immune complex disease. The remaining patients have negative immunofluorescence.

Treatment with corticosteroids, immunosuppressive agents, and anticoagulants is generally ineffective. The immunologic nature of the disease is further revealed when the frequent development of the identical pathologic lesion is seen following renal transplantation.

Goodpasture's Syndrome

Perhaps the best-known example of antiglomerular basement membrane disease is the syndrome of pulmonary hemorrhage and glomerulonephritis. Pathologically, the kidneys resemble those seen in idiopathic rapidly progressive glomerulonephritis, although all the patients have circulating antiglomerular basement membrane antibodies and linear fluorescent staining in the glomerular capillary wall. Recurrent brisk hemoptysis associated with respiratory insufficiency and severe anemia is followed by an abnormal urinary sediment and progressive renal failure. Patients are usually young or middle-aged; men are more often affected than women. Goodpasture's original description was in a paper dealing primarily with the influenza pandemic of 1918; the syndrome has been seen in association with influenza, exposure to hydrocarbons, and other infectious diseases, although most have no identifiable precipitating factor.

Since hemoptysis usually occurs before renal abnormalities develop, it is possible that some exogenous factor alters the antigenicity of pulmonary basement membrane, leading to the production of antibodies that cross-react with the glomerular basement membrane. Death frequently occurs from the pulmonary hemorrhage, hemosiderin deposition, and pulmonary fibrosis rather than from the renal disease. Knowledge about this condition is still fragmentary, however. While it is usually considered to be a rapidly progressive disorder, McPhaul and Mullins recently reported that 10% of all patients evaluated with renal biopsy had evidence of antibasement membrane antibodies, indicating considerable variability in clinical expression. Further confusion has arisen with the occasional occurrence of Goodpasture's syndrome in patients with immune-complex disease.

Treatment of the rapidly progressive form of Goodpasture syndrome is disappointing. Combined therapy of corticosteroids, cyclophosphamide, azathioprine, and plasma exchange may hold some promise. The latter presumably reduces circulating antibody, complement, and fibrinogen.

IgG-IgA Nephropathy (Berger's Disease)

This relatively mild form of acute glomerulonephritis, occurring in up to 20% of adults and observed mainly in individuals between the ages of 16 and 35, is classified as focal glomerulonephritis. Only a small number of glomeruli are involved by a process that involves mesangial proliferation and a deposition of IgG, IgA, and complement within the mesangium. There is frequently a history of a viral upper respiratory infection. Patients present with gross hematuria and mild proteinuria (50%); hypertension and signficant proteinuria is rare. Serum IgA levels are elevated in some patients; renal function is usually normal.

Berger's initial description and subsequent observations suggested that the disease is generally benign and may be a major cause of idiopathic hematuria. More recent observations, however, have demonstrated occasional progressive renal failure with IgG-IgA nephropathy. Notably, IgA deposits are found in about one-third of patients with idiopathic hematuria.

No effective treatment has yet been described. Hypertension and proteinuria are treated in the manner described in other sections of this chapter.

The Nephrotic Syndrome

The glomerular diseases described may produce proteinuria but usually present as an acute nephritic syndrome. Certain glomerular lesions and a group of systemic diseases produce massive proteinuria. In almost all children and in two-thirds of adults, the nephrotic syndrome is due to primary glomerular disease; in one-third of adults it is secondary to one of a group of diseases including diabetes, systemic lupus, and amyloidosis (see Table 4-3).

The nephrotic syndrome (or nephrosis) is characterized by three cardinal findings: proteinuria greater than 3.5 gm/24 hours, hypoalbuminemia, and lipiduria. Most patients present with generalized edema particularly involving the face and hands,

TABLE 4-3—CAUSES OF NEPHROTIC SYNDROME IN ADULTS

Nephrotic syndrome (primary to kidney), 75%
    Minimal change disease (lipoid nephrosis), 15%
    Membranous glomerulopathy, 23%
    Membranoproliferative glomerulonephritis, 8%
    Focal sclerosis, 8%
    Proliferative glomerulonephritis 23%

Secondary nephrotic syndrome 25%
    Diabetes mellitus, 5-10%
    Systemic lupus, 5-10%
    Lymphomas and solid tumors, 5-10%
    Amyloidosis
    Multiple myeloma
    Sickle cell anemia
    Malaria
    Syphilis
    Inorganic mercury and mercurial compounds
    Bismuth, gold
    Insect stings
    Poison ivy
    Tridione
    Paradione
    Snake bites

anasarca, ascites, pleural and pericardial effusions, and joint effusions. An increase in hepatic lipoprotein synthesis accompanying the increase in albumin synthesis accounts for the elevated cholesterol level (which is usually in excess of 300 mg %), the elevation of other lipid fractions, and the lipiduria; associated with these changes is the early development of atherosclerosis. A "reflex" increase in hepatic synthesis of other proteins also occurs, leading to elevated levels of hepatic-derived procoagulants, perhaps partially accounting for the hypercoaguable state and increased incidence of thromboembolic phenomena.

The urinary sediment contains hyaline, granular and waxy casts. A characteristic finding is the oval fat body, an epithelial cell filled with cholesterol esters, which produces a birefringent Maltese cross in polarized light.

Fluid retention in the nephrotic syndrome may reach 10-20 excess liters of water. The reduction in plasma oncotic pressure leads to a shift of fluid from vascular to extravascular compartments; the associated contraction in plasma volume leads to increased reabsorption of salt and water by stimulation of the renin-angiotensin system and other regulatory forces.

Glomerular selectivity may be estimated from electrophoresis of the urinary protein or by measuring the clearance ratio of IgG to that of transferrin. The more selective the proteinuria (IgG/transferrin ratio less than 0.15 or urine protein consisting mainly of albumin with small peaks of alpha-1 and gammaglobulin), the better the prognosis.

Treatment is nonspecific and primarily symptomatic. Sodium and fluid restriction are generally necessary; however, sudden fluid shifts may occur, and the patient may be at risk of sudden hypotension from intravascular hypovolemia despite massive edema. Diuretics should be used only if significantly symptomatic edema or effusions develop.

The acute treatment of hypovolemia, effusions (compromising respiratory status), or edema (compromising perfusion or resistance to local infection) may be treated with intravenously administered albumin (preferably with a Swan-Ganz pulmonary arterial catheter). Aggressive use of diuretics may deplete the intravascular space more rapidly than the edema can be mobilized.

Adrenal corticosteroids and/or immunosuppressive agents such as azothioprine or cyclophosphamide may be useful in the treatment of marked proteinuria when the biopsy demonstrates a lesion known to be responsive to such intervention, such as lipoid nephrosis (minimal change disease) or SLE. Massive proteinuria, with a marked catabolic state may require medical (iatrogenic renal artery embolization) or surgical nephrectomy.

Lipoid Nephrosis or Minimal Change Disease

Seventy to 80% of children and less than 20% of adults with the nephrotic syndrome have near normal kidneys by light microscopic examination. Lipid accumulation in tubular cells because of hyperlipidemia is observed, but glomerular structures are normal and neither immunoglobulins nor complement are seen on immunofluorescence. Electron microscopy, however, reveals fusion of the foot processes that arise from the visceral epithelial cells and extend to the basement membrane of the capillary. The precise relationship between this, the only identified abnormality, and increased protein filtration is not clear. The epithelial cells and their foot processes are coated with a sialoprotein that confers a negative charge on the capillary wall. This negative charge is believed to oppose filtration of the negatively charged albumin; in some manner, foot process disease interferes with this mechanism. The cause of minimal change disease is not known but may be a defect in cell-mediated immune responses; the occurrence of the nephrotic syndrome with Hodgkin's disease supports this hypothesis.

About 90% of patients with this disease will respond to corticosteroid therapy. While many subsequently relapse, further remissions may usually be obtained by reinstituting therapy. Refractory cases may respond to the addition of immunosuppressive therapy with cyclophosphamide or chlorambucil. Despite frequent relapses, progression to chronic renal failure is uncommon.

Membranous Glomerulonephropathy

More than one-third of adults with the idiopathic nephrotic syndrome have a glomerular lesion characterized by diffuse thickening of the capillary basement membrane with little increase in cellularity. Progressive disease obliterates the capillary lumina. Subepithelial deposits are seen on electron microscopy; immunofluorescence reveals granular collections of IgG (IgM and IgA to a more variable extent) and the C3 component of complement. These deposits are believed to be immune complexes containing either exogenous antigens such as hepatitis virus or endogenous antigens such as DNA. The nephrotic syndrome accompanying malignant disease may represent tumor-associated antigen-antibody complexes.

Patients with membranous glomerulonephropathy usually develop slowly progressive renal failure, but prognosis in reported series varies widely. Fifteen to 38% have spontaneous remissions or significant improvement. Ten-year survival ranges from 25-76%. Renal vein thrombosis occurs in 30-40% of patients and may be prevented by anticoagulant therapy. There is conflicting evidence whether treatment with steroids or immunosuppressive drugs promotes preservation of renal function and improves survival.

Membranoproliferative Glomerulonephritis

The problems associated with relating structural abnormalities to clinical manifestations are emphasized by this form of glomerulonephritis; 50% of these patients present with the nephrotic syndrome, and 10% of adults with the idiopathic nephrotic syndrome have this lesion. Thirty percent have proteinuria and hematuria, and the rest have a frankly nephritic syndrome with red cell casts and gross hematuria. Hypertension and azotemia are common. Characteristically, mesangial cell proliferation is seen with mesangial interposition between endothelium and basement membrane, producing a thickened and split capillary wall. Coarsely granular IgG, C3, and properdin in a lumpy-bumpy pattern along capillary walls are found with immunohistologic study.

Two subgroups with different clinical profiles and peripheral complement concentrations are observed. Type I exhibits subendothelial electron-dense deposits and is associated with fluctuating levels of C3 and depressed C1q, C2, and C4. Electron-dense deposits within the glomerular basement membrane (GBM) are seen in type II; C3 is consistently depressed, while C1q, C2, and C4 are normal. In these patients, a circulating nephritic factor capable of cleaving C3 (C3NeF) may be present.

Ten-year survival without the need for dialysis or transplantation is less than 50%. The use of steroids is controversial, although alternate-day programs may preserve renal function. While recurrence has been reported in transplanted kidneys, recent studies have suggested that transplantation may substantially improve life expectancy.

Focal Sclerosing Glomerulopathy

Many adult patients with idiopathic nephrosis and the pathologic findings of minimal change disease may actually have focal sclerosis of juxtamedullary glomeruli located deep within the kidney (missed by a more superficial biopsy). These segmental lesions contain IgM and C3; the appearance of the kidney is otherwise similar to that of minimal change disease. Prognosis in these patients is generally unfavorable; they respond poorly to steroid therapy, and the disease may recur with renal transplantation.

TUBULO-INTERSTITIAL DISEASES

Interstitial renal disease is suggested by a urinary sediment without cellular casts, urinary protein excretion less than 2 gm/day, and evidence of disproportionately severe tubular dysfunction such as sodium wasting, defects in concentration leading to nocturia and polyuria, and a non-anion gap hyperchloremic acidosis.

Acute and Chronic Pyelonephritis

Significant bacteriuria, the hallmark of renal infection, may occur without tissue invasion, with asymptomatic ("silent") invasion, or as symptomatic pyelonephritis. While bacteria may reach the kidney by lymphatic or hematogenous spread, present thought suggests that most infections reach the kidneys by retrograde ascent from urethra, bladder, and ureter. Infection limited to the bladder produces urinary frequency, dysuria, and hematuria, and is termed cystitis.

A statistical approach, the presence of more than 100,000 colony-forming units per ml of urine, defines significant bacteriuria; concentrations lower than this usually suggest contamination from lower urinary structures. One catheterized specimen provides 95% confidence that significant bacteriuria is present; one voided, clean midstream specimen is probably associated with close to 90% accuracy.

Although 3-6% of presumably normal women exhibit bacterial colonization, colonization with invasion is much more common in the presence of urinary obstruction. Pathologic studies reveal that invasion produces inflammation of renal pelvis and calyces with microabscess formation in wedge-shaped areas within the medulla. Reduction in medullary blood supply by inflammation may lead to papillary necrosis. Papillary necrosis is particularly common in the diabetic woman with pyelonephritis and presents with high fever, severe back pain, and occasionally with the finding of medullary fragments in the urine.

Petersdorf and Turck have proposed the following clinical classification for urinary tract infection:

Uncomplicated urinary tract infections. The sudden onset of shaking chills, fever, flank pain, and costovertebral angle tenderness together with pyuria and white blood cell casts makes the diagnosis of acute pyelonephritis. Acute pyelonephritis is considered asymptomatic when it is episodic and occurs in the normal female urinary tract. Although 75-90% of all urinary tract infections are due to *E. coli*, almost all uncomplicated infections are due to that agent.

Any of the following are usually effective for *E. coli*; however, sensitivity of the particular organism should guide therapy. Treatment should be continued for 10-14 days. A repeat urinalysis (and culture if indicated) should be performed 1-2 weeks following the cessation.

- Ampicillin, 250-500 mg four times daily.
- Tetracycline, 250 mg four times daily.
- Sulfisoxazole, 1 gm four times daily.

Complicated urinary tract infections. Acute pyelonephritis in a male at any time or recurrent infection in a female suggests the presence of congenital or acquired urinary tract obstruction. While the involved organism may still be *E. coli*, others are commonly isolated. Multiple organisms regardless of the count also suggest contamination, although this may also be seen with renal abscesses. Table 4-4 shows the frequency of organisms in a hospitalized population representing both nosocomial and recurrent urinary tract infections.

Treatment and prognosis are determined by the organism

TABLE 4-4—ETIOLOGY OF URINARY INFECTIONS IN 448 HOSPITALIZED PATIENTS (PAZIN AND BRAUDE)

Escherichia coli	35.8%
Proteus mirabilis	16.4%
Enterobacter aerogenes	16.3%
Klebsiella pneumoniae	10.1%
Pseudomonas aeruginosa	5.8%
Enterococci	4.0%
Citrobacter spp.	3.3%
Proteus excluding *mirabilis*	3.0%
Alcaligenes faecalis	2.2%
Staphylococcus epidermidis	2.0%
Staph. aureus	1.1%

responsible. A high percentage of patients grow out organisms susceptible to either of the following antimicrobial agents; the general treatment guidelines given above also apply in these cases: cephalexin, 500 mg four times daily; trimethoprim (160 mg)-sulfamethoxazole (800 mg), two to four times daily.

CHRONIC ASYMPTOMATIC BACTERIURIA
Three to 6% of women and less than 1% of men have asymptomatic bacteriuria. Women who become pregnant may develop acute pyelonephritis. Other studies show that a significant proportion of others with asymptomatic bacteriuria may also develop renal infections.

CHRONIC PYELONEPHRITIS
Pathologic and epidemiologic studies cast doubt on whether chronic infectious pyelonephritis is an actual disease entity. A number of other etiologic agents produce the identical clinical and pathologic picture and may also be associated with bacteriuria (see below). Blunted calyces and cortical scars have often been considered as pyelographic evidence of chronic infection, but recent studies suggest that vesicoureteral reflux may produce

renal damage without infection (reflux nephropathy). Thus, other morphologic abnormalities with associated infection, rather than infection alone, are probably the cause of this syndrome; most nephrologists would prefer the term chronic interstitial nephritis to chronic pyelonephritis. Table 4-5 taken from Murray and Goldberg shows the frequency of etiologic factors in one series of newly diagnosed chronic interstitial nephritis.

Multiple causes were present in 7% of the group. The table supports the belief that infection is not a major cause of interstitial nephritis, since none had urinary tract infections as the first evidence of renal disease. The importance of specific risk factors is emphasized, however, since 27% subsequently became infected. Fifty-two percent of those who developed UTI had anatomic abnormalities, and 26% had nephrolithiasis.

Acute Ischemic Necrosis

Acute renal failure following circulatory shock, trauma, CNS injury, or other cause must be differentiated from acute prerenal failure (see acute renal failure). Acute tubuloischemic necrosis (shock kidney, ATN, lower nephron nephrosis, etc.) is character-

TABLE 4-5—ETIOLOGIC FACTORS IN CHRONIC INTERSTITIAL NEPHRITIS

Factor	Frequency
Anatomic abnormalities	30%
Analgesic abuse	20%
Hyperuricemia	11%
Hypertensive nephrosclerosis	10%
Nephrolithiasis	9%
Sickle cell disease (SS)	1.0%
Renal tuberculosis	1.0%
Bacterial urinary tract infection	Not present
Idiopathic	11%

From Murray and Goldberg. Ann Intern Med 82:453, 1975.

ized pathologically by relatively normal glomeruli with congestion of the medullary pyramids and damage of the renal tubules. Patients exhibit oliguria with isosthenuria and urinary sodium concentrations of 30-60 mEq/liter. The initial oliguria is often interrupted by a dramatic diuretic phase during which serum creatinine levels may continue to rise. Restriction of intake during the oliguric phase and careful replacement of electrolytes and water during the diuretic phase should minimize complications. Dialysis may be indicated (see acute renal failure), but mortality is high because of the underlying condition.

Renal Tubular Acidosis

Renal tubular acidosis (RTA) is a descriptive term for several types of defective renal acidification (Table 4-6). The acidosis present in uremia is secondary to diminished acid excretion paralleling diminished renal function and is of the anion gap type. Renal tubular acidosis differs in that it is secondary to the "wasting" of bicarbonate in the urine (defective bicarbonate resorption and/or generation).

Of the several types, the two most common are proximal RTA (type II) and distal RTA (type I) (Tables 4-7 and 4-8).

The proximal tubule normally resorbs 80-90% of the filtered bicarbonate, causing the pH of the tubular fluid to decline from 7.4 to 6.5. The remainder is normally resorbed in the distal tubule but is limited to a maximum of about 1500 mEq of bicarbonate per day (15-20% of the usual daily production of bicarbonate). This distal resorptive process allows the final acidification to proceed from 6.5 to as low as 4.4.

Bicarbonate resorption requires carbonic anhydrase and is increased with decreased vascular volume, hypokalemia, hypercapnia, and increased mineralocorticoids.

In type II or proximal RTA, bicarbonate is not resorbed appropriately. Because up to 90% of the filtered bicarbonate is normally resorbed here and the distal tubule is limited to no more than 20% of the normal daily bicarbonate production, bicarbonate losses may be substantial. Preservation of distal tubular function and excretion of titratable acid allows the common finding of an early morning urine pH below 6.0. The huge losses,

TABLE 4-6—FINDINGS IN RENAL CAUSES OF ACIDOSIS

	Proximal R.T.A. (type II)	Distal R.T.A. (type I)	C.R.F.
STONE FORMATION	Rare	Common (Calcium)	Uncommon
ASSOCIATED TUBULAR DEFECTS	Common*	Rare	Rare
BICARBONATE AND pH	↓	↓	↓
ANION GAP	None	Nl	↑
SERUM CHLORIDE	↑	↑	Normal or ↓
SERUM POTASSIUM	↓	↓	↑
BUN	Normal (initially)	Normal (initially)	↑
URINE pH	Commonly <6.0	Never <5.5	Commonly <6.0
EASE OF REPLACEMENT	Resistant	Sensitive	Sensitive

* Represents Fanconi's syndrome.

TABLE 4-7—CAUSES OF PROXIMAL OR TYPE II R.T.A.

Primary
　　Congenital
　　Adult

Secondary or acquired
　　Disorders of carbohydrate metabolism
　　Disorders of amino acid metabolism
　　Disorders of protein metabolism
　　　　Nephrotic syndrome (rarely)
　　　　Multiple myeloma
　　　　Amyloidosis
　　　　Hypergammaglobulinemia

　　Heavy metal toxicity
　　　　Lead
　　　　Copper's (Wilson's disease)
　　　　Mercury

　　Drugs
　　　　Acetazolamide
　　　　Outdated tetracycline

　　Hyperparathyroidism

however, make the patient resistant to treatment; the more bicarbonate administered, the more it is excreted.

Fanconi's syndrome is proximal RTA when seen in association with other proximal renal tubular defects (congenital or acquired) such as aminoacidurias or chronic lead toxicity.

Type I or distal RTA is associated with less bicarbonate wasting but defective final acidification, so the pH of the urine never falls below 5.5.

Differentiation in the absence of significant acidosis may be made by evaluating the response of the urine pH to acid load (ammonium chloride) or to bicarbonate loading administration.

Toxic Nephritis

Analgesic abuse nephritis. Ingestion of ten or more analgesic tablets daily for 8-10 years has been implicated as a major cause of interstitial nephritis. Phenacetin was originally emphasized as

TABLE 4-8—CAUSES OF DISTAL OR TYPE I R.T.A.

Primary
  Congenital
  Adult

Secondary or acquired
  Disorders of protein metabolism
    Amyloidosis
    Hypergammaglobulinemia

  Disorders of calcium metabolism
    Hyperparathyroidism
    Hypervitaminosis D
    Hyperthyroidism

  Drugs
    Lithium
    Amphotericin B

the major offender, but aspirin and other ingredients may also be important. Patients frequently have associated gastrointestinal symptoms from mucosal irritation and commonly attribute their drug abuse to musculoskeletal or psychologic symptoms. Arrest of the disease usually follows discontinuation of the analgesics.

Antibiotic nephritis. Aminoglycosides injure renal tubules, producing albuminuria and azotemia, which are usually reversible if diagnosed early. Age, dose, and underlying renal disease appear to increase the chances of developing gentamicin nephrotoxicity. All aminoglycosides appear to have toxic potential for the kidney; differences may not be clinically significant. *Amphotericin B* produces both glomerular and tubular damage by affecting sterols; renal abnormalities frequently limit the duration of therapy. *Methicillin* has recently been implicated as an important cause of interstitial nephritis; 17% of 52 patients receiving methicillin compared to 3% of 29 patients receiving a cephalosporin developed hematuria and proteinuria. *Demeclocycline* can produce nephrogenic diabetes insipidus, and outdated *tetracycline* can produce Fanconi's syndrome with a disturbance of proximal tubular function and loss of amino acids, glucose, phospate, potassium, bicarbonate and water.

Heavy metal nephritis. Gold salts used for the treatment of rheumatoid arthritis may produce hematuria and proteinuria. Both *mercury* and *lead* produce tubular damage.

Radiation nephritis. Following a latent period of at least 6 months after large doses of abdominal radiation, a diffuse nephropathy with damage to tubules, glomeruli, and arterioles may be observed. Minimal proteinuria without hematuria, hypertension, and progressive renal failure are common in this syndrome, which has a variable prognosis.

SYSTEMIC DISEASES INVOLVING THE KIDNEYS
Primarily Glomerular Involvement

Systemic lupus erythematosus. Nephritis secondary to SLE is probably the most common form of adult glomerular disease. Over 90% of patients have pathologic evidence of renal disease, and it is symptomatic in at least two-thirds. Renal biopsy with pathologic classification has added considerably to the understanding of the natural history of lupus nephritis; the classification in Table 4-9 has been proposed by Baldwin et al.

Unfortunately, both mesangial and focal proliferative can change to either diffuse proliferative or membranous forms of lupus nephritis.

Patients with mesangial and focal proliferative nephritis are treated with steroids when indicated for the control of other manifestations of SLE. Steroids and cytotoxic agents such as azathioprine, cyclophosphamide, or nitrogen mustard are suggested for diffuse proliferative disease. Steroids alone for prolonged periods are suggested for membranous nephritis. Baldwin et al. recommend the early "prophylactic" use of steroids (or even immunosuppressive agents) once the diagnosis of lupus nephritis is made.

Vasculitides. Renal involvement in periarteritis nodosa may be due to the classic medium-sized arterial inflammation or, more commonly, to diffuse proliferative and necrotizing changes within the glomeruli. Eighty to 90% of patients show some renal abnormality, which may include mild proteinuria, microscopic

TABLE 4-9—RENAL ABNORMALITIES IN SYSTEMIC LUPUS ERYTHEMATOSUS

	Mesangial	Proliferative		Membranous
		FOCAL	DIFFUSE	
FREQUENCY	14%	14%	50%	27%
HYPERTENSION	25%	40%	66%	54%
NEPHROTIC SYNDROME	8%	8%	70%	67%
RENAL FAILURE	25%	8%	80%	50%
LIGHT MICROSCOPY	Frequently normal	Focal proliferative Small crescents	Diffuse proliferative Many crescents Sclerotic glomeruli	Similar to membranous nephritis
IMMUNOFLUORESCENCE	IgG, C3 IgA	Granular IgG in mesangium and capillary walls	Diffuse coarse granular IgG, IgM, and C3	Finely granular IgG in capillary walls
COMPLEMENT LEVELS	Normal	Normal	Low	Normal
5-YEAR MORTALITY	—	30%	71%	30%

hematuria, and the presence of red blood cell casts. Early treatment with steroids seems to preserve renal function.

The necrotizing vasculitis of Wegener's granulomatosis may produce either a chronic or an acute glomerulonephritis. Early treatment with cytotoxic agents is indicated. Patients with either periarteritis or Wegener's usually have normal blood pressures and serum complement levels.

Diabetic glomerulosclerosis. Diffuse or nodular glomerular lesions with associated arteriolar and arterial disease occur in most patients with juvenile onset diabetes. Proteinuria is an early sign; the nephrotic syndrome may occur later. Hypertension is common. Pyelonephritis and occasionally papillary necrosis may complicate the underlying disease process. The Kimmelstiel-Wilson lesion—the presence of relatively acellular mesangial nodules—is seen in 10-15% of patients.

Although the lesion is considered to be nonimmunologic in nature, IgG and IgM deposits have been found in 50% of patients. While this may relate to a defect in mesangial and basement membrane function, the possibility exists that immunologic responses to exogenous agents including insulin might be responsible. To further support this thesis, some juvenile onset diabetic children have responded to steroid treatment.

Amyloid disease. Proteinuria or the nephrotic syndrome in a patient with normal size kidneys and without hypertension should suggest amyloid glomerulopathy. This is even more likely if malignant disease, osteomyelitis, regional enteritis, tuberculosis, multiple myeloma, or rheumatoid arthritis are present. IgG, but not complement, is found in the amorphous material scattered throughout the glomerulus. Fifty to 60% of patients with amyloid involvement of the kidney will have positive rectal biopsies. Treatment in secondary amyloid involvement of the kidney must be directed at the underlying condition; no treatment is available for primary renal amyloidosis (see Amyloidosis, page 291).

Henoch-Schoenlein syndrome. Ballard et al. performed renal biopsies in seven adults with this syndrome. History of ingestion of medications was found in most. Hematuria and proteinuria were observed in all, and biopsy revealed diffuse glomerular proliferation. Five died, and this outcome was correlated with crescent formation. There is no known effective treatment.

Primarily Interstitial or Tubular Involvement

Multiple myeloma. Precipitation of abnormal proteins within the renal tubules appears to lead to azotemia and isosthenuria without hypertension. Frequently, anemia is disproportionate to the elevation of urea or creatinine. Amyloidosis occurs in approximately 15% of patients with myeloma and may produce a nephrotic syndrome, which does not occur in its absence. Myeloma is a monoclonal gammopathy with plasma cell proliferation of either IgG, IgA, IgD, or IgE; free light-chain production leads to excretion of Bence-Jones protein. Since tubular protein forms obstructive casts readily, procedures that lead to dehydration must be carefully avoided in these patients.

Hypercalcemic and hypokalemic nephropathies. An early sign of both varieties of nephropathy is impairment of urinary concentrating ability. Hypercalcemia may lead to irreversible renal damage with progressive azotemia. Hypertension occurs when nephrocalcinosis develops and may not abate even if the calcium is restored to normal. Hypokalemia may lead to sodium retention and edema; urinalysis may reveal minimal proteinuria and a small number of hyaline or granular casts. Nitrogen retention does not occur, and the nephropathy responds to potassium replacement.

Gouty nephropathy. Mild proteinuria, decreased creatinine clearance, slowly progressive nitrogen retention, and impairment of concentration ability are characteristic. Up to 50% of patients with gout may die from renal disease; 15% have urate calculi. Inhibition of uric acid formation by administration of allopurinol should prevent and partially reverse gouty nephropathy. Controversy over the precise nature of the renal disease found in patients with gout still exists.

Sarcoid nephropathy. Widespread granulomatous involvement of the kidney is usual; hypercalcemia with hypercalciuria is responsible for most cases of renal involvement. Sarcoid granuloma have been found in 7-19% of patients but are difficult to identify by renal biopsy because of their scattered distribution throughout the kidney. Rarely, direct granulomatous involvement leads to hypertension and uremia. Steroids may be beneficial.

Scleroderma kidney. Almost half of patients with scleroderma show fibrinoid necrosis with intimal proliferation of arteries and arterioles and/or glomerular and mesangial proliferation. Fifty percent of patients with scleroderma die from renal disease. No successful treatment has yet been elucidated.

VASCULAR DISEASES OF THE KIDNEY
Nephrosclerosis

Almost all patients who die with hypertension exhibit arterial and arteriolar changes in their kidneys; 10% of patients without hypertension also reveal such changes. In about 10% of patients with hypertension, the lesions are severe enough to produce marked renal insufficiency with azotemia, proteinuria, and hematuria. While anemia may occur, it is not universal, so that the occurrence of hypertensive retinopathy and azotemia without anemia suggests renal vascular disease. Progressive arteriolar disease with necrotizing intimal changes is frequently associated with accelerated hypertension and papilledema; this syndrome is usually termed "malignant hypertension."

Renal Artery Occlusion

Embolic occlusion of a major or branch renal artery produces severe flank or upper abdominal pain. There are usually fever and leukocytosis; microscopic hematuria is present in more than half of the patients. Incomplete occlusion, usually due to an atheromatous plaque, may produce rapidly progressive hypertension. Intravenous pyelography, with films exposed at 1 and 2 minutes, usually shows differences in filling time between the involved and uninvolved kidney. However, 20% of patients with moderately severe renal artery narrowing will not have an abnormal IVP. Measurement of renal function is helpful, but renal arteriograms are definitive.

Renal Vein Thrombosis

Renal vein thrombosis may occur with malignant invasion of renal veins (particularly in hypernephroma), thrombophlebitis with inferior vena cava extension, congestive heart failure, periarteritis, following trauma or surgery, and with dehydration. It may complicate a variety of primary renal diseases but is especially common in papillary necrosis and renal amyloidosis. Sudden thrombosis presents with severe flank pain, proteinuria, and hematuria. If it is gradual, collateral venous channels may appear, which are seen as ureteral notching on the intravenous pyelogram. Rarely, the nephrotic syndrome may result.

NEPHROLITHIASIS

Almost 90% of renal calculi are composed of calcium salts. Calcium stones may be associated with hyperparathyroidism, hypervitaminosis D, sarcoidosis, acute demineralization following immobilization, Cushing's syndrome, renal tubular acidosis, and idiopathic hypercalciuria. Uric acid stones are formed only in an acid urine and when there is increased excretion of uric acid in patients with gout or certain hematologic diseases.

Traditionally, reduction of calcium and increase of water intake reduce the frequency of calcium stones; recent studies have suggested that thiazide diuretics and sodium phosphate may also reduce stone formation. Urate stones may be prevented by alkalinization of the urine with bicarbonate and carbonic anhydrase inhibitors, increased water intake, and inhibition of urate production with allopurinol.

HYPERNEPHROMA (RENAL CELL CARCINOMA)

Hypernephroma or renal cell carcinoma is the most common of renal malignancies. Gross hematuria is seen in 18-20% of patients, flank pain in 15-42% and palpable masses in 37-63%. The classic triad of all three is uncommon. The tumor usually presents as a hormonal syndrome. The varied presentation has earned it the name of "the internists' tumor." These syndromes include: (1) fever of unknown origin, (2) hypercalcemia, (3) peripheral neuropathy, (4) secondary amyloidosis, (5) refractory anemia, usually normochromic and normocytic, (6) polycythemia due to increased erythropoietin production, (7) congestive heart failure due to increased arteriovenous shunting through the tumor, (8) Cushing's syndrome, (9) nonmetastatic liver malfunction, (10) association with von Hippel-Lindau disease (heredofamilial disease with cerebellar hemangioblastoma and retinal angioma), and (11) metastatic lesions of lung, liver, or brain. The only known cure for renal cell carcinoma is surgical resection.

BLADDER CANCER

Ten percent of malignancies in adults are of the renal pelvis, ureter, and urinary bladder. Multicentric with a tendency to recur, they are derived from transitional epithelium and have been related etiologically to exposure to aromatic amines in the dye, chemical and rubber industry, tobacco, and ingestion of artificial food sweeteners. Squamous cell carcinoma is much less common, has a poorer prognosis, and is associated with renal calculi and chronic infestation with *Schistosoma hematobia.*

Hematuria is an almost universal manifestation and should be evaluated by cytoscopy with appropriate biopsy. Both cell type and degree of extension determine prognosis; 30% of those with tumor beyond the bladder wall live for 5 years.

CYSTIC DISEASES OF THE KIDNEY
POLYCYSTIC KIDNEY DISEASE (PKD)

Adult PKD (autosomal dominant inheritance) is present in one of 500 autopsies. It must be considered in the differential diagnosis of hypertension, proteinuria, renal failure, flank pain, and microscopic hematuria. Ten percent have renal calculi, the kidneys are frequently palpable, there is a high incidence of renal infection, and up to a third also have cysts involving the liver.

The cystic disease may also involve lungs, spleen, pancreas, and other intraabdominal organs. Ten percent develop subarachnoid hemorrhage secondary to intracranial aneurysm. Diagnosis is confirmed by intravenous pyelography, ultrasound, and radioisotope techniques. Treatment centers around management of associated hypertension and urinary infections and the prevention of analgesic neuropathy. Nephrectomy is sometimes indicated.

An infantile form (autosomal recessive inheritance) is frequently associated with liver disorders, which are usually the cause of death.

MEDULLARY SPONGE KIDNEY

The terminal collecting ducts that connect the renal pelvis to the lower nephrons are dilated and frequently contain calculi; damage to the renal parenchyma occurs secondary to the obstruction produced by the calculi. Infection and hematuria are frequent complications; hypertension is not present. Diagnosis is made by IVP. Many patients are asymptomatic and require no treatment. Dehydration should be avoided and infection promptly treated.

ABNORMALITIES OF BODY FLUIDS
Distribution of Water and Electrolytes

Body water may constitute as little as 45% of total body weight in the obese and up to 75% in the lean. Thirty to 40% of total body water is intracellular, 14-16% interstitial, 4-5% intravascular, and 2% within the lymphatic system. These compartments are delimited by the cell membrane, which is selectively permeable to ions, and the capillary wall, which is freely permeable to electrolytes and water. Although the ionic composition differs, the compartments are normally in osmotic equilibrium as water passes from areas of higher water concentration to those of lower concentration. Alterations in plasma osmolarity reflect alterations in intracellular osmolarity, except in disequilibrium states. Usually, osmolarity (solute per volume of solution) and osmolality (solute per volume of water) are similar. Freezing point depression measurements reflect osmolality and may be greater than predicted from electrolyte measurements in lipemic serum because of greatly diminished plasma water content.

Osmolarity may be calculated from the formula

$$2[Na^+] + 2[K^+] + \frac{[glucose]}{18} + \frac{[BUN]}{2.8}$$

Urea diffuses freely across cell membranes and does not affect water equilibrium. Acute alcoholic intoxication may increase osmolarity, since the alcohol itself becomes an unmeasured osmotically active substance not identified in the formula.

Plasma proteins raise plasma osmotic pressure by 25 mm Hg (plasma oncotic pressure), a level close to capillary pressure which tends to oppose the diffusion of water into the interstitial space (Starling forces). The interstitial space measured by bromide dilution is decreased in early hypovolemic shock, but decreased plasma protein concentration due to alterations in permeability in many critically ill patients produces vascular contraction with interstitial expansion. Colloids expand the vascular space by water transfer from the interstitium, while sodium-rich crystalloids expand the interstitial space and may produce pulmonary edema.

Osmolarity is maintained at 280-285 mOsm/liter by appropriate secretion of antidiuretic hormone (ADH) in response to concentration changes in fluids reaching the supraoptic nuclei of the hypothalamus. ADH increases the permeability of the distal convoluted and collecting tubules, water passes into the hypertonic interstitium of the renal papillae, and a concentrated urine is excreted. In the absence of ADH (or with diseased distal tubules), less water passes into the interstitium despite the osmotic gradient, and a dilute urine is excreted.

The regulation of body water is somewhat more complex. Volume receptors in the left atrium and great vessels reflexively stimulate the production of ADH in response to volume contraction. Fluid volume is also regulated by regulating sodium stores. Aldosterone secretion by the zona glomerulosa leads to parallel retention of sodium and water. This integrated and sensitive control is demonstrated by the response to blood loss of less than

10%; increased ADH and aldosterone secretion are promptly observed.

Hyponatremia

A low serum sodium concentration may reflect either excess body water (dilutional hyponatremia) or sodium loss in excess of water loss (depletional hyponatremia). The distinction is of great importance: use of 5% sodium chloride solution in a patient with congestive heart failure and dilutional hyponatremia might produce acute pulmonary edema. As a general rule, depletional hyponatremia almost never occurs in patients with edema; dilutional hyponatremia is common in the critically ill patient, depletional hyponatremia relatively rare.

Sodium depletion. Found in patients who have been starved or who have severe gastrointestinal fluid losses. It may also be seen in adrenal insufficiency and occasionally in patients who have been vigorously treated with diuretics and salt restriction. *Dilutional hyponatremia* is believed due to excessive ADH secretion and is seen in such edematous states as congestive heart failure, liver disease, and renal disease. Fluid restriction to 1200 ml daily usually increases sodium concentration.

Inappropriate secretion of ADH (SIADH). Results in water retention even though plasma osmolarity is lower than normal and should inhibit ADH secretion to produce water diuresis. Patients are hyponatremic and hypoosmotic; urine osmolarity almost always exceeds plasma osmolarity. Plasma creatinine is normal, and evidence of renal, cardiac, or hepatic disease is absent. Hyponatremia is due in part to urinary salt wasting, which decreases when hyponatremia is severe. The diagnosis is confirmed by observing correction of hyponatremia with fluid restriction and reappearance of characteristic abnormalities when daily fluid administration is increased to 2-3 liters.

SIADH is found in patients with oat cell carcinoma and other intrathoracic tumors and in CNS disease including meningitis and encephalitis. Drugs such as chlorpropamide, tolbutamide, carbamazepine (Tegretol), amitriptyline (Elavil), and clofibrate either stimulate ADH secretion or augment its action on the tubules. Hyponatremia with diuretics may be due to sodium depletion or to direct limitation of renal water excretion.

Differential diagnosis is aided by measurement of urinary sodium excretion and estimation of extracellular volume by clinical means or by measurement of central venous pressure. (Table 4-10)

Hypernatremia

Water depletion in excess of sodium loss results in hypernatremia (increased serum sodium concentration). The usual causes include insufficient water intake or excessive loss due to diarrhea, polyuria secondary to renal disease or diabetic acidosis, or lack of ADH (diabetes insipidus). The prolonged use of high doses of the newer potent diuretics may also cause this type of dehydration.

Clinically, the skin is dry and flushed; the mucous membranes are dry and the skin turgor is normal. Laboratory findings are compatible with a state of dehydration. The blood urea nitrogen level, hematocrit, serum sodium level, and serum osmolality are elevated. Urine volume is decreased, with a high specific gravity and osmolality.

TABLE 4-10—DIFFERENTIAL DIAGNOSIS OF HYPONATREMIA

Spot Urinary Sodium Excretion	Hypervolemia	Hypovolemia
More than 15 mEq/ liter	SIADH	Hypoadrenalism, renal salt wasting, Bartter's syndrome, diuretics (early)
Less than 15 mEq/ liter	Cardiac Renal Hepatic	GI or skin loss of sodium, diuretics (late)

excess, have been advocated but most clinicians today prefer the use of bicarbonate measurements calculated from determinations of pH and Pco_2. The interpretation of bicarbonate concentration is aided by reference to in vivo carbon dioxide or acid titration curves, which show the expected alterations in bicarbonate or Pco_2 when one or the other is deliberately altered.

Figures 4-1 and 4-2 show data from published whole-body titration curves plotted with pH as the dependent variable in order to facilitate clinical use. Figure 4-1 shows changes in pH that would occur with changes in Pco_2; the heavy line identifies values that would be seen if physiologic compensation did not occur while the hatched area shows the confidence limits for renal compensation. Patients with alterations in carbon dioxide tension would be expected to fall in the hatched area if they achieve maximum renal compensation; pH values approach the

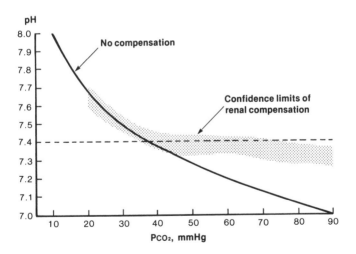

Figure 4-1. Change in pH obtained from whole body titration curve when carbon dioxide tension is altered. Note blunting of pH changes in acute or chronic situations compared to effect without shifts in buffer capacity.

solid line if maximum compensation has not yet occurred. Figure 4-2 shows similar changes in pH with changes in bicarbonate concentratio.

P_{CO_2} Change for a 5 mEq change in HCO_3^-
Decrease in $H_{CO_3}^-$ – 8 mm Hg decrease in P_{CO_2}
Increase in $H_{CO_3}^-$ – 5 mm Hg increase in P_{CO_2}

$H_{CO_3}^-$ change for a 10 mm Hg change in P_{CO_2}
Increase in P_{CO_2} – 0.6 mEq increase in $H_{CO_3}^-$
Chronic P_{CO_2} increase – 6 mEq increase in $H_{CO_3}^-$
Decrease in P_{CO_2} – 4 mEq decrease in $H_{CO_3}^-$

Changes in arterial P_{CO_2} are related to changes in alveolar ventilation and carbon dioxide tension. The latter increases with

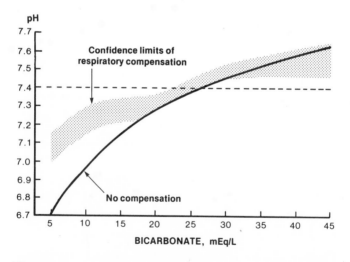

Figure 4-2. Change in pH obtained as in Figure 4-1 when bicarbonate concentration is changed. A change in pH is blunted because of changes in ventilation.

fever and other causes of hypermetabolism, decreases with decreased tissue oxygenation.

Changes in body buffer stores are somewhat more complex. Calculation of anion gap assists in determining whether a low bicarbonate is due to decreased bicarbonate reabsorption with hyperchloremia or to the presence of acidic unmeasured anions in the plasma.

$$\text{Anion gap} = [Na^+] - [Cl^-] - [Hco_3^-]$$

Causes of buffer deficits with or without anion gaps are shown below.

Low bicarbonate with anion gap

- Diabetic ketoacidosis
- Alcoholic ketoacidosis
- Lactic acidosis
- Renal failure
- Intoxication with salicylates, methanol, paraldehyde, or ethylene glycol

Low bicarbonate without anion gap

LOW PLASMA POTASSIUM

- Diarrhea
- Renal tubular acidosis
- Carbonic anhydrase inhibition

HIGH SERUM POTASSIUM

- Ammonium chloride administration
- Chronic interstitial nephritis
- Obstructive uropathy

Bicarbonate reabsorption is enhanced by potassium depletion, volume contraction, and elevation in Pco_2. Buffer excesses that ordinarily lead to alkalosis can be divided on the basis of their response to saline infusion and their urinary chloride excretion.

High bicarbonate with decreased urinary chloride (respond to saline)

- Vomiting with gastric losses
- Diuretic therapy
- Posthypercapnic state

High bicarbonate with increased urinary chloride (no saline response)

- Hyperaldosteronism
- Bartter's syndrome
- Cushing's syndrome
- Severe potassium depletion
- Licorice ingestion

Treatment of Fluid and Electrolyte Disturbances

Estimation of a total electrolyte deficit requires knowledge of the plasma concentration, body weight, and distribution space of that electrolyte expressed as a percentage of total body weight. Such estimates are usually extremely inaccurate, and good clinical practice usually suggests administration of half of the calculated deficit followed by repeat measurement.

Rapid restoration of plasma bicarbonate is frequently desirable, although sudden return of pH to normal may lead to potassium depletion or to increased cerebral acidosis. While extracellular fluid constitutes 20% of total body weight, recent studies have suggested that the bicarbonate space is actually increased in patients with acidosis. The use of a 30% estimate of bicarbonate space, aiming for 20-22 mEq/liter of plasma bicarbonate rather than complete normality, and initial administration of half the calculated dose is a reasonable clinical approach.

For example, calculate the bicarbonate deficit in a 70-kg patient with a plasma bicarbonate of 15 mEq/liter. Bicarbonate space is probably 30% of 70 kg, or 21 liters. Bicarbonate deficit is $22 - 15$, or 7 mEq/liter (aiming for 22 mEq/liter after replacement). Total calculated deficit is 7 mEq/liter × 21 liters, or 147 mEq. Good clinical practice would suggest administration of 50-70 mEq of bicarbonate solution. Since bicarbonate may be consumed rapidly during periods of acidosis, bicarbonate concentration following administration of bicarbonate could be unchanged or actually lower than before replacement.

The calculation of sodium deficit in a patient with depletional hyponatemia further illustrates the problems associated with calculation of total body deficits. This example also demonstrates how infused solutions may shift water from one body compartment to another. Before infusion of sodium, tissue and extracellular osmolarity are identical. Infusion of sodium chloride raises the plasma osmolarity; since water moves from regions of low osmolarity to high osmolarity, pure water flows from the intracellular space to the extracellular space. This water does not contain sodium, and thus it dilutes the infused sodium. Calculations of this type have shown that the calculation of the total sodium deficit in such a patient requires the assumption that the sodium space is actually total body water. Good clinical practice would be the administration of half the calculated dose—the sodium space might be estimated at 30% of body weight.

The composition of certain commonly used replacement fluids is shown in Table 4-11.

Colloid solutions such as albumin are indicated in hypotensive patients when it is impossible to raise central venous pressure by the infusion of crystalloid solutions or if there is evidence of an increased pulmonary interstitial space (interstitial or alveolar edema clinically). The ability of infused albumin to remain in the intravascular space and pull in water from an expanded interstitial space was recently demonstrated by Hauser et al. One thousand ml of Ringer's lactate solution increased plasma volume by only 194 ± 18 ml, while 25 gm of albumin in 100 ml of fluid increased it by 465 ± 47 ml. The colloid solution produces substantial increases in cardiac output and arterial blood pressure. There is no evidence that colloids leak into the interstitial space and aggravate hypoxemia, but there is evidence that they can improve oxygen transfer.

TABLE 4-11—ELECTROLYTE REPLACEMENT FLUIDS

Composition	Concentration (mEq/liter)			
	NA	CL	HCO₃	mOSm
0.85% NaCl	145	145		290
0.45% NaCl	77	77		154
5% D/W				280
Hypertonic sodium bicarbonate	45 mEq of Na and HCO₃ each in 50 ml ampules			
Sodium bicarbonate solution			595	1190
Example of a "balanced" salt solution: Lactated Ringer's solution (Hartmann's modified solution) NaCl, 0.6%, KCl, 0.03%, CaCl₂, 0.022%, Na Lactate, 0.3%				
Na	130	Cl	111	
K	4	HCO₃	27	
Ca	4			

252

REFERENCES

Renal Failure

Anderson RJ, Linas SL, Berns AS, Henrich WL, Miller TR, Gabow PA, Schrier RW: Nonoliguric acute renal failure. N Engl J Med 296:1134, 1977.

Bennett WM, Muther RS, Parker RA, Feig P, Morrison G, Golper TA, Singer I: Drug therapy in renal failure: dosing guidelines for adults. Part I: Antimicrobial agents, analgesics. Ann Intern Med 93(Part 1):62, 1980.

Bauer JH, Brooks CS: The long-term effect of propranolol therapy on renal function. Am J Med 66:405, 1979.

Maher JJ: Principles of dialysis and dialysis of drugs. Am J Med 62:475, 1977.

Glomerular Disease

McPhaul JJ Jr, Mullins JD: Glomerulonephritis mediated by antibody to glomerular basement membrane: immunologic, clinical and histopathologic characteristics. J Clin Invest 57:351, 1976.

Lockwood CM, Rees AJ, Pearson TA, Evans DJ, Peters DK, Wilson CB: Immunosuppression and plasma exchange in treatment of Goodpasture's syndrome. Lancet 1:711, 1976.

Van der Peet J, Arisz L, Brentjens JRH, Marrink J, Hoedemaeker PhJ: Clinical course of IgA nephropathy in adults. Clin Nephrol 8:335, 1977.

Nissenson AR (moderator), Baraff LJ, Fine RN, Knutson DW: Poststreptococcal acute glomerulonephritis: fact and controversy. Ann Intern Med 91:76, 1979.

Noel LH, Zanetti M, Droz D, Barbanel C: Long-term prognosis of idiopathic membranous glomerulonephritis. Study of 116 untreated patients. Am J Med 66:82, 1979.

Curtis JJ, Wyatt RJ, Bhathena D, Lucas BA, Holland NH, Luke RG, Forristal J: Renal transplantation for patients with type I and type II membranoproliferative glomerulonephritis. Serial complement and nephritic factor measurements and the problem of recurrence of disease. Am J Med 66:216, 1979.

Collaborative Study of the Adult Idiopathic Nephrotic Syndrome: A controlled study of short-term prednisone treatment in adults with membranous nephropathy. N Engl J Med 301:1301, 1979.

Kupor LR, Mullins JD, McPhaul JJ Jr: Immunopathologic findings in idiopathic renal hematuria. Arch Intern Med 135:1204, 1975.

254 MEDICAL RESIDENT'S MANUAL

Tubular and Interstitial Disease

Murray T, Goldberg M: Chronic interstitial nephritis: etiologic factors. Ann Intern Med 82:453, 1975.

Goldberg M, Murray TG: Analgesic-associated nephropathy. An important cause of renal disease in the United States? N Engl J Med 299:716, 1978.

Nolan CM, Abernathy RS: Nephropathy associated with methicillin therapy: prevalence and determinants in patients with staphylococcal bacteremia. Arch Intern Med 137:997, 1977.

Petersdorf RG, Turck M: Some current concepts of urinary tract infections. DM, December 1970, pp 3-30.

Kunin CM, McCormack RC: An epidemiologic study of bacteriuria and blood pressure among nuns and working women. N Engl J Med 278:635, 1968.

Pazin GJ, Braude AI: Immobilizing antibodies in urine. II. Prevention of ascending spread of *Proteus mirabilis.* Invest Urol 12:129, 1974.

Baldwin DS, Gluck MC, Lowenstein J, Gallo GR: Lupus nephritis. Clinical course as related to morphologic forms and their transitions. Am J Med 62:12, 1977.

Systemic Disease

Mauer SM, Barbosa J, Vernier RL, Kjellstrand CM, Buselmeier TJ, Simmons RL, Najarian JS, Goetz FC: Development of diabetic vascular lesions in normal kidneys transplanted into patients with diabetes mellitus. N Engl J Med 295:916, 1976.

Ballard HS, Eisinger RP, Gallo G: Renal manifestations of the Henoch-Schoenlein syndrome in adults. Am J Med 49:328, 1970.

Vascular Diseases

Lessman RK, Johnson SF, Coburn JW, Kaufman JJ: Renal artery embolism: clinical features and long-term follow-up of 17 cases. Ann Intern Med 89:477, 1978,

Llach F, Arieff AI, Massry SG: Renal vein thrombosis and nephrotic syndrome. A prospective study of 36 adult patients. Ann Intern Med 83:8, 1975.

Nephrolithiasis

Pak CYC, et al.: Ambulatory evaluation of nephrolithiasis. Classification, clinical presentation and diagnostic criteria. Am J Med 69:19, 1980.

Hypernephroma

Clayman RV, Williams RD, Fraley EE: The pursuit of the renal mass. N Engl J Med 300:72, 1979.

Acid Base

Oh MS, Carroll HJ: The anion gap. N Engl J Med 297:814, 1977.

Arbus GS: An in vivo acid-base nomogram for clinical use. Can Med Assoc J 109:291, 1973.

Hauser CJ, Shoemaker WC, Turpin I, Goldberg SJ: Oxygen transport responses to colloids and crystalloids in critically ill surgical patients. Surg, Gynecol Obstet 150:811, 1980.

5

Diseases of Joints, Bones and Connective Tissue

POLYARTHRALGIAS OF UNKNOWN ETIOLOGY
Rheumatoid Arthritis

Rheumatoid arthritis (RA) is a multisystem connective tissue disease (CTD) of uncertain etiology. Women are affected two to three times as often as men. It is the second most common arthritic syndrome (with osteoarthritis first) and has a prevalence of 0.3%-2.5% of the adult population, depending on the criteria used for diagnosis.

Autoantibodies (IgG and IgM) directed against IgG are found in patients with RA; however, immune complex formation does not alone account for the manifestations of the disease. Tissue invasion by lymphocytes (T cells particularly) and local proliferation of phagocytic macrophage-like (type A) cells and secretory fibroblast-like (type B) cells may be more important. Cell-mediated (type IV) immune reaction thus becomes a major factor. A significant component of the inflammatory process involves activation of complement via both the classical and alternate pathways. Collagenases and proteases produced by local cells and the invading white cells result in connective tissue destruction (of collagen and proteoglycans). Developing acidity and release of prostaglandins cause local resorption of bone.

The etiology is not understood, but the interaction of environmental (infectious) agents and unusual immunologic response is suspected in RA and other connective tissue diseases. A familial pattern exists for RA; in one study, HLA DW4 was positive in 36% of patients.

Pathologic changes in the joint are nonspecific, but include thickening of the synovium, which encroaches on and covers the articular cartilage, producing a pannus. Erosion of cartilage and bone is followed by fusion of adjacent bones across the articular space. Decreased motion due to chronic inflammation, thickened synovium, pannus formation, and ankylosis leads to disuse atrophy of local muscles. Tendon inflammation and weakening of points of insertion produces laxity, with resultant displacement (subluxation). Small vessel vasculitis, positive by immunofluorescence for immunoglobulin and complement, produces skin or mucosal ulcers, neuritis, and cerebral or coronary arteritis and Raynaud phenomenon. Rashes and petechiae are infrequent. The rheumatoid nodule is a response to localized microvasculitis. Serial layers of lymphocytes and macrophages form a pallisaded appearance, with eventual fibrinoid necrosis of the center. Although classically noted to occur in subcutaneous tissues, particularly over the elbow, they may occur anywhere in the body, including connective tissues, lung, and myocardium.

CLINICAL MANIFESTATIONS

RA is a slowly developing illness, usually heralded by morning stiffness and ill-defined joint complaints and often associated with malaise and weakness. The hands (MCP and PIP) and feet (MTP) are most commonly affected, but involvement of peripheral large joints is frequent. Gradually, the arthralgias become more defined and arthritis develops. Multiple joints are often affected simultaneously, and the distribution is usually symmetric. Synovial thickening is apparent on examination. Ankylosis, subluxation, and contractures lead to joint deformities such as "ulnar deviation of the proximal phalanges on the metacarpals, "swan-neck deformity with flexion of the DIP joints and hyperextension of the PIP joints, and the "boutonniere" deformity with the flexed PIP joint protruding through the overlying extensor tendons.

Involvement of the vertebrae with laxity of ligaments may result in subluxation. Life-threatening impingement on the spinal cord or vertebral arteries, particularly with involvement of C_1-C_2, may produce sensory losses and upper motor neuron denervation. Early changes of separation or minor subluxation are demonstrable in more than two-thirds of patients with RA—three time more frequently than is seen in ankylosing spondylitis. Arthritis of the cricoarytenoid joint of the larynx may diminish vocal cord mobility, resulting in hoarseness or even laryngeal obstruction when fixed in adduction. Osteoporosis is common later in the disease and may relate to corticosteroid therapy. Joint effusions may escape, and extend, producing "cysts." The most common cyst forms in the popliteal area (Baker's cyst). This cyst may produce discomfort and limitation of motion. It may dissect up or down the leg, and if it ruptures, inflammation suggesting thrombophlebitis may occur.

Neurologic abnormalities include the rare focal cerebral arteritis, the uncommon symptomatic vertebral subluxation and the focal neuritis already noted, and nerve entrapment. The "carpal tunnel syndrome" is an example of paresthesia and ensuing loss of motor function due to entrapment and compression of the median nerve in the thickened flexor sheath of the wrist. The carpal tunnel syndrome may occur in up to one-fourth of all patients and is often an early finding that may even precede clinical recognition of the disease.

Rheumatoid nodules are typically subcutaneous and found over extensor surfaces such as the elbow. One of the many organs in which these same nodules may form is the lung. Caplan's syndrome is the association of large, roentgenographically apparent nodules in the lungs of patients with RA and pneumoconiosis. These nodules may also form in the dura mater and rarely produce a focal cerebritis. Occasionally, nodules form on the cardiac valves, principally the aortic valve.

Serositis of the pleura or pericardium may occur. Although small pericardial effusions or a thickened pericardium may be noted in half the patients, they are usually asymptomatic and rarely lead to tamponade. Occasional pleural effusions require treatment because of restriction of pulmonary function or secondary infection leading to empyema. Although symptomatic myositis is uncommon, electromyographic abnormalities are demonstrable in most patients before steroid therapy; clinical myopathy occasionally follows corticosteroid administration. Renal disease is uncommon, noted primarily in the elderly, and consists of a mild reduction in function due to some combination of obliterative microvasculitis, interstitial nephritis, and amyloid deposition. The role of chronic analgesic and nonsteroidal antiinflammatory use is unsettled. Gold and D-penicillamine are both nephrotoxic.

Splenomegaly is noted in approximately 5% of patients with RA. Many of these patients have Felty's syndrome—the triad of RA and splenomegaly with leukopenia. Virtually all patients with RA have antibodies to immunoglobulin attached to the granulocyte membrane. Patients with Felty's syndrome also have antibodies directed at the granulocyte membrane. Lysis and reticuloendothelial phagocytosis result, leading to neutropenia and splenomegaly. Marrow production is normal or increased. Patients with RA have an increased susceptibility to infections, which may relate to diminished leukocytic phagocytosis, decreased antigen-specific IgM production, and increased turnover of endogenous immunoglobulins. In addition, patients receiving corticosteroids seem to be at an even greater risk for infection.

LABORATORY STUDIES

Rheumatoid factor (RF) is a circulating antibody (principally IgG and IgM) to endogenous IgG. Only IgM RF produces IgG-coated latex or RBC agglutination; with this method, RF is found in only 75% of patients with RA. Positive reactions may also be noted in almost all diseases associated with immune complex formation and increase with age in the "normal" population. After the first 2 years, the titer varies with disease activity; before that the titer may fluctuate widely, and even become negative with no relationship to the course of the disease.

LE cells are noted in up to 20% of patients and a positive ANA in up to half; anti-DS-DNA and anti-Sm are always negative unless the syndrome is mixed with SLE. The ESR (erythrocyte sedimentation rate) is frequently elevated. Serum complement is normal except with very active disease. Cryoglobulins may be found in patients with active rheumatoid vasculitis. A nonspecific increase in all immunoglobulins may be noted. Polymers of IgG RF may lead to increased viscosity and a hyperviscosity syndrome similar to that described in Chapter 7.

A normochromic, normocytic anemia of chronic disease is almost always present with chronic RA. Coomb positive hemolytic anemias occur infrequently. Either mild leukocytosis or neutropenia may be present, and mild thrombocytopenia is not uncommon. Mild eosinophilia with normal IgE levels may be noted in some patients with multisystem disease.

Examination of synovial fluid reveals 10,000-50,000 white blood cells, about 50% neutrophils, with few red blood cells. The viscosity is decreased, and the mucin clot formation is poor. Mucin clot formation, dependent on polymerization of hyaluronic acid, is tested for by adding 1% acetic acid to the fluid after the fibrin clot has already formed (if it does). Complement levels in the synovial fluid are characteristically less than one-third of the serum levels (similar to SLE and distinct from all other arthritides). Rheumatoid factor is useful only if the normally agglutinating hyaluronic acid is removed by hyaluronidase. Ragocytes or "RA cells" are granulocytes that have ingested immune complexes visible as bright red granules, but these are nonspecific unless the granules are shown to be RF complexes. Glucose is usually low.

Effusions from serous surfaces such as the pleura or pericardium are typically exudative with a high specific gravity, LDH (effusion to serum ratio), and total protein (greater than 3.5 gm/dl). The white and red cell counts are usually low. The glucose is characteristically less than 25% of the serum value, but as many as 10% of patients have normal glucose levels.

DIAGNOSTIC CRITERIA

As with each of the connective tissue diseases, RA is manifest as a multisystem disease with no specific diagnostic technique available. The rheumatoid factor is present in only 75% of patients and may be positive in other CTD. Diagnosis thus rests on demonstrating common manifestations that cannot be ascribed to other causes.

The abridged ARA criteria for making the diagnosis of RA are given in Table 5-1. Criterion 1 is the only acceptable historical finding. Criteria 2-6 must be observed by a physician, and 1-5 must have been present for at least 6 weeks. The diagnosis of RA is classical if seven criteria are met, definite if five are met, and probable if three are met. However, if any one of the exclusions listed in Table 5-2 is present, the diagnosis cannot be made.

TREATMENT

Maintenance of function using physical therapy and sequential drug therapy is the *mainstay of management*. Salicylates remain the cornerstone of drug therapy. Up to 3-5 gm/day of aspirin should be administered in incremental doses to control pain and inflammation. The limit to treatment is occurrence of toxic symptoms such as tinnitus or the development of gastrointestinal bleeding. Aspirin decreases platelet aggregability, whereas other salicylates, such as choline salicylate, do not.

TABLE 5-1—DIAGNOSTIC CRITERIA FOR RHEUMATOID ARTHRITIS

Morning stiffness
Pain or tenderness in one or more joints
Synovial thickening or joint effusion in at least one joint
Same as the above in at least one other joint
Symmetrical involvement, excluding DIP
Subcutaneous nodules
Typical roentgenographic changes
Positive rheumatoid factor
Poor mucin precipitate from synovial fluid
Characteristic histologic changes in synovium
Characteristic histologic changes in nodule

TABLE 5-2—EXCLUSIONS TO THE DIAGNOSIS OF RHEUMATOID ARTHRITIS

Clinical picture
  Gout
  Demonstrable tophi
  Infectious arthritis
  Joint tuberculosis
  Hypertrophic osteoarthropathy
  Neuroarthropathy
  Shoulder-hand syndrome
  Dermatomyositis
  Reiter's syndrome
  Rheumatic fever
  Scleroderma
  SLE butterfly rash

Histologic picture
  Periarteritis nodosa
  Sarcoidosis

Laboratory abnormalities
  High titer of ANA*
  Homogentisic aciduria

* Originally described as a high concentration of LE cells.

A wide variety of other nonsteroidal antiinflammatory (NSAI) agents are available; unfortunately, no critical, large-scale, prospective study directly comparing efficacy has yet been performed. Serial attempts of trials of some of these for minimum periods of 6 weeks often results in successful control of the disease.

Although moderate doses of antimalarials such as chloroquine and hydroxychloroquine are said to be safe, the occurrence of reversible rashes and irreversible ocular keratopathy limits the choice of this agent as a *second step* therapy to those physicians experienced with this agent and capable of ensuring careful ophthalmologic screening.

The *third step* in the management of chronic RA is gold. Two-thirds of patients refractory to aspirin, NSAI, and chloroquine derivatives will respond. Its mechanism of action is unknown. Weeks to months of gradually increasing doses may be necessary before a response is observed. Skin rashes, thrombocytopenia, or proteinuria may limit its use. Aplastic anemia occurs in less than 0.02 % of patients treated with gold.

The *fourth step* is the use of D-penicillamine. Up to 70% of patients refractory to prior measures will improve with penicillamine. Slowly increasing increments of dose are necessary, and response may be delayed. Like gold, penicillamine may produce significant proteinuria or thrombocytopenia, but skin rashes are less severe. Loss of taste is noted in about 5% of patients.

The *final step*, reserved for patients with rapidly progressing disease associated with severe systemic manifestations, is immunosuppression with azathioprine or cyclophosphamide. Improvement occurs in some patients, but there may be increased risk of lymphoreticular malignancies.

Corticosteroids are used with other agents for treatment of both acute exacerbations and rapidly progressive disease. Acute exacerbations can generally be controlled with 0.2-0.5 mg/kg/day of prednisone for short periods of time, followed by rapid tapering and withdrawal when possible, although frequently lower doses must be continued for several weeks to avoid relapses. Higher or more chronic dosages offer no advantages unless the course is rapidly progressive.

Intraarticular injections of corticosteroids provide rapid, short-term relief in the patient with disabling pauciarticular disease. Risks include introduction of infection as well as subsequent occurrence of a traumatic arthropathy due to overuse of a damaged joint in the absence of pain.

Synovectomy may control symptoms in some patients and is essential in the management of carpal tunnel syndrome and Baker cyst. Total joint replacement is becoming increasingly available and should be considered in all patients with severe arthropathy that is limiting function. The best results have been with hip and M-C joints, somewhat less reliable results with knee and elbow. Symptomatic instability of C_1-C_2 must be stabilized surgically.

Treatment of Felty's syndrome is necessary when the granulo-cytopenia is severe or an increasing occurrence of infections is noted. Corticosteroids, to limit the immune reaction, have met with little success. Lithium or androgens may occasionally increase granulocyte production. Splenectomy will result in an acute granulocytosis in all patients, but this is sustained in only about two-thirds.

Juvenile Rheumatoid Arthritis

Juvenile rheumatoid arthritis, (JRA), or Still's disease, is a variant of RA seen primarily in children but also in adults. The peak onset is between 1 and 5 years, and girls are more commonly affected than boys.

Three clinical forms of the disease are each noted with similar frequencies. With all forms, about half of the patients have retarded growth. Also, about one-fourth have little or no pain in the affected joints.

Systemic form. Typically, this presents with high spiking fevers and is more common in boys. Concomitant arthralgias/arthritis are noted in only about one-third of patients at the onset of the disease. Rashes, generalized lymphadenopathy, and hepatosple-nomegaly are very common. Pleuritis and pericarditis are each noted in about one-third of patients. Most patients develop polyarthritis; however, a chronic deforming arthritis develops in about half of these patients. Myocarditis may occur. This form is the one Still described originally, although the eponym is now applied less specifically to all forms of JRA.

Polyarticular form. This form is more common in females and has a presentation and clinical manifestation similar to adult RA. Chronic joint deformities are not common and are mild. Systemic amyloidosis occasionally develops.

Mono- or pauciarticular disease. The third form affects fewer than five joints and is also more common in girls. Systemic manifestations are less common with this form; however, iridocyclitis, uncommon with the other forms, develops in about one-fourth of these patients. Except for iridocyclitis, which may lead to cataracts and blindness, the prognosis is good.

Leukocytosis and an elevated ESR occur commonly and generally in proportion to the clinical manifestations. Rheumatoid factor occurs in less than 20% of all patients with JRA—being present in up to two-thirds of patients with the polyarticular adult form and usually absent in the other two forms. The ANA is positive in about one-third of patients with the pauci- and polyarticular forms and usually negative in the systemic form; in the pauciarticular form, patients with a positive ANA are the most likely to develop chronic iridocyclitis. Diagnosis of JRA is clinical and particularly difficult in patients with the systemic form of the disease. For this reason, other causes must be excluded. To prevent complications, iridocyclitis should be detected early through the use of periodic slit lamp examination.

Treatment for all forms continues to remain symptomatic, using nonsteroidal, anti-inflammatory agents (particularly aspirin). Signs of developing hepatotoxicity should be carefully monitored. Local mydriatics and steroids are used to treat iridocyclitis. Systemic steroids should be reserved for life-threatening complications of myocarditis or severe vasculitis and for progressive iridocyclitis.

ACQUIRED CONNECTIVE TISSUE DISORDERS
Systemic Lupus Erythematosus

Systemic lupus erythematosus (SLE) is a prototype multisystem connective tissue disease (CTD) that (like many other similar diseases) may result from the interaction of an environmental factor and an abnormal host response. A hyperactive antibody response, perhaps due to deficiency of suppressor T cells, produces antibodies to a variety of tissue substances. Support for an abnormal immune system comes from the increase in HLA-DRw2 and HLA-DRw3 antigens, a high incidence of antilymphocyte antibodies, and deficiencies of C2 or C4 (and in other patients, of C5 and C8). An attractive hypothesis might be that an inherited deficiency of the complement system results in attempted compensation by other components of the immune system as some sort of negative feedback or inhibitory control fails.

Studies from New Zealand black/New Zealand white hybrid mice in which females develop anti-DNA antibodies and die from immune complex glomerulonephritis provide an animal model for SLE. All New Zealand mice carry type C oncornavirus, but only the NZB/NZW hybrids exhibit a deficiency in suppressor T cells and develop anti-DNA antibodies.

Regardless of the stimulus, SLE seems to be an immune complex disease with DNA-anti-DNA complexes trapped in basement membranes of blood vessels and producing complement activation with release of a variety of toxic mediators. Anti-DNA of the IgG class has great avidity for kidney tissue and is probably an important determinant of renal disease. Type II cytotoxicity also occurs as killer lymphocytes with Fc receptors for immunoglobulins are activated.

Pathologic changes vary with organ involvement and activity of the disease. The underlying lesion is deposition of immune complexes within the subendothelium or basement membrane, resulting in an inflammatory reaction, which may be diffuse or localized. These changes include the nonspecific cellular components of inflammation and fibrinoid deposits and the more specific presence of hematoxylin bodies (rounded masses that represent degenerated nuclei). Localized disease is common and may affect any combination of systems with variable composition over time and space. Systems affected include serosal surfaces (joints, pleura, pericardium, or peritoneum), skin, kidneys (glomeruli), and the central (ventriculitis or diffuse vasculitis) and peripheral (neuritis) nervous system. Positive immunofluorescent studies may be obtained in "normal" skin in over half the patients with SLE. Histologic and immunochemical abnormalities tend to be noted in other organs only when clinical manifestations suggest an abnormality. Renal involvement is a glomerulopathy which may be focal, diffuse, or membranous (see page 235); progression from focal to diffuse or membranous disease tends to occur only with active, uncontrolled disease. In addition, similar changes in the tubular basement membrane produces an interstitial nephritis.

CLINICAL MANIFESTATIONS

SLE may affect persons of any age, race, or sex, but most often affects females (85%) between the ages of 20 and 45. With the advent of more specific therapy, median survival has improved from less than 2 years to over 8 years during the past 25 years. Over this same period, the causes of death have shifted with the relative frequency of infection and malignancy increasing and uremia and central nervous system disease decreasing.

The most common symptoms, arthralgias and arthritis, are nondeforming, symmetrical, and often evanescent. Involvement tends to be of the wrists, hands, proximal interphalangeal (PIP) joints, metacarpophalangeal (MCP) joints, elbows, knees, and ankles. Bony erosions, pannus formation, and synovial thickening are uncommon; although subluxation, Swan-neck deformities, and aseptic necrosis of bone may be noted, their occurrence relates in part to corticosteroid therapy. Skin involvement may include the classic butterfly or malar rash (with erythema, telangiectasia, and keratotic plugging), a similar diffuse eruption, vitiligo (in blacks), periungual telangiectasias, patchy alopecia, short broken scalp hair ("lupus hairs"), and mucosal ulceration. Urticaria or angioedema rarely occurs. Raynaud's phenomenon is infrequent. Discoid lupus is a variant of SLE that is chronic, confined to the skin, and infrequently progresses to active SLE. Skin lesions are similar to those noted with the butterfly eruption, however, and are spread over the head, neck, upper trunk, and arms. Scaling and atrophy with scarring are prominent.

Clinically apparent renal involvement is noted in over half of all patients and is manifested as proteinuria (minimal to massive) and/or hematuria (microscopic to gross). The nephrotic syndrome, renal insufficiency, or interstitial nephritis may develop and progress to chronic renal failure. Abnormalities of the renal biopsy may be noted in up to 80% of all patients. Nontender lymphadenopathy is frequent and due to a nonspecific proliferative response associated with the disease. Although splenomegaly with or without hemolytic anemia is uncommon, pathologically most patients have an intimal proliferation ("onion skin" appearance) of the splenic microvasculature. Hepatomegaly is more common, but the cause is unclear. Chronic active hepatitis, when associated with lupus erythematosus (LE) cells (20% of patients) or a positive ANA (up to 50%), has been termed "lupoid hepatitis," but is an immune complex disease associated with hepatitis B virus. Gastrointestinal manifestations are principally oral mucosal ulcerations, anorexia, and nausea.

Cardiac involvement is frequent and consists primarily of pericarditis, although occasionally myocarditis is noted. The pericardial effusion is usually mild, and tamponade occurs infrequently. Libman-Sacks (nonbacterial verrucose) endocarditis may occur rarely. Coronary atherosclerosis appears to be accelerated by corticosteroid therapy. Rarely, acute myocardial infarction due to vasculitis occurs. Pulmonary involvement may include evanescent sterile parenchymal infiltrates or pleural effusion or infiltrate. Neurologic abnormalities may be acute and intermittent or chronic, subjective (neurosis or psychosis), or objective (seizures or organic brain syndrome), focal or diffuse, and central or peripheral (mononeuritis simplex).

Hematologic manifestations include anemia and leukopenia commonly and thrombocytopenia occasionally. Although the Coombs test may be positive, the anemia is usually normochromic, normocytic, and secondary to diminished erythropoiesis rather than hemolysis. Defects in coagulation may be due to antibodies to factors VII, IX, or X or the inhibition of prothrombin activation (the "lupus anticoagulant"), as well as diminished production of procoagulants.

Diminished production of other proteins including albumin is frequently noted, although the levels of immunoglobulins are usually elevated.

LABORATORY ABNORMALITIES

The ANA is very sensitive and is present in virtually all patients with SLE but may be negative in the late stages of severe multisystem disease. Unfortunately, it is nonspecific, because a number of other connective tissue diseases as well as some older "normal" people may have a positive ANA. The titer (greatest dilution at which the test remains positive) is important and, using a minimum of 1:32 as the definition of normal and 1:100 as unquestionably significant, will screen out the low titer "normals" occasionally noted. The ANA technique most commonly used determines the presence of circulating antibodies to nuclear elements by reacting the patient's serum with heterologous (rat or mouse) nucleated cells (liver or kidney) and then introducing fluorescein-tagged antibody to human immunoglobulin. A number of nuclear elements are antigenic, so that the staining pattern of the ANA may vary. Circulating antibodies to ribonucleic acid (RNA) produce a *nucleolar pattern,* which is never noted in benign conditions but may be found in scleroderma (PSS) and Sjögren's syndrome (SS) as well as SLE. The *rim (shaggy or membranous) pattern* represents antibody to resting cell deoxyribonucleic acid (DNA) and may be either immunoglobulin IgM (noted in rheumatoid arthritis and other CTD) or IgG (noted in SLE, RA, and drug-induced SLE). Subtypes of DNA include *single-strand (S-DNA)* and *double-strand (DS-DNA),* of which anti-S-DNA has a low specificity and anti-DS-DNA is only seen in SLE. The *speckled pattern* represents antibodies formed to extractable (nonhistone, acidic) nucleoproteins (ENA) and usually suggests a diagnosis of mixed connective tissue disease, in which it is virtually always present. The *diffuse (or homogenous) pattern* results from antibody directed to the DNA-histone complex (deoxyribonucleoprotein) and is the least specific for all the patterns, being found in RA, SS, drug-induced SLE, other CTD, and even in normal individuals. The diffuse pattern may mask other patterns, and to detect each of them, when more than one is present, it is essential to perform serial dilutions. The diffuse pattern reaction accounts for the LE phenomenon, in which the patient's serum is mixed with heterologous nuclei and then polymorphonuclear leukocytes (PMN) are added; these PMNs then engulf the antibody-coated nuclei, producing a characteristic LE cell. The LE phenomenon is less sensitive and less specific than the ANA and almost never positive in SLE with a negative ANA, so that it is not useful as a screening test. *Anti-Sm (soluble nuclear) antibody* is quite specific for SLE and is found particularly in patients with renal involvement. Both the titer of the

ANA and the presence or absence of LE cells are poorly correlated with disease. Antilymphocyte antibodies are found in more than three-fourths of patients, and their presence correlates directly with disease activity.

Serum complement, both total and components (C_3 and C_4), is decreased in active disease. The fall in serum complement may precede clinical flare-ups in days to weeks and will rise a few days after the abatement of symptoms. Other abnormalities include the frequent presence of hypergammaglobulinemia and the occasional occurrence of a positive Coombs test or a false-positive VDRL. Here the pattern is important, because a false-positive VDRL has a "beaded" appearance rather than the usual homogenous pattern. False-positive serologic tests for syphilis may occasionally precede any other clinical or serologic manifestations of SLE.

Skin biopsies may be useful, since up to 70% of patients have characteristic histologic and immunofluorescence findings, even in uninvolved skin. Serial skin biopsies may be useful in following the patient.

Clinical evidence of renal involvement should be followed immediately by renal biopsy (preferably closed) to determine the type of renal pathology and thus the choice of therapy. The value of renal biopsy at the time of SLE diagnosis in the absence of clinical renal disease, and the value of serial renal biopsy in following these patients, remain to be determined. (Table 4-9)

Patients with neurologic manifestations may be evaluated with technetium brain scans, which may show focal uptake; electro-encephalograms (EEG), which may show focal abnormalities; and cerebrospinal fluid (CSF) examination, which may show increased protein, increased lymphocytes, and decreased C_4— each of which correlates better with disease duration than disease activity.

Diagnosis of SLE may be quite difficult because of its multisystem nature and the lack of specific serologic tests. A positive ANA should virtually always be present. The remainder of the diagnosis rests on evidence of multisystem disease with no other identifiable etiologies. Useful but not uniformly accepted criteria are those proposed by Cohen, which are abstracted in Table 5-3;

TABLE 5-3—CRITERIA FOR THE DIAGNOSIS OF SLE

Butterfly rash

Discoid lupus

Raynaud's phenomenon

Alopecia

Photosensitivity

Mucosal ulceration

Nondeforming arthritis

LE cells (or ANA)

Chronic false-positive VDRL

Proteinuria (3.5 gm/day)

Cellular renal tubular casts

Pleuritis or pericarditis

Psychosis or seizures

Hemolytic anemia or leukopenia or thrombocytopenia

four or more of these are necessary to make the diagnosis of SLE—each in the absence of other identifiable causes. Clearly, the diagnosis remains clinical.

Discoid lupus has the characteristic facial eruption associated with a positive ANA. If other systems are involved, the diagnosis of SLE should be applied.

Drug-induced SLE. This is the occurrence of the manifestations of SLE following the administration of medications known to cause such syndromes: procainamide, hydralazine, isoniazid, and others. Procainamide is the best characterized of the group. A positive ANA may be noted in up to 75% of patients receiving 2 gm/day for 2-6 months; up to one-third of these patients develop an SLE-like syndrome, which characteristically has more pulmonary involvement, less skin involvement, and no renal involvement. The occurrence of a positive ANA occurs in half of patients receiving hydralazine and one-third of patients receiving isoniazid; the rate of occurrence is about doubled in slow acetylators compared to fast acetylators. Each of these probably requires a genetic predisposition to manifest the disease. Each produces a positive ANA by different mechanisms: hydralazine, which induces antibodies that cross-react with DNA; procainamide, which complexes to DNA and results in antigenicity to the complex; and isoniazid, which denatures native DNA. Anti-DS-DNA and anti-Sm are always negative with the drug-induced positive ANAs.

Treatment of SLE. Treatment is guided by symptomatology. Even though the underlying abnormalities cannot be specifically corrected, appropriate therapy may significantly prolong life and increase functional abilities. Management begins with reassurance, support, and establishment of continuity. Physical therapy and rehabilitation are important. Attempts should be made to encourage a normal lifestyle without undue restrictions. Rest and salicylates may control manifestations of serositis and arthritis, although when more than 3 g/d of aspirin is required, other nonsteroidal anti-inflammatory agents should be used. Hydroxychloroquine has been used successfully in the management of the skin lesions; however, the occurrence of ophthalmologic complications mandates careful serial eye examinations. Active renal or CNS disease may respond to high doses of corticosteroids (1-2 mg/kg/day of prednisone in divided doses) and then tapered to lower daily or every other day doses for control. Withdrawal should be attempted intermittently. Diffuse and membranous forms of renal involvement may require even higher doses and, in cases that do not respond, consideration should be given to adding immunosuppressive agents (azathioprine or cyclophosphamide) to the regimen. End-stage renal disease has been treated successfully with dialysis and renal transplantation.

The occurrence of fever and organ-specific manifestations of inflammation are characteristic of SLE, but underlying infection must always be considered particularly because of the increased susceptibility to infections incurred by virtue of both the disease and its treatment.

Prognosis has improved, and presently the median survival is well above 8 years. Pregnancy may be associated with exacerbations of the disease. Predictors of a poor prognosis are a high rim titer, a high anti-DS-DNA titer, a low complement, and worsening renal function.

Progressive Systemic Sclerosis
(Scleroderma)

Scleroderma or progressive systemic sclerosis (PSS) is a chronic multisystem disease. The onset is typically between 20 and 50 years, and females are affected two to three times as often as males.

Widespread microscopic inflammation of the vascular system is followed by increased numbers of fibroblasts and an overproduction of normal collagen. The microvascular pathologic process includes a marked decrease in the number of normal arterioles and capillaries, with fibrinoid necrosis and intimal proliferation of the arterioles and widely dilated capillary loops. Ultimately, widespread fibrosis ensues. The skin is involved initially in one-third and develops clinically in over two-thirds of patients, and microscopically in virtually all patients. Pathologic changes in the skin include thinning of the epidermis, with marked dermal fibrosis (and atrophy of the dermal appendages) fixing the skin to subcutaneous tissues. Edema (scleredema) is followed by sclerosis, which produces a thickened, leathery appearance. With progression, the skin becomes atrophic. These changes are usually initially confined to the fingers and hands (acrosclerosis) and later spread to involve the arms, torso, and face. Involved areas have limitation of motion due to the extensive fibrosis, which may result in flexion contractures. Skin ulcers and hypo- or hyperpigmentation are each noted in about one-third of patients. Alopecia is noted occasionally. Telangiectasias and subcutaneous calcinosis each develop in 10-15% of patients.

Sclerodactyly represents the combination of taut skin with tapering of the digits distally from the MCP joints. Polyarthritis, particularly of the large joints, and migratory arthralgias are noted in 20-50%. Pathologically, the synovium undergoes changes similar to those of the skin, with early mild inflammatory changes followed by fibrosis, which may become extensive. The arthritis is nonerosive and nondeforming, although abnormal appearance and function may result from the extensive fibrosis. Tendinous and periarticular calcinosis are noted in about 10% of patients.

Myalgias are common, and myositis (similar to that seen in polymyositis) with proximal muscle weakness and elevated muscle enzymes develops in 10-20%. Generalized muscular atrophy develops in 50-60%. Raynaud's phenomenon develops in 80-98% and is the presenting manifestation in about one-third. The combination of calcinosis, Raynaud's phenomenon, esophageal involvement, sclerodactyly, and telangiectasia is known as the CREST syndrome, a variant of scleroderma that often has a relatively mild clinical course.

The esophagus is involved in more than three-fourths of patients, with pathologic changes similar to those seen in the skin including diffuse fibrosis, thinned mucosa often with ulceration, and atrophy of the smooth muscle (lower two-thirds). Manifestations of esophageal hypomotility include dysphagia, retrosternal fullness, and symptoms of reflux esophagitis. Other common areas of gastrointestinal involvement include the proximal small bowel and the large intestine. Manifestations may include obstructive or paralytic ileus, malabsorption, constipation, and diverticulosis which may progress to pneumatosis intestinalis. Microvascular obliteration or obstruction may produce infarction.

The lungs are involved in up to half of patients. Diffuse interstitial fibrosis with occasional cystic formation is the common pathologic lesion. The pulmonary arteries, particularly the smaller branches, are involved, with intimal proliferation and muscular hypertrophy leading to pulmonary hypertension. Patients often have a nonproductive cough and dyspnea on exertion. Recurrent pneumonias are common. Pulmonary function tests characteristically show a decreased vital capacity, decreased diffusion of carbon monoxide (DL_{CO}), and a decrease in arterial oxygen content with exercise. The restrictive element may be compounded by decreased chest wall motion due to overlying skin fibrosis. Cor pulmonale may develop.

The heart is involved in 40-80% of patients. Myocarditis may occur, and fibrous replacement of the myocardium with resultant cardiomyopathy is common. Small vessel coronary arteritis occasionally occurs. Valvular disease is uncommon. Arrhythmias and heart block, reflecting fibrous replacement of conduction tissues, occurs in about 10%. Chronic fibrinous pericarditis is frequently seen in patients with cardiomyopathy. Less commonly, acute pericarditis may occur, but tamponade is rare.

Kidney abnormalities are found in more than one-third of patients and usually occur early. The lesions include thickening of the glomerular basement membrane (glomerulosclerosis), with intimal proliferation and fibrinoid necrosis of the smaller arteries and arterioles. Concomitant hypertension and proteinuria are common manifestations. About one-third of these patients develop a malignant hypertensive phase, frequently accompanied by acute renal failure.

Neuropathies are uncommon but may include cranial (particularly trigeminal), peripheral, and autonomic nerves (in decreasing order of occurrence). Seizures occur rarely. Carpal tunnel syndrome may result from fibrous involvement of the tendon sheaths of the wrist.

The ESR is elevated in up to two-thirds of patients. Hypergammaglobulinemia (particularly IgG) is noted in half. Fifty to 90% have a positive ANA; the speckled pattern (ENA) is the most common (see mixed connective tissue disease); anti-DS-DNA and anti-Sm are absent. Twenty-five to 35% have a positive RF. False-positive serologic tests for syphilis are noted in up to 5%. Serum complement is usually normal. Eosinophilia is infrequently noted (see eosinophilic fasciitis). Elevated muscle enzymes and abnormal electromyography and biopsy are noted with active myositis, and the findings are similar to those noted in polymyositis. Nailbed and nailfold capillaroscopy demonstrates dilated capillaries characteristic of PSS and polymyositis, the degree of which correlates closely with extent and activity of disease.

Other connective tissue diseases (particularly Sjögren's syndrome) are noted in up to one-fourth of patients. Because many of these have an immunologic basis, further support is given for an immune-related pathophysiology for PSS.

Variants of PSS include localized linear scleroderma or morphea, CREST, mixed connective tissue disease (MCTD), and eosinophilic fasciitis.

MCTD represents one of the "overlap syndromes," in which features are seen that are common to PSS, SLE, and polymyositis. MCTD affects patients in the fourth and fifth decades of life. Clinical features include Raynaud phenomenon, scleroderma-like skin changes, telangiectasias or swollen hands, and esophageal hypomotility as seen in PSS. Polyserositis and a nondeforming polyoarthritis/polyarthralgia are common. An inflammatory myositis similar to polymyositis with myalgias, proximal muscle weakness, elevated muscle enzymes, and abnormal electromyography is frequent. Heliotrope discoloration of the eyelids similar to dermatomyositis is occasionally seen. Nephritis and CNS involvement are rare, but neuropathies (especially of the trigeminal nerve) are common. Occasionally, pulmonary fibrosis with decreased DLco occurs. Fever, rash, lymphadenopathy, splenomegaly, and hepatomegaly are common. Laboratory features include anemia, leukopenia, hypergammaglobulinemia, LE cells, and a positive ANA. The ANA pattern is characteristically speckled and composed of an extremely high-titer of anti-ENA (specifically anti-RNP). Antibodies to DS-DNA or Sm are absent or low-titer; if high-titer, the diagnosis is SLE. Execpt for pulmonary or renal involvement, the disease typically responds well to corticosteroid therapy.

Another scleroderma-like syndrome is *eosinophilic fasciitis* (EF), or Shulman's syndrome, which affects the middle-aged, with men predominating slightly. In this variant, manifestations of swollen, painful extremities composed of thick indurated skin, myositis, and fasciitis are pathologically characterized by eosinophil infiltrates and edema. Hypergammaglobulinemia, elevated ESR, and marked eosinophilia are common. Attacks often follow strenuous exercise. Corticosteroids are beneficial; spontaneous remissions may occur. In addition, scleroderma-like syndromes have been noted in people with polyvinyl chloride exposure or silicosis.

Except for MCTD and EF variants, PSS does not usually respond to corticosteroids. Penicillamine or cytotoxic immunosuppressives may eventually prove beneficial. Management is essentially limited to careful monitoring and vigorous symptomatic treatment of associated phenomena. Although up to two-thirds of patients are alive at 5 years, the disease progresses relentlessly to death. Causes of death include malignant hypertension, acute renal failure, myocardial infarction or failure, and pulmonary insufficiency. The disease is milder when visceral involvement is limited and more severe in males, blacks, and the elderly.

Polymyositis and Dermatomyositis

These entities may occur individually or together and may be associated with other CTD (particularly SLE, RA, or PSS) or with malignancy. Their frequent occurrence together, or initial symptoms of one with later manifestations of the other and similar pathology, causes them to be considered to represent a spectrum of the same disease process. Adults are typically affected from the ages of 30-60, although a childhood polymyositis also occurs. Females are affected twice as often as males.

The etiology remains unknown, but the most popular theory is that the syndrome results from cell-mediated (T cell) destruction of target tissue. Derepression and/or cross-antigenicity have been suggested as initiators, and the association with malignancy suggests a hypersensitivity response to tumor antigens, which cross-react with muscle antigens. Humoral mechanisms have also been implicated, since a mild immunodeficiency is occasionally noted and antibodies to myosin and nuclear antigens are frequently noted. Similar diseases in animals have been produced by injecting extracts of normal muscle or antithymus antibodies. In addition, the role of infectious agents has not been eliminated, and some investigators have found virus-like particles in involved muscle.

Pathologic changes in polymyositis (PM) are characterized by lymphocytic infiltrates, particularly perivascular, with focal or diffuse necrosis and vacuolization of muscle fibers and evidence of regenerative activity. Both type I and II fibers are involved. Whether 10% of patients have a normal appearing biopsy or do not have PM is debated. Immunofluorescence studies occasionally demonstrate immunoglobulin and complement, particularly in children. Electron microscopy is nonspecific, although occasionally virus-like particles may be noted. Dermatomyositis (DM) is characterized pathologically by a lymphocytic infiltration of the dermis with necrosis of the basal cells and epidermal atrophy.

Eighty to 90% of patients with PM initially present with a gradually (weeks to months) progressive symmetrical proximal muscle weakness, which is generally painless; however, aching myalgias are noted in about one-fourth. Occasionally, the onset is acute over 1-2 weeks. In addition, the neck, pharyngeal, and laryngeal muscles may be affected, leading to an inability to hold the head erect, dysphagia, dysphonia, and occasionally dysarthria. The distal muscles are affected in 25% of patients. The ocular muscles are rarely affected. Rashes and arthralgias are each noted in about one-fourth of patients early in the disease process. Typical skin changes of DM occur in one-third. Raynaud's phenomenon is seen in about 20% of patients but is rarely present when PM is associated with malignancy. Subcutaneous calcifications occur, particularly in children. Muscle contractures and atrophy are late features of the disease. There may be hypomotility of the gastrointestinal tract similar to PSS, although it is frequently limited to the lower esophagus (30% of patients).

Skin manifestations of DM include erythema, maculopapular rashes, or scaling or exfoliative dermatitis, and may occur separately or together; they may be noted anywhere, but particularly over the joints. Pruritis is common. A characteristic purplish periorbital discoloration of the skin (heliotrope) is frequently seen, and periorbital edema is common. Diffuse muscle weakness occurs in about half of all patients. Esophageal involvement and Raynaud's phenomenon are each present with frequency equal to that observed in pure PM.

Up to 10% of patients with PM-DM have an associated malignancy. The type of tumor roughly parallels the occurrence in the general population, although gastric and ovarian carcinoma may be more common and colon carcinoma less common. These patients are older than the average of those with DM-PM and younger than the mean age of people with malignancy. The sex ratio has been variously given as 1:1 to 2:1, with a female preponderance. Except for the rarity of Raynaud's phenomenon, there are no clinical or pathologic differences from PM-DM not associated with malignancy. Etiologic hypotheses have already been discussed.

The diagnostic procedure of choice is biopsy of involved skin or muscle. Routine stains should be diagnostic. Fluorescent studies and EM offer no diagnostic benefit at the present time. Muscle enzymes, particularly CPK, are usually elevated and fluctuate directly with, and preceding by 1 month, the clinical course, although exceptions have been noted. Electromyography characteristically demonstrates short polyphasic potentials, fibrillation, and repetitive high-frequency discharges. The ESR may be elevated but often does not parallel the clinical course. Although almost half of patients have antimyosin antibodies, 80% have immunoconglutinin, and almost 40% have ANA, these are not useful discriminators because neurogenic atrophy and the muscular dystrophies are associated with similar findings. Fifty % of patients with PM-PSS have an antibody to PM-1, an antigen derived from the thymus. Other serologic abnormalities often reflect the presence of other CTD.

Etiologic considerations in the differential diagnosis include trichinosis, toxoplasmosis, and pentazocine (Talwin) abuse. The diagnosis of PM-DM must always be accompanied by a careful search for underlying malignancy.

The mainstay of treatment remains corticosteroids (up to 1 mg/kg/day of prednisone tapered in parallel with serum enzymes). Maintenance therapy of 0.1-0.3 mg/kg/day should continue for months to years. True remissions are uncommon, and relapses occur frequently after discontinuation of therapy, although disease-free intervals of several months between discontinuation and flare-up may occur. Pure DM and PM seem to be more responsive to steroids than the combined syndrome or DM or PM in association with malignancy or other CTD. The earlier treatment is instituted, the more likely response will occur. The addition of immunosuppressive agents (particularly methotrexate) may allow control of symptoms (after 3 months of high-dose steroid therapy) or reduction of steroid dosage when necessary. Unfortunately, myopathy (atrophy of type II muscle fibers with normal muscle enzyme levels) is not an infrequent complication of chronic high-dose steroid therapy.

The Vasculitides

The syndromes of vasculitis are all characterized by inflammation and degrees of necrosis of the blood vessel wall. Classification is by both clinical manifestations and histopathologic changes.

Vasculitis is caused by immunologic abnormalities, which may be limited to blood vessels or secondary to other conditions. Immune complexes, formed in antigen excess and aided by increased vascular permeability, are deposited along vascular basement membrane. Subsequently, complement is activated and an inflammatory infiltrate develops. Giant cells may form. Ultimately, fibrinoid necrosis and/or weakness of the vascular connective tissue develop as a result of enzymes released from the inflammatory cells. These mechanisms then result in the syndrome of vascular inflammation, increased vascular permeability, focal fibrinoid necrosis, aneurysmal formation, and intimal proliferation.

POLYARTERITIS NODOSA

The polyarteritis nodosa group of vasculitides includes classic polyarteritis nodosa (PN), allergic granulomatosis (AG), and an "overlap syndrome" combining features of both. Segmental necrotizing lesions are noted in the small muscular arteries, particularly near bifurcations, with occasional distal spread to involve arterioles or transverse spread to involve adjacent veins. Lesions of various stages of inflammation are present, and the lesion often progresses to vessel wall degeneration with intimal proliferation and thrombosis. Allergic granulomatosis differs pathologically by more involvement of smaller vessels and the presence of giant cells and granulomas.

Both PN and AG tend to involve virtually every organ system, although PN is said not to involve the lungs, which AG frequently does. AG is characteristically associated with marked eosinophilia, with tissue infiltration and granulomatous changes in the lesions. Patients generally have a history of atopy (particularly asthma). Organs frequently involved include the kidneys, liver, and visceral vasculature.

Symptoms of both may be nonspecific (malaise and weight loss); organ-specific symptoms are often the presenting manifestations. Men are more commonly affected than women, and the peak occurrence is during the third and fourth decades of life.

The most common manifestations are abdominal pain, nausea, diarrhea, or gastrointestinal bleeding due to mesenteric vasculitis. Arthralgias and myalgias are common. The kidneys are involved in up to 80% of patients (with both glomerulosclerosis and large vessel vasculitis), and renal angiography is diagnostic (noting medium vessel segmental aneurysmal formation). Proteinuria or hematuria are common early manifestations. Hypertension frequently occurs early. Renal involvement may progress to renal failure. Skin involvement (subcutaneous nodules or vasculitic ulcers) affects half of patients. Peripheral neuropathy is noted in one-third of patients. CNS changes are uncommon. Pleuritis, pericarditis, myocarditis, and coronary arteritis may each affect about one-fourth of patients.

Leukocytosis and an elevated ESR are noted in most patients. Hepatitis B surface antigen is frequently present (in more than one-third), and may have a pathophysiologic role in that it has been found in immune complexes within vascular lesions. Histologic examination of clinically involved tissue is essential for diagnosis. The highest yield is obtained from testicular biopsy. Classic changes may be noted on renal angiography in patients with renal involvement; however, similar appearances may be noted with other syndromes, for example, in persons who are chronic intravenous drug abusers (heroin addicts).

Diagnostic difficulties in separating classic PN from AG have resulted in a third diagnosis (the "overlap syndrome"), with features intermediate between the two.

Treatment with corticosteroids (0.5-1.0 mg/kg/day) have improved 5-year survival from less than 15% to about 50%. Immunosuppressive therapy should be added if the patient does not improve with steroids. Chronic heparin therapy may decrease the incidence of thromboocclusive events.

WEGENER'S GRANULOMATOSIS

Although the etiology of Wegener's granulomatosis (WG) remains unknown, clinical and pathologic distinctions that separate it from the other vasculitides include the classic triad of a necrotizing granulomatous vasculitis of the upper and lower respiratory tract, focal glomerulonephritis, and a generalized, focal, small-vessel, necrotizing vasculitis. The granulomatous reaction may involve pulmonary parenchyma, resulting in large masses which may cavitate. Involvement may be limited to the lungs or other organs, sparing the kidneys, and this is known as limited Wegener's.

The peak age of onset occurs from 30-50 years with no sex predilection; the limited form is seen much more commonly in females. All patients have lung involvement, and more than 90% have involvement of the nasopharynx or sinuses. Twenty percent of all patients have no renal involvement (limited Wegener's). Transient arthralgias, vasculitic skin ulcers, and serous otitis media are each seen in over one-third. Peripheral neuropathy, pericarditis, and coronary arteritis are each noted in about one-fourth.

Diagnosis rests on histologic examination of affected tissue. Nonspecific manifestations include mild anemia, mild leukocytosis, and an elevated ESR. Renal involvement may manifest initially as hematuria or proteinuria before progressing to renal failure. Bony erosions may occur in conjunction with sinus involvement, and "saddle nose" may result.

Rapidly fatal courses (mean survival less than 6 months) have been observed in untreated patients and patients treated only with corticosteroids. The addition of cytotoxic immunosuppressives to the regimen markedly improves survival (particularly in patients with limited Wegener's), with the mean survival well over 2 years and occasional permanent remissions.

GIANT CELL ARTERITIS

Giant cell arteritis is a generic term encompassing both temporal (or cranial) arteritis and Takayasu's disease. Both are panarteritides, segmentally involving medium and large arteries, and both characteristically have electron microscopic evidence of degeneration of the internal elastic lamina of the vessels, which may be immune-mediated. Both may involve the aortic arch and its cranial branches; the cranial vessel involvement is more prominent and characteristic in temporal arteritis, whereas Takayasu's disease may involve any of the major arteries.

Temporal arteritis. This disease almost always occurs after the age of 55, with females predominating. Classic manifestations include fever, very high ESR (usually greater than 100 mm/hour), anemia, and headaches with tender, enlarged temporal arteries. Early symptoms may be vague and nonspecific, such as malaise, anorexia, and weight loss. Sudden blindness may occur in up to 50% of untreated people. Aortic aneurysms or claudication of the extremities may occur. Aside from the marked elevation of the ESR, anemia is frequently seen. Tests of liver function are often abnormal (despite no characteristic histologic picture) and revert to normal with treatment. Early temporal artery biopsy should be performed when the diagnosis is considered, noting that involvement may be segmental and that multiple or bilateral biopsies may be necessary. The manifestations of temporal arteritis are exquisitely sensitive to corticosteroids (0.5-1.0 mg/kg/day of prednisone), which should be continued at a lower maintenance level (0.1-0.2 mg/kg/day) for at least 1-2 years.

Polymyalgia rheumatica (PMR). PMR is so frequently associated with temporal arteritis that many consider them part of the same syndrome. Twenty to 50% of those with PMR have temporal arteritis. Manifestations include proximal muscle morning stiffness, myalgias, and low back pain. Serum muscle enzymes and electromyograms are normal. Only mild atrophy without inflammation is seen on muscle biopsy. The ESR is characteristically greater than 50. Consideration should always be given to performing one or several temporal artery biopsies in patients diagnosed as having PMR, even in the absence of classic symptoms of temporal arteritis. Isolated PMR characteristically responds to low doses of corticosteroids (0.2 mg/kg/day of prednisone).

Takayasu's disease. "Pulseless disease" is a less common arteritis (particularly of the aortic arch) more often seen in younger individuals (second or third decade), females, and Orientals. Nonspecific manifestations of fever, anorexia, and weight loss often precede symptoms of pain specifically referrable to the areas of involvement. Bruits are frequently noted, and ultimately symptoms of decreased or absent blood flow occur owing to intimal proliferation and thrombosis of the narrow lumen. Renal artery involvement may lead to hypertension. Although occasionally spontaneous remissions occur, the disease generally follows a progressive downhill course to death within 2-4 years. Although steroids may be tried, no clear benefit has yet been demonstrated.

HYPERSENSITIVITY VASCULITIS

Hypersensitivity vasculitis (HV) is a group of immune complex-mediated small vessel vasculitides in which the response results from a hypersensitivity reaction to an antigen. Other terms include small vessel vasculitis, allergic vasculitis, and leukocytoclastic (from the fragmented neutrophils commonly observed in the lesion) angiitis. The lesions typically involve small vessels (arterioles and venules) with necrotizing inflammation. No granulomas form. All lesions are characteristically at the same histologic stage, reflecting the single point antigen challenge and response characteristic of the pathophysiology. Any age and both sexes may be affected. A history of recent drug exposure (particularly penicillin or sulfa) or viral illness is often elicited. Often, the patient has a malignancy (particularly lymphoreticular) or connective tissue disease (particularly RA or SLE). The skin is involved in almost all. Palpable purpura is classic, but vesicles, ulcers, nodules, or urticaria may be noted. Occasionally, other organs are involved, with manifestations similar to those described for other vasculitides.

Distinct syndromes encompassed by hypersensitivity vasculitis include serum sickness, Henoch-Schoenlein purpura, essential mixed cryoglobulinemia, vasculitis associated with connective tissue diseases, and vasculitis associated with malignancy. Mild anemia, moderate leukocytosis, and an elevated ESR are common. A broad evaluation should search for other organ involvement as well as for possible associated conditions. Histologic examination of affected tissues is essential. Treatment hinges on removal of the offending antigen or treatment of the underlying disease. High-dose corticosteroids (0.5-1.0 mg/kg/day of prednisone) may limit the severity of the manifestations.

SJÖGREN'S DISEASE

Sjögren syndrome is a chronic systemic inflammatory disease of autoimmune origin. Mikulicz (1892) first described the parotid gland features of the syndrome, and Sjogren (1933) the ocular features.

The syndrome is one of dry, inflamed mucous membranes (sicca syndrome), particularly of the eyes (keratoconjuctivitis sicca) and mouth (xerostomia); both result from decreased exocrine gland secretions and associated atrophy. Mucous membranes may be involved. Arthritis, usually rheumatoid, is the third feature of the syndrome, and two of the three features are required for diagnosis. Terminology in this disorder has become increasingly confusing, and presently the dry mucous membranes feature is termed sicca syndrome (SS), the association with RA is called SS-RA, and the association of SS with other arthritides is called Sjogren. When RA is associated, it precedes the onset of SS by an average of 10 years in three-fourths of patients.

The peak age incidence is 40-60, and 90% of the patients are female. Although the etiology is not known, autoimmunity mediates the pathophysiology. Association with HLA-B8 and HLA-Dw3 suggest genetic predisposition. Elevated immunoglobulin levels, IgM-RF, ANA, antithyroid antibodies, and others, are abnormalities suggesting an autoimmune basis. Almost half of patients without rheumatoid arthritis have antibodies to a lymphoid nuclear antigen (SS-B or Ha), while an antisalivary duct antibody is found with SS-RA but less commonly in pure SS. SS-RA may represent a secondary form in which the course is more gradual and less deranging than pure SS.

Pathologic features include early lymphocytic infiltrates around exocrine gland ducts with inflammation, increasing infiltrates, and atrophy of the glandular tissue. During the process, intermittent obstruction of the duct from dried secretions and narrowing (from periductal inflammation and hypertrophy of the lining cells) result in dilatation of the proximal ducts and glandular swelling. Changes are present in minor glands as well, and a lip biopsy is highly sensitive. In addition, widespread lymphocytic infiltrates form in most organs and may produce a picture of pseudolymphoma. This disease provides a link between autoimmunity and the lymphoproliferative diseases, since these patients are at a more than 40-fold increased risk of developing lymphoma.

Ocular manifestations include burning, itching, or a "gritty" sensation in the eyes; however, up to one-half of those with pathologic abnormalities have no ocular complaints. Xerostomia is accompanied by dry cracked mucosa and a red, smooth tongue. Salivary gland enlargement, usually parotid, is usually bilateral and noted in up to half of patients; enlargement may be acute, painful, and recurrent, or chronic and painless. Recurrent painful acute episodes of enlargement are observed in over three-fourths of patients with pure SS, but are infrequent with SS-RA.

Purpura and lymphadenopathy are each seen in about half of people with SS alone and infrequently in SS-RA. Other clinical manifestations in one-fourth to one-third of patients with SS alone and uncommonly in SS-RA include Raynaud's phenomenon, splenomegaly, myositis, renal involvement (renal tubular acidosis, nephrogenic diabetes insipidus, or chronic interstitial nephritis), and pulmonary involvement (commonly a fibrosing alveolitis). Waldenstrom's macroglobulinemia is occasionally seen, particularly with pure SS.

The frequency of various conditions in patients with Sjögren's syndrome and the frequency of Sjögren's syndrome in various conditions provides insight into its immunologic basis.

Frequency of various diseases in patients with Sjögren's: RA, 35-55%; PSS, 5-8%; primary biliary cirrhosis or chronic active hepatitis, 6%; SLE, 4-5%; polymyositis, 2-4%.

Frequency of Sjögren's in patients with various diseases: SLE, 50%; RA, 25-30%; PSS, 40-50%; chronic active hepatitis, 35%; primary biliary cirrhosis, 50-100%; fibrosing alveolitis, 22%.

DIAGNOSIS

All patients with SS-RA have elevated titers of RF, but 80% with SS alone have similar elevations. Anti-SS-B may be useful but is also positive in 12% of patients with SLE and no SS. The

Schirmer test, a rough estimate of tear production, has numerous variables that decrease its reliability, although combined with Rose Bengal staining, stimulation with ammonia, and slit lamp examination for keratitis, the test becomes quite useful. Parotid flow measurements, sialography, and even radionucleide (^{131}I or ^{91}Tc) scintigraphy may be useful. Regardless of results, precise diagnosis continues to rest on histologic examination. Lip biopsy is accessible, simple, sensitive, specific, and a good index of the severity of the disease process. Beta-2-microglobulin is a protein component of cellular membranes. It is increased in quantities in the serum and exocrine secretions of these patients in proportion to the severity of the disease process, and has been implicated as possibly playing a role in the pathophysiology.

Treatment for limited disease is symptomatic and consists of lubricants such as artificial tears to avoid irritative and damaging keratitis especially of the cornea. Frequent fluids, chewing gum, and adequate hydration will minimize symptoms of xerostomia. Salivary duct calculi should be diagnosed early and removed promptly. Analgesics may be necessary for acute glandular enlargement. Surgical removal of salivary glands for chronic enlargement or frequent acute episodes must be avoided; this only reduces salivary secretions further. Steroids or immunosuppressive agents should be reserved for life-threatening systemic involvement.

DEGENERATIVE JOINT DISEASE

Degenerative joint disease (DJD, or osteoarthritis) is the most common of the arthritides. By age 40, over 85% of people have radiologic changes. Under the age of 50 men are more commonly affected, but after 50 the prevalence is greater in women. By age 70, virtually all individuals are affected.

DJD, traditionally an expected accompaniment of aging, has been called "wear-and-tear" disease. It is a disease of cartilage. The chronic trauma of weight bearing, as well as acute trauma and infection, may result in loss of cartilage. The proteoglycan component of ground substance in cartilage is gradually lost. Subchondral and marginal bone proliferates. Chondrocytes increase in number but eventually become ineffective in maintaining proteoglycan and collagen production. As the process continues, cartilage thins, flakes, and cracks. Continued use of the joint denudes the cartilage surface, and subchondral sclerosis and cyst formation occur. Characteristic joint space narrowing (from loss of cartilage) and osteophytic spurs (from marginal bone proliferation) are noted.

Inflammation is typically absent; however, hydroxyapatite crystals may be deposited and may then lead to a mild inflammatory response.

DJD is usually noninflammatory and chronic, and it affects joints subjected to chronic or subacute stress. Secondary DJD may also occur as a sequela to infection or acute trauma to a joint. Any joint may be affected with aching on motion or stress, stiffness, and bony enlargement. The disease is usually oligoarticular at the onset and insidiously involves other joints. Early joints frequently involved include the metacarpophalangeal and interphalangeal joints as well as the hips and knees. Heberden's nodes, lateral bony enlargement of the base of the terminal phalanx at the DIP, are common, and Bouchard's nodes, with similar findings in the PIP, may also occur.

An acute inflammatory form of DJD known as erosive osteoarthritis may occasionally develop, particularly in the hands and the DIP joints. Acute pain, swelling, and erythema occur, and Heberden nodes frequently develop subsequently.

Diagnosis is made by excluding the inflammatory arthritides. The ESR is typically normal. Radiologic changes include joint space narrowing and osteophytic spurring occasionally with subchondral cyst formation. Radioopaque cartilage fragments may be free in the joint space. Effusions are clear and viscous and usually have less than 3000 white cells per cu mm.

Treatment begins with rest of the involved joint and application of heat locally. Gradually progressive exercise with the avoidance of strain is important. Despite the general noninflammatory character of the disease, nonsteroidal antiinflammatory agents may frequently be of benefit. Debridement of loose deforming cartilage or joint replacement may be necessary for intractable discomfort or loss of normal motion. Total replacement of hips, knees, and other joints has remarkably changed the outlook for these patients.

DISEASES ASSOCIATED WITH ARTHRITIS
Sarcoidosis

Joint involvement is noted in 10-15% of patients with sarcoidosis. Another 5% of patients have bone cysts, particularly in the hands and feet. Acute migratory polyarthritis of large joints is noted with acute flare-ups of sarcoidosis and usually lasts less than 6 weeks. A chronic large and small joint polyarthritis may develop owing to granulomatous involvement of the synovium and articular surfaces. Swollen painful fingers, sarcoid dactylitis, show diffuse osteitis on x-ray examination. Granulomatous tenosynovitis may also occur. Joint destruction is unusual with both forms unless bone cysts erode through articular surfaces. Although hyperuricemia and a positive rheumatoid factor are occasionally present, gout and RA are generally not. Treatment of the arthritis is symptomatic.

Erythema nodosum, a frequent accompaniment of sarcoidosis, may also be noted with streptococcal infections, infectious granulomatous diseases, inflammatory bowel disease, and drugs such as oral contraceptives and sulfonamides. Most often, however, there is no associated or underlying disease. Patients develop painful nodular lesions of the lower extremities and frequently have an inflammatory arthritis.

Relapsing Polychondritis

This is a rare inflammatory destructive disease of cartilage, which most commonly involves the ears and nose. It is noted most often in middle-aged persons. Loss of cartilagenous support leads to collapse of involved tissue. Fever, iritis and episcleritis, and hearing loss are relatively common. Cataracts or aortic insufficiency may develop. When the tracheobronchial tree is involved, collapse results in death. Involvement of articular cartilage leads to an inflammatory erosive arthritis. Anemia and elevated ESR are common. Biopsy of involved cartilage is recommended for diagnosis. Corticosteroids will effectively control the disease.

Familial Mediterranean Fever

Familial Mediterranean fever (FMF, or familial paroxysmal polyserositis) is a disorder seen particularly in Sephardic Jews, Arabs, and Armenians. It occurs in autosomal recessive and sporadic patterns, and the etiology and pathophysiology are not known. Manifestations usually begin in childhood and consist of episodic fever, peritonitis, pleuritis, and arthritis (in decreasing order of frequency), with occasional painful erythematous skin lesions or associated amyloidosis. The attacks generally last 1-2 days and recur every 2-4 weeks. Fever is almost always present, may reach 40°C, and is often preceded by a chill. Abdominal pain is also almost always present, becoming generalized after several hours of localized symptoms. Findings are consistent with peritonitis. Nausea, vomiting, and abdominal distention usually occur. Radiographs reveal an edematous small intestinal wall and paralytic ileus. Pleuritis, often unilateral, is observed in three-fourths of patients, and transient pleural effusions are occasionally seen. Three-fourths of patients develop episodic nondestructive monoarticular arthritis of the large joints, which lasts from a few days to 3 weeks. Large painful erythematous lesions of the lower extremities and feet are noted in one-third of patients and last only 1-2 days. Systemic amyloidosis is not uncommon.

Leukocytosis and elevated ESR are almost always present during exacerbations. Radiographic changes are usually nonspecific, although generalized and subchondral osteoporosis may be seen. Synovial biopsies are equally nonspecific; amyloid deposits may occasionally be noted.

The only agent found useful has been colchicine, which may be used both acutely (0.6 mg hourly for 4 doses, q2h for 2 doses, then q12h for 4 doses) or prophylactically (0.6 mg two or three times a day). Recently, hemodialysis has been effective.

Amyloid Deposits and Amyloidosis

Amyloid was first described by Virchow (1853); he thought it was of polysaccharide composition; it was later classified by Reimann into four types: (1) *primary,* involving mesenchymal organs, (2) *secondary,* involving parenchymal organs, (3) *amyloid associated with myeloma,* and (4) isolated organ amyloidosis that embraced *senile cerebral and cardiac involvement.* Recent studies have shown that the distinctive Congo red staining property is related to an unusual protein that has a beta-pleated sheet structure and has been called a beta-fibril; this unusual protein is found in invertebrates (silkworm) but not in healthy vertebrate tissue. It is highly insoluble, making in vivo removal a major problem.

The amyloid in primary amyloidosis is derived from immunoglobulin light chains and designated AL; that in secondary amyloidosis may contain immunoglobulin fragments but is composed primarily of a unique fibrillar protein designated as AA protein. AA protein isolated from patients has an almost identical N-terminal amino acid sequence. A circulating protein antigenically related to the AA protein (SAA), found in human serum, may be a precursor of tissue AA protein, and seems related to both the genetic background and the type of amyloidogenic stimulus (rheumatoid arthritis, osteomyelitis, etc.) in a given individual. Glenner has used this new information (Table 5-4) to revise the Reimann classification.

Immunocyte-derived amyloidosis. The "primary" or monoclonal protein type occurs in middle-aged and older individuals; almost all have evidence of monoclonal Bence-Jones protein in urine or serum (or both) and excessive plasma cells on bone marrow examination (see Amyloid Cardiomyopathy, page 33).

Reactive amyloidosis. The "secondary" type has been reported in 14-26% of patients with rheumatoid arthritis and with ankylosing spondylitis, Reiter's syndrome, psoriatic arthritis, chronic rheumatic heart disease, dermatomyositis, scleroderma, Behcet's syndrome, and systemic lupus. It is also seen with chronic infections such as tuberculosis, leprosy, paraplegia with decubitus ulcers and pyelonephritis, bronchiectasis, osteomyelitis, syphilis, ulcerative colitis, regional enteritis, malaria, and chronically infected burns. It involves liver, spleen, kidneys, and adrenals and may present as the nephrotic syndrome.

Organ limited amyloidosis. This is common in the elderly; cerebral deposition seems associated with dementia, while cardiac deposition can produce ventricular dysfunction, conduction defects, and arrhythmias.

TABLE 5-4—NEWER CLASSIFICATION OF AMYLOID

Clinicopathologic Process	Major Fibril Protein
Acquired systemic amyloidosis	
Immunocyte dyscrasias with amyloidosis (primary of Reimann)	
Monoclonal gammopathy (not overtly neoplastic)	AL
Plasma cell myeloma	AL
Waldenstrom macroglobulinemia	AL
Heavy chain disease	AL
Agammaglobulinemia	AL
Other immunocytic neoplasms	AL
Reactive systemic amyloidosis (Secondary of Reimann)	
Acute recurrent and chronic suppurative or granulomatous	AA
Infections (tuberculosis)	
Chronic inflammatory conditions (rheumatoid arthritis)	AA
Hodgkin's disease	AA
Solid tumors such as renal and bladder adenocarcinoma	?
Heredofamilial systemic amyloidosis	
Familial Mediterranean fever	AA
Other neuropathic and non-neuropathic forms	?
Organ Limited	
Immunocyte derived	AL
Cardiovascular (senile)	ASc_1
Cerebral	?
Cutaneous	?
Localized deposition	Varies with location
Adapted from Glenner	

SERONEGATIVE SPONDYLOARTHRITIDES (HLA-B27-ASSOCIATED ARTHROPATHY)

Tissue compatibility factors in animals were discovered early in this century. Human antibodies (leukoagglutinins) to foreign white blood cells were noted in 1954, resulting in the term human leukocyte antigens (HLA). Subsequently, these protein antigens were found to reside on the surface of all cells. They interact with either humoral immunoglobulin (serologically detectable, or SD, antigens) or lymphocytes (lymphocyte detectable, or LD, antigens). The genetic locus (H-2 complex) that codes for these antigens is found in a short region of chromosome 6 and very near loci coding for synthesis of C_2, properdin factor B, and beta 2 microglobulin. Four distinct loci are present in the H-2 complex for coding LD (HLA-D) and SD (HLA-B, HLA-C, and HLA-A) antigens (given in the sequence of location away from the chromosome's centromere). In addition, immune response gene (Ir genes), which regulate lymphocyte immune recognition and cell-cell interaction, are thought to reside between the HLA-D and HLA-B loci. Whether the antigens themselves or nearby tightly linked genes result in the expression of disease directly or by predisposing to abnormal responses to a trigger is unknown. Although four loci are present, the A and B loci are considered most important for tissue typing. These two genes are assumed to be codominant, and the presence of two chromosomes results in a potential of four major HLA antigens. Each antigen (or allele) is given a number relating to the HLA locus. Identified, but not yet internationally approved, antigens are given a prefix of w.

An increased occurrence of certain HLA antigens has been noted with several diseases. HLA-A2 has been associated with congenital heart disease, and A3 with hemochromatosis. HLA-Dw2 has been associated with multiple sclerosis, and Dw4 with RA. Increased occurrence of HLA-Dw3 has been seen in patients with Sjögren's syndrome, chronic active hepatitis, and celiac disease. SLE is associated with HLA-DRw2 and HLA-DRw3. The best-studied and most homogenous group of HLA-associated diseases are the B27-associated arthropathies. These include ankylosing spondylitis, Reiter's syndrome, and psoriatic arthritis as well as intestinal (inflammatory bowel disease) arthropathy and JRA (particularly when associated with spondylitis or sacro-ileitis).

Ankylosing Spondylitis

Ankylosing spondylitis (AS), previously also known as rheumatoid spondylitis and Marie-Strumpell disease, is a chronic insidious inflammatory disease of the axial skeleton associated with pain and stiffening of the sacroiliac joints and spine. The disease most commonly affects young, white males. The onset is usually in the 20s, 90% of patients are male, and blacks are infrequently affected.

Up to 95% of Caucasians with AS have the HLA-B27 antigen versus about half of black Americans with AS. These figures compare to the normal prevalence of B27 in the population of 7% among whites, 4% for black Americans, and a virtual absence in black Africans. Because B27 is codominant and autosomal, it will be found in half of first-degree relatives of patients with AS. Radiographic evidence of AS develops in 20% of males who have the B27 antigen, even though most have either no symptoms or only mild backaches.

Pathologically, the synovial inflammation in AS appears identical to that seen in RA. The predilection for progressive stiffening of the axial skeleton with ossification of ligaments and syndesmophyte formation resulting in bony ankylosis appears related to the presence of inflammation at the sites of attachment of ligaments to bones. The heavy calcification immediately surrounding the spine may lead to the characteristic radiographically apparent "bamboo spine."

The onset is insidious and, although frequently asymptomatic, may manifest as aching low back pain and morning stiffness. The age and morning stiffness are important clues for early diagnosis; nonetheless, about half the patients are misdiagnosed at this stage, and AS is not recognized for months to years. Large peripheral joint arthritis (particularly the knees) is noted early in about 20%, and eventually in about one-third. Two-thirds of patients have arthritis of the hip joints. Gradually, restriction of motion of the entire spine develops, with an associated restriction of motion of the thoracic cage. A stooped-over posture is adopted for comfort, and fixed thoracic kyphosis results. Other associated manifestations include acute anterior uveitis (in 25% and often recurrent). Much less commonly observed are aortic regurgitation (due to focal medial necrosis of the proximal aorta and resultant dilation of the aortic ring) and conduction defects (due to fibrous or amyloid deposition), the cauda equina syndrome (lumbosacral sensorimotor loss due to nerve entrapment and posterior diverticular herniation of dura), a peculiar bilateral upper lobe pulmonary fibrosis, and amyloidosis with renal involvement leading to renal failure. Older patients previously treated with x-ray therapy have occasionally been found to have a cauda equina syndrome resulting from sarcoma.

Symmetric bilateral sacroiliitis is common and seen early. Atlantoaxial subluxation may be demonstrated in up to 20% of patients. Radiographs of peripheral joints demonstrates an erosive arthritis similar to that seen with RA. The diagnosis remains clinical and should be considered in patients with chronic low back pain and stiffness, which usually responds to antiinflammatory agents, but not to rest and limited motion of the spine or thoracic cage. Typical radiographic appearance is quite helpful. The presence of HLA-B27 antigen should be regarded as a confirmatory test with primary utility when the clinical complex is not typical. It may have a role in the genetic counseling of families with members who have AS.

Reiter's Syndrome

Reiter's syndrome (RS) is classically considered to represent a triad of arthritis, urethritis, and conjunctivitis; however, mucocutaneous lesions are frequently present, and any component may be absent for variable periods of time.

Young males between 20 and 40 are most frequently affected. The etiology is uncertain, but attacks may follow attacks of amebic, bacillary, or nonspecific dysentery or venereal diseases due to *Chlamydia* or *Mycoplasma.* The dysenteric form occurs in an epidemic pattern, whereas the venereal form has an endemic pattern. The pathophysiologic basis for systemic expression of the disease is unknown. Males account for more than 90% of patients with the epidemic form and 98% of those with the endemic form. HLA-B27 is present in well over half (up to 96%) of patients with the endemic form, over 90% of those with the epidemic form, and virtually all patients regardless of type when there is associated spondylitis or sacroiliitis.

Pathologically, there is a dense lymphocytic infiltration of the dermis, with overlying epidermal hyperkeratosis and microabscesses of the skin known as keratoderma blenorrhagica, histologically indistinguishable from pustular psoriasis. Onycholysis and subungual keratosis are common. Similar dermal changes occur in the mucous membranes (particularly of the palate and tongue); however, the overlying mucosal epithelium is denuded and generally painless. Small (2-3 mm) superficial ulcers form on the glans penis and may coalesce, forming circinate balanitis. Synovial changes are nonspecific, erosive, and similar to those of RA.

Clinical manifestations are generally first seen 1-4 weeks after sexual exposure or diarrhea. Urethritis is usually the first symptom and is followed days to weeks later by the other components of the syndrome. Aside from arthritis, which may be pauci- or polyarticular, other rheumatologic complaints include arthralgias, tenosynovitis, and fasciitis. The arthritis is asymmetric and tends to affect the lumbar vertebrae, sacroiliac joints, knees, ankles, and toes. Synovitis of the PIP and DIP joints may produce "sausage" digits. The mucocutaneous lesions and urethritis may be painless. Prostatitis may be observed in three-fourths of patients. Conjunctivitis occurs in most patients; some develop iridocyclitis. Conjunctivitis, urethritis, and prostatitis tend to subside in several days. Mucocutaneous lesions may persist for weeks, and arthritic complaints may last from 2-6 months before spontaneous remission. Diarrhea frequently precedes the other clinical features, even in the endemic venereal form. Aortic regurgitation and conduction defects may occur (by the same mechanisms noted with AS), and myocarditis and pericarditis occasionally develop. Conjunctivitis or iridocyclitis may recur much later in the absence of other manifestations. Some patients develop a chronic polyarthritis, and these have periodic recurrences of other components of the syndrome.

Elevated ESR and mild leukocytosis are common. HLA-B27 may be helpful if the syndrome is not classic. Reiter cells, macrophages that have ingested polymorphonuclear leukocytes, are nonspecific. The synovial fluid is cloudy with increased white cells (50,000/cu mm), poor mucin clot, and sterile cultures. Complement levels are normal in the synovial fluid in distinction to RA. Serologic autoantibodies are absent.

Treatment of the urethritis is as recommended for nongonococcal urethritis (NGU) and probably does not affect the occurrence or course of RS. The arthritis may be treated with nonsteroidal antiinflammatory agents. Intraarticular steroids may benefit persistent pauciarticular disease. Conjunctival lesions may require artificial tears. Iridocyclitis, when it occurs, may require intraocular steroids. Systemic steroids or immunosuppressive agents should be avoided.

Psoriatic Arthritis

Psoriatic arthritis is the occurrence of arthritis in about 7% of patients months to years following the onset of psoriasis. Females are affected slightly more often than males, and the peak onset is between 20 and 40. The etiology is unknown; however, 20% have the HLA-B27 antigen, and if the arthritis includes spondylitis the incidence approaches 90%.

Synovial inflammation (which is nonspecific and may be chronic), ankylosis of joints, and contractures are noted. The arthritis clinical activity does not parallel the skin lesions.

Clinical manifestations range from an asymmetric oligoarticular disease (70% of patients) involving the small joints (often associated with "sausage" digits), through symmetrical polyarticular disease (similar to RA), to a destructive polyarthritis known as arthritis mutilans. Sacroiliitis or spondylitis is found occasionally. Anemia and elevated ESR are common. Hyperuricemia is seen in up to 20% of patients. Radiographs reveal destruction and ankylosis; the "pencil in cup" deformity of the digits results from "whittling" resorption of bone distally, which appears radiographically to set in a "cup" formed by erosion of the proximal surface of adjacent bone. Treatment is similar to that for RA, except for antimalarials, which may produce an exfoliative dermatitis and are contraindicated in psoriasis. Methotrexate may be beneficial in persons with arthritis mutilans.

Arthritis of Inflammatory Bowel Disease

Approximately 20% of patients with regional enteritis (Crohn's disease) or ulcerative colitis develop an associated arthritis. Either of two types of arthritis may develop. The most common is an acute inflammatory pauciarticular arthritis, which generally involves large joints particularly of the lower extremities. Attacks tend to slightly follow and parallel the clinical course of the enteritis or colitis and usually last up to 6 weeks. Joint destruction is unusual. Erythema nodosum and uveitis may be noted. Ankylosing spondylitis is the second type, and accounts for about 40% of the arthritis in these patients. Both sexes are affected equally. HLA-B27 antigen is found in 50-70%.

Arthralgias or migratory nondestructive arthritis may be seen in up to 90% of patients with Whipple's disease and frequently precede other manifestations of the disease. The PAS-staining granules and bacteria-like particles frequently observed in the bowel lesions are not found in joint fluid or synovial tissue.

Behcet's Syndrome

This triad of recurrent oral and genital ulcers and uveitis is common in men (2:1) in their 20s or 30s and particularly in persons with Mediterranean or Japanese ancestry. Other frequently associated features include polyarthritis, cutaneous vasculitis and erythema nodosum or multiforme, colitis, and phlebitis (associated with decreased fibrinolytic activity). Involvement may also include the CNS, pericardium, or lung. The underlying pathologic lesion is diffuse vasculitis of the capillaries and venules. An immune-mediated cause is probable. Renal vasculitis or glomerulonephritis are uncommon, although renal amyloidosis occasionally occurs. The arthritis is common, pauci- or polyarticular (particularly the large joints), intermittent, and nondeforming. Anemia, leukocytosis, elevated ESR, and polyclonal gammopathy are common. A mild elevation of neutrophils and mononuclear cells in the CSF is noted, with active CNS involvement. About 20,000/cu mm neutrophils are usually found in synovial fluid from arthritic joints. Synovial biopsy reveals nonspecific inflammation. Radiographs are unremarkable. The diagnosis is clinical. Steroids may improve the uveitis and neurologic disturbances, but not the arthritis. Immunosuppressive agents may be considered in the management of progressive multisystem disease.

DISEASES CAUSED BY INFECTIOUS AGENTS
Infectious Arthritis

Infectious arthritis may be either acute or chronic, is generally monoarticular, and is frequently metastatic from another focus but may also result from penetrating trauma or direct spread from contiguous areas. Agents involved include bacteria (and mycobacteria), fungi, *Treponema pallidum,* and viruses.

Acute bacterial (septic or pyogenic) arthritis. May result from bacteremia with organisms such as *Neisseria gonorrheae, S. aureus, Strep. pyogenes, Strep. pneumoniae, H. influenzae, E. coli,* and *Pseudomonas, Proteus,* and *Salmonella* species. An acute monoarticular arthritis is common, but multiple joints may be involved. Large joints are usually affected, although joints in which arthritis or prosthetic surfaces have been present are particularly frequent sites. Predisposing factors include debilitation, diabetes, alcoholism, congenital or acquired immune deficiencies, and treatment with immunosuppressive agents. Arthrocentesis for culture and sensitivity is mandatory. The preexistence of other arthritic conditions should not mislead the physician. The fluid is generally cloudy or purulent, with white counts exceeding 50,000/cu mm and glucose less than 50% of the serum glucose. Radiographs may show only evidence of an effusion. Prompt treatment with appropriate antibiotics given intravenously should continue for a minimum of 2 weeks. Gonorrhea, the most common bacterial arthritis in adults, may be treated with oral agents after the acute infection appears controlled. Frequent joint aspiration to remove all purulent material and rest of the involved joint will usually prevent restrictive sequelae. Open surgical drainage may be required for hip infections or other joints when poorly responsive to therapy.

Tuberculous arthritis. This disease is usually metastatic in children. The large joints of the lower extremities and the vertebral bodies, particularly thoracic (Pott's disease), are most commonly affected. A destructive deforming arthritis may ensue. Atypical mycobacteria may produce a similar picture. The effusion demonstrates a moderately elevated white count, and synovial biopsy may be necessary for diagnosis. Specific skin tests may be suggestive. Surgical debridement or synovectomy may be necessary.

Fungi. Fungi may produce oligo- or polyarticular disease, which when untreated may result in joint destruction. Synovial biopsy may be required for diagnosis. Systemic antifungal therapy is necessary, and occasionally surgical exposure is required.

Syphilis. This may produce several syndromes. Congenital syphilis may result in osteochondritis in infancy and a synovitis in the teenage years. Polyarthritis may occur in secondary syphilis and tertiary syphilis may produce gummatous involvement of the synovium. Syphilitic denervation may result in a neuropathic (Charcot) joint (discussed separately).

Viruses. May produce migratory polyarthritis through infection or immune complex disease. Both rubella and hepatitis B virus produce migratory polyarthralgias or polyarthritis, and similarly may be observed following immunization with live attenuated rubella virus.

Osteomyelitis

Infection of bone may occur from direct spread (penetrating trauma or contiguous infection) or hematogenous seeding. Rapidly growing bone and bone with poor vascular supply are the most susceptible. The metaphyses of long bones are particularly susceptible. Children account for more than 80% of cases of osteomyelitis, and *Staph. aureus* is the etiologic agent in almost two-thirds. Involvement of multiple sites is noted in 7% of patients. Virtually any organism, including *Mycobacteria* and fungi, may produce osteomyelitis. Patients with sickle cell disease or postsplenectomy are prone to *Salmonella* osteomyelitis, although the most common organism is still *Staphylococcus.* The majority of patients present with the subacute development of pain, fever, chills, and malaise. Over one-third may present with only vague symptoms, which progress insidiously. Radiographic evidence includes focal osteolytic lesions, new bone formation, and periosteal elevation, but these findings follow the clinical onset by 1-3 weeks. Initial management must be determined by analyzing clinical circumstances. A focus of origin should always be sought and antibiotic therapy guided by bacteriologic information. Parenteral therapy should be given for 3-6 weeks. Progression or unresponsiveness may require surgical drainage, extirpation, or even amputation to avoid chronic bacteremia and sepsis.

TRAUMATIC AND NEUROGENIC DISORDERS
Traumatic Arthritis
Direct noninvasive injury of any joint may result in acute inflammation, which often persists several days. The more hemorrhagic the effusion, the longer the arthritis persists. Gross hemorrhage into joints, particularly when recurrent, may result in joint destruction, fibrosis, and a deformed appearance with chronic swelling and synovial thickening. Hemophiliacs are particularly at risk and may develop arthritis with only walking or minimal trauma when factor levels are extremely low. Regardless of the cause, once developed a painless effusion may persist or recur over the ensuing several weeks or months. Treatment is with symptomatic analgesics. Arthrocentesis followed by elastic bandage wraps is recommended for hemorrhagic effusions to limit resultant joint damage.

Avascular Necrosis of Bone
Avascular necrosis of bone occurs more commonly in regions of limited collateral blood supply such as the femoral and humeral heads, the navicular and lunate bones of the wrist, and the talus

of the foot. Interference with vascular supply to these regions results in painless, insidious infarction and osteonecrosis. As fragmentation and joint deformity develop, pain and limitation of motion are manifested. Interruption of vascular supply may result from traumatic causes such as fracture (femoral or humeral heads) or dislocation (hip).

Atraumatic causes include hemoglobinopathies, vasculitides, infections, and Cushing syndrome. Occasionally, revascularization occurs; however, arthroplasty is necessary when destructive changes are severe.

Neuropathic Joint Disease

Neuropathic joint disease (Charcot joints) results from instability of the joint and insensitivity to chronic, recurrent minimal daily trauma. Neurologic disorders resulting in this progressive arthropathy include syphilis (tabes dorsalis), diabetes, syringomyelia, meningomyelocele, and other central and peripheral neuropathies. Depending on the region of neurosensory loss, weight-bearing joints are principally affected. Destruction of cartilage and subchondral bone, development of large marginal osteophytes, and the occurrence of fractures of the articular surface lead to disorganized joints. Pain, swelling, warmth, and sanguinous effusions are common. On examination, the joint is unstable, hypermobile, and crepitant; roentgenograms demonstrate these characteristics. Treatment consists principally of external stabilization of the joint and avoidance of trauma and weight bearing.

Carpel Tunnel Syndrome

Carpel tunnel syndrome, a classic entrapment neuropathy, is a distal neuropathy of the median nerve arising as a result of impingement of fluid or other structures within the flexor tendon sheath of the wrist. The disorder is most common in middle-aged women. Causes include edema, osteophytes, arthritis, and tenosynovitis. Thickening of tendon sheaths may occur from granulomata (tuberculosis or RA), amyloid deposition, myxedema, gout, and acromegaly. Lipomas or benign ganglionic cysts are also frequent causes. Bilateral involvement is frequent. Symptoms include numbness, tingling, and burning in the distribution of the median nerve, particularly at night. With progression, atrophy of the thenar eminence develops and is accompanied by decreased abduction and opposition of the thumb. Tinel's sign is an increase in symptoms elicited by percussion of the median nerve at the wrist or forced flexion of the wrist. Treatment of the underlying cause or injection of steroids locally (for inflammatory syndromes) may be temporarily beneficial. Surgical decompression is often necessary.

Myasthenia Gravis

Myasthenia gravis (MG) is a neuromuscular disorder which produces weakness and easy fatigability, particularly of muscles innervated by the cranial nerves. Females are affected three times as often as males. Although the disease affects patients of any age, the greatest prevalence is in the third decade, with a second peak occurring in elderly men. It appears to be an autoimmune disease, since most patients have IgG antibodies against the muscular acetylcholine receptor and also against the sarcoplasmic reticulum of skeletal muscle. Ten percent of patients have or develop thymoma (young women with this frequently have HLA-B8), and most have lymphoid follicle hyperplasia. An increased occurrence of other autoimmune phenomena (SLE, PSS, PA, RA, Hashimoto's thyroiditis, and Addison's disease) is observed. The disorder generally presents as gradually progressive weakness. Muscle groups frequently involved include ocular (90% develop double vision or ptosis), facial and pharyngeal (65% develop difficulty speaking, chewing, or swallowing), and occasionally proximal muscle weakness late in the course of the disorder. Respiratory muscle involvement may be heralded by the onset of progressive dyspnea. Clinical findings may be asymmetric. Rapid fatigability with repetitive motion is characteristic, and the patient states that strength improves with rest and gradually lessens during the course of the day. The pupils are virtually never involved. The more confined the distribution and the slower the earlier progression, the better the prognosis and response to therapy.

The Mary Walker phenomenon is the occurrence of increased muscle weakness in patients with MG when a humoral substance, probably lactic acid, is released into the circulation following ischemic exercise. Similar symptomatology accompanying certain malignant tumors, particularly oat cell carcinoma of the lungs, is known as the Eaton-Lambert syndrome. Muscle weakness and aching in this syndrome may occur before diagnosis of the tumor, involve the proximal muscle groups, and improve with each of the first few muscle contractions. The diagnosis of MG is made when strength is returned to fatiguing muscle groups following injection of edrophonium chloride (10 mg I.V.) or neostigmine (0.5 to 2.0 mg I.M.). The Eaton-Lambert syndrome is unresponsive to these agents. The short duration of action of edrophonium makes neostigmine preferable for managing acute attacks. Maintenance therapy usually consists of divided daily doses of pyridostigmine bromide orally. Excessive doses of any of these agents may produce paradoxical muscle weakness in addition to other cholinergic effects. Two-thirds of patients with thymoma will improve after thymectomy, and one-third of these have a complete remission. Progressive MG, despite the above measures, warrants a trial of high-dose corticosteroid therapy, which produces improvement in over three-fourths of patients. Unfortunately, protracted therapy with corticosteroids has many adverse effects, including steroid myopathy. Nondepolarizing muscle relaxants must be avoided because of the marked increase in the activity of these agents. Sedatives and antiarrhythmic agents may exacerbate the disorder.

DISORDERS OF BIOCHEMICAL AND ENDOCRINE ABNORMALITIES
Gout

Gout, first described by Hippocrates, is an acute or chronic arthritis due to urate crystal-initiated inflammation. More than 90% of patients are men; its onset is most common in the fourth decade, and its prevalence is about 3 in 1000.

Hyperuricemia results from increased uric acid production or decreased excretion. An important substrate, phosphoribosyl pyrophosphate (PRPP), is involved in the initial synthesis of uric acid precursors and also in its recycling by the enzyme phosphoribosyl transferase. Gout is frequently due to an increased production of PRPP; a congenital absence of the recycling transferase produces the Lesch-Nyhan syndrome (hyperuricemia with severe neurologic disturbances). Allopurinol blocks uric acid production from either hypoxanthine or xanthine, while probenecid decreases urate resorption.

The total body pool of urate is normally 1200 mg in males and 600 mg in females. On a purine-free diet, about half the pool turns over; two-thirds of urate excretion is renal (proximal resorption with distal secretion and reabsorption), the remainder gastrointestinal. The total pool may be increased 25-fold in tophaceous gout.

The incidence of gout rises progressively with increasing urate concentration. Seven mg/day, the concentration where physiochemical saturation occurs, is a useful upper limit of normal, but one-third of patients with gout will have lower concentrations, and many individuals with higher concentrations do not have gout.

Decreased excretion may occur with decreased filtration (global decrease in renal function) or decreased tubular secretion (specific tubular defects or competitive blockade of the organic acid secreting mechanism). Such competitive inhibition occurs in the presence of ketones or low levels of salicylate. *Increased excretion* occurs with cholecystographic contrast agents, guaiaphenesin, uricosuric agents (probenecid and sulfinpyrazone), or high levels of salicylate. Tubular defects in urate reabsorption are seen occasionally with carcinoma, Fanconi's syndrome, Wilson's disease, and rarely as an isolated defect.

More than 80% of men with serum urate levels exceeding 9 mg/day have or will develop gout, whereas only about 1% of the population with levels below 6 mg/day have or develop gout. In addition, the risk of nephrolithiasis rises from about 10% of men with excretion of 300 mg/day to about half of those excreting more than 1100 mg/day. Even with similar degrees of uricosemia or uricosuria, the risk of nephrolithiasis is markedly less in women. Eighty percent of patients with uric acid stones who do not have clinical gout have normal serum urate levels.

Regardless of the cause, as urate concentrations rise and saturation is exceeded, urate precipitates as a negatively birefringent crystal and is deposited in tissues, principally periarticular and renal. Polymorphonuclear leukocytes phagocytose these crystals and release enzymes, inciting inflammation. Colchicine inhibits PMN phagocytosis of urate crystals, and the anti-inflammatory agents inhibit the inflammatory response accompanying enzyme release.

Urate deposition and accompanying inflammation in the joint results in degeneration and destruction of cartilage and subchondral bone with proliferation of synovium and marginal bone, pannus formation, and occasionally fibrosis or ankylosis. Punched-out bony lesions and erosions may occur. Sodium urate deposits in the kidney tend to occur in the medulla, producing interstitial inflammation and uniform glomerulosclerosis. Gouty tophi, deposits of urate with surrounding inflammation, may develop in other cartilaginous or fibrous tissues including the ears, tendons, large joint bursa, and even the skin, eyelids, and sclera. Involvement of the myocardium or cardiac valves is infrequent. In idiopathic gout, acute gouty arthritis generally follows a period of asymptomatic hyperuricemia. Although neither predictive nor diagnostic, the higher the asymptomatic serum urate level, the more likely it is that gout or nephrolithiasis will occur.

Acute gouty arthritis characteristically involves peripheral joints. The initial joint involved in 50% of persons is the metatarsophalangeal joint of the great toe (podagra), occasionally is bilateral, and ultimately develops in 90% of patients. More than 80% of involved joints are in the lower extremities and include joints in the feet, ankles, and knees. There is generally no clear correlation between the occurrence of an attack and the serum urate level, which may possibly be secondary to the actions of endogenous hormones. Attacks may be triggered by dietary indiscretion (alcoholic binges or excessive meals), psychologic stress, or physical stress (inordinate exertion, trauma, or surgery).

After its onset, gout tends to occur spontaneously every several months to a few years with increasing frequency, increasing involvement of other joints, and decreasing response to therapy.

Several years of untreated, continuing hyperuricemia in persons with gout leads to visible tophaceous deposits and joint deformities in more than half. Effective early control of hyperuricemia in the patient with gout reduces the incidence of these chronic gouty changes to less than 20%. The tophi are generally painless; however, stiffness, chronic aching, and deformity of the joints may be noted. The later process of fragmentation of large tophi results in crippling and often bizarre deformities. Ulceration of the stretched skin over large tophi leads to drainage of the chalky material composed of monosodium urate crystals. Here again, the lower extremities are most often involved. Involvement of the hip or spine is distinctly uncommon.

Hypertension and albuminuria are each seen in one-third of patients with gout. Common defects in renal function include decreased concentrating ability, decreased renal ammonia generation, mild hyperchloremic metabolic acidosis, and mild degrees of nitrogen retention. Up to one-fourth of patients die of uremia.

Nephrolithiasis develops in one-third of patients with gout and is correlated with both the serum and urinary urate levels. Of those with stones, 20% have symptomatic nephrolithiasis preceding the first gouty attack. More than 80% of these stones are uric acid, and the remainder are calcium oxalate or phosphate alone or combined with uric acid. Uric acid stones are radiolucent.

Secondary gout is noted with conditions that increase the uric acid level secondary to increased production or decreased excretion. Increased nucleic acid turnover is observed in the myeloproliferative diseases, leukemias, other malignancies, and psoriasis. Destruction of tumor with chemo- or radiotherapy will increase uric acid by rapidly increasing the free purine load. Decreased urate excretion is seen in persons receiving thiazide diuretics and in those with chronic renal failure.

The diagnosis of gout is definitely made when negatively birefringent monosodium urate crystals are demonstrated in fluid from the affected joint.

The cornerstone of therapy of the acute gouty attack is

colchicine, which will relieve the attack within 48 hours in over 90% of patients. The oral dose is 0.5-1.0 mg initially, then 0.5 mg every hour for 8 hours, then 0.5 mg q2h; the regimen is stopped when pain relief or severe gastrointestinal intolerance (nausea, vomiting, cramping, or diarrhea) occurs. Less GI irritation is noted with the intravenous regimen of 1-2 mg (diluted and given over 20-30 minutes) every 4-6 hours until pain is relieved, intolerance occurs, or the total 24-hour intravenous dose reaches 4 mg. Short-term high doses of phenylbutazone, indomethacin, or ibuprofen are also often very effective. Unless the patient is already taking them, drugs that lower the serum uric acid level should be avoided since they exacerbate or prolong the attacks. Rest of the involved joint is important. Following initial control, maintenance colchicine (0.5 mg 3 times daily) should be begun for 2-3 weeks. In patients with frequent attacks, 1 or 2 weeks after an attack allopurinol (300 mg/day) should be instituted. Uricosuric agents may be used in patients intolerant of allopurinol. Gout is frequently associated with obesity and hypertriglyceridemia, and gradual weight reduction should be planned. Alcoholic beverages should be avoided.

Chronic gouty arthritis with visible or radiographically apparent tophi should be treated with allopurinol in an attempt to lower the serum uric acid concentration to below 6 mg/day.

The treatment of asymptomatic hyperuricemia is still debated. Allopurinol should probably be used in all patients with serum uric acid levels above 9 or 10 mg/day and in patients excreting more than 1000 mg of uric acid in a 24-hour period.

Secondary gout should be treated with the addition of high fluid intake and alkalinization of the urine. Prophylactic administration of allopurinol may be beneficial in patients with psoriasis or malignancy, particularly when chemo- or radiotherapy is to be instituted.

Pseudogout (Chondrocalcinosis Articularis)

Pseudogout, also known as chondrocalcinosis, pyrophosphate arthropathy, or CPPD crystal deposition disease, is caused by intraarticular deposition of calcium pyrophosphate dihydrate

(CPPD) crystals, which are weakly positively birefrigent under polarized light.

Pseudogout is an oligoarthritis found in elderly patients, associated with crystals in synovial fluid and radiographically apparent intraarticular calcification and calcification of articular cartilage. More appropriate terminology may be CPPD disease, since such findings may also mimic other arthritides and are known as pseudorheumatoid arthritis, pseudoosteoarthritis, and pseudo-Charcot joint. Joints affected tend to be of the lower extremity. Subchondral cyst formation and degeneration are common. Attacks are sudden, acute, and usually intermittent. Symptoms may be confused with other arthritides. The diagnosis rests on demonstration of CPPD crystals in the joint fluid and is supported by typical radiographic changes. In addition, chondro-calcinosis may occur in a familial pattern or be associated with metabolic diseases such as ochronosis, hemochromatosis, and primary hyperparathyroidism. Acute CPPD disease may be treated with phenylbutazone or other nonsteroidal anti-inflammatory agents. Colchicine is less reliable here than it is in the treatment of gout. Existent disease is not reversible.

BONE DISEASE
Paget's Disease
Paget's disease (osteitis deformans) affects 3% of individuals over 45 years old. Increased osteoclastic activity accompanied by an inadequate increase in osteoblastic activity results in osteolysis. Localized osteolytic lesions develop within the body of long bones and the axial skeleton and gradually extend with accompanying bony fibrosis and sclerosis. Increased vascularity results in a marked increase in skeletal blood flow. Bony enlargement is a common accompaniment of the disease. Radiographs of the skull may demonstrate multiple areas of radiolucency known as osteoporosis circumscripta. Lesions in long bones include osteoporosis and expanding lytic lesions accompanied by marginal sclerosis and complicated by fractures. Thickening of involved bone, particularly the cortex, is common. Although the majority of patients are asymptomatic, bony enlargement, bone pain, and

skeletal deformity are the most common symptoms. Bony over-growth may impinge on cranial nerves or the spinal cord, and fractures may occur. Osteoarthritis may develop in the hips or knees. Widespread involvement may result in a high cardiac output state and symptoms of heart failure. Less than 1% of patients develop sarcoma of the skull, pelvis or long bones; occasionally these are multicentric. The degree of bony turnover is reflected by an elevated serum alkaline phosphatase and elevated urinary hydroxyproline excretion. The serum calcium and phosphate levels are usually normal although hyperuricemia may develop. Treatment begins with analgesics and, when necessary, non-steroidal anti-inflammatory agents. Advancing disease may require suppression of bone resorption with high dose corticosteroids, sodium etidronate (EHDP), or calcium. Calci-tonin and cytotoxic agents such as mithramycin may be useful in certain cases.

Osteopenia

Osteoporosis is a decrease in bone mass with a parallel decrease of supporting matrix or osteoid. *Osteomalacia* is demineralization with replacement by osteoid tissue. Since the two processes are frequently associated, the clinical term osteopenia is frequently preferred. The disorder is generalized and may result from either increased resorption or decreased production of bone. A certain degree of osteoporosis appears to be a normal accompaniment of aging, and is particularly accelerated in women after the meno-pause.

Aside from the primary varieties, osteoporosis may be associated with systemic diseases such as hypogonadism, diabetes mellitus, hyperparathyroidism, hyperthyroidism, hyperadreno-corticism, malabsorption and malnutrition, alcoholism, deficiencies of calcium or ascorbic acid, and chronic immobilization. Chronic administration of heparin may produce osteoporosis. Heritable disorders of connective tissue such as Ehlers-Danlos syndrome, osteogenesis imperfecta, homocystinuria, and Marfan's syndrome are often associated with osteoporosis.

Clinical manifestations include easy fractures and deformities (such as kyphosis), particularly of the spine and long bones. Vertebral collapse may result in pain and, rarely, cord or nerve compression. Radiographs demonstrate generalized demineralization. "Codfish" vertebrae result from weakening of bone with concave deformities corresponding to the intervertebral disks. Serum levels of calcium and phosphate are normal, but hypercalciuria may be noted. Urinary hydroxyproline levels are usually normal. The serum alkaline phosphatase is normal except after fractures or shortly after immobilization, when it may be elevated. When the degree of osteoporosis appears out of proportion to the age of the patient, the metabolic causes discussed above should be considered. In addition, generalized osteoporosis may be seen as a feature of carcinomatosis, multiple myeloma, leukemia, and lymphoma.

Therapy consists of avoidance of even minor trauma and exercises to increase muscle strength and compensate for deformities. Acute fractures are treated with immobilization. Vertebral fractures or collapse are treated with bed rest and analgesia but not traction. Further therapy should warrant thorough evaluation for secondary causes first. Although estrogens may be beneficial prophylactically in postmenopausal women, the risks must be weighed. Recent studies have shown that estrogen therapy reduces the severity of established osteoporosis in this group; combined use of progesterones and estrogens appears to reduce the increased incidence of uterine carcinoma seen with estrogen therapy alone. Fluoride may also be beneficial when combined with calcium and vitamin D supplements.

Osteomalacia (called rickets in children) occurs with vitamin D deficiency or "resistance" (renal insufficiency or renal tubular acidosis) resulting from decreased renal conversion of 25-OH D_3 to the 1,25-dihydroxy form. Several of the anticonvulsants inhibit vitamin D absorption or 1-hydroxylation. Hypophosphatemia from any cause may result in rickets or osteomalacia.

Clinical manifestations consist of easy fractures and deformities. Rickets includes classic manifestations of bowing of weight-bearing long bones, "rachitic rosary" (prominent costochondral junctions), and Harrison's groove (notching of the ribs at the site of the attachment of the diaphragm). Irritability, muscle weakness, and hypotonia may accompany osteomalacia, and hypocalcemia, when present, may produce tetany.

Treatment with phosphate, calcium, or vitamin D depends on the cause. Renal "unresponsiveness" should be treated with the active form of vitamin D (1,25-dihydroxycholecalciferol).

MISCELLANEOUS DISORDERS
Cryoglobulinemia
Cryoglobulins are immune complexes recognized by cold precipitation (room temperature or colder). Three classes of cryoglobulins have thus far been described: isolated monoclonal IgM, IgG, or IgA (type I); antibodies to polyclonal IgG (type III); or mixed, with polyclonal and a monoclonal component (type II). The antigens in cryoglobulin precipitates may be antibodies such as antinuclear antibodies, rheumatoid factors, cold agglutinins, and antiviral antibodies.

Cryoglobulinemia has been noted in (1) hematologic disorders (multiple myeloma and Waldenstrom's macroglobulinemia, lymphoma and chronic lymphocytic leukemia, polycythemia and hemolytic anemias), (2) connective tissue diseases (systemic lupus erythematosus, rheumatoid arthritis, polyarteritis nodosa, Sjögren's syndrome, ankylosing spondylitis, and particularly Raynaud's disease), (3) infectious diseases (infective endocarditis, infectious mononucleosis, cytomegalovirus infection and malaria), (4) glomerulopathies (poststreptococcal glomerulonephritis, Goodpasture's syndrome, and Berger's disease), (5) granulomatous diseases (leprosy and sarcoidosis), (6) malignancy, and (7) idiopathically.

Symptoms do not correlate well with the quantity of cryoglobulin in plasma, but are related to the type of cryoglobulin. Symptoms are primarily cutaneous and vasomotor with type I. Types II and III are associated with Raynaud phenomenon (often atypical), vasculitis and purpura, neurologic involvement (peripheral neuropathy), and renal involvement. Other common manifestations are anemia, bleeding tendency, and arthritis. Less commonly, a hyperviscosity syndrome may occur.

Essential mixed cryoglobulinemia is a syndrome in which

manifestations (in decreasing order of frequency) include weakness, purpura, arthralgia or arthritis, liver involvement, renal involvement, pulmonary involvement (dyspnea and increased alveoloarterial oxygen difference), and splenomegaly. Hepatitis B virus antigen complexed with IgM or IgG is found in 75% of patients, suggesting a viral etiology.

Other common laboratory findings include rouleaux formation and an increased erythrocyte sedimentation rate at 37°C, which is normal at room temperature and decreased at 4°C.

Blood must be carefully collected in syringe and tube warmed to 37°C and clotted at 37°C before placing the resultant serum at 4°C for several days of observation.

Treatment is presently limited to plasmapheresis for symptomatic hyperviscosity.

Raynaud's Phenomenon

Raynaud's phenomenon is characterized by episodic attacks of reversible vasospasm characteristically triggered by cold or emotional stimuli.

Involvement is typically of the extremities, particularly the fingers. The classic sequence following a trigger is a demarcated pallor of the involved region resulting from vasospasm; this is often accompanied by burning or tingling. Reduced venous flow then leads to cyanosis. Minutes to hours later, a reactive hyperemia ensues, frequently associated with throbbing pain. Although uncommon, fingertip ulcers may occur when the vasospasm is frequent, severe, and sustained.

More than 85% of patients have the idiopathic variety (Raynaud's disease). Known causes include connective tissue diseases (particularly scleroderma, SLE or RA, in that order), the paraproteinemias (such as multiple myeloma), dysproteinemias (such as cryoglobulinemia), malignancy, obstructive arterial disease (particularly thromboangiitis obliterans), thoracic outlet syndromes, freeze injury, use of vibrating instruments, heavy metal poisoning, exposure to vinyl chloride, and use of vasoconstrictors (ergot alkaloids) or propranolol. Raynaud's phenomenon not infrequently precedes other manifestations of these conditions.

Treatment is limited to symptomatic therapy. Centrally acting sympatholytics (particularly reserpine) seem to be much more effective than peripheral sympatholytics or direct vasodilators. Cervical sympathectomy does not offer sustained benefit, although lumbar sympathectomy may relieve lower extremity symptoms in refractory cases.

Hypertropic Osteoarthropathy

Although clubbing of the fingers and toes and hypertrophic osteoarthropathy are not synonymous, they frequently occur together. Clubbing of the digits represents enlargement of the distal portion of the digits resulting from periostitis. The swelling is often insidious and painless but may develop acutely or be painful intermittently. The acquired form of the disease is often seen with carcinoma of the lung (5-10% of patients), chronic lung disease, congenital cyanotic heart disease, biliary cirrhosis, and inflammatory intestinal diseases. The idiopathic form has no associated diseases. The heritable form is transmitted as an autosomal dominant with low penetrance in females.

Hypertrophic osteoarthropathy (HO) is found with the same relationships noted for clubbing. These two processes may occur together, precede each other, or occur independently. Similar pathologic changes in other joints result in arthralgias or polyarthritis particularly of the knees, ankles, elbows, wrists, and metacarpophalangeal joints. The synovial fluid is noninflammatory in nature. Radiographs reveal periostitis. Underlying diseases must be thoroughly looked for. Treatment is limited to symptomatic analgesics. Regression may be noted with improvement in the underlying disorder or with unilateral intrathoracic vagotomy.

Pachydermoperiostosis is a rare familial variant of HO in which marked clubbing in young boys is associated with marked thickening of the skin of the face and scalp.

Lower Back Pain

Lower back pain frequently has no readily identifiable cause. A constellation of genetically predetermined, poor supporting structures, poor posture, recurrent strain (high heels), or mild trauma may all be important. Radicular pain or a positive straight leg raising sign suggest neurologic involvement and warrant myelography. Symptomatic treatment with rest, firm bed mattress, analgesics, muscle relaxants, and local mild heat may be tried. Cutaneous nerve stimulation may be beneficial in some patients. Although generally not inflammatory, a positive bone scan may predict patients who might respond to nonsteroidal antiinflammatory agents. Sacroileitis and ankylosing spondylitis should always be considered in young patients.

REFERENCES

Rheumatoid Arthritis

Feigenbaum SL, Masi AT, Kaplan SB: Prognosis in rheumatoid arthritis. A longitudinal study of newly diagnosed younger adult patients. Am J Med 66:377, 1979.

Bywaters EGL, Curwen M, Dresner E, et al.: Ten year follow-up of rheumatoid arthritis. Lancet 2:1381, 1960.

Moutsopoulos HM, Webber BL, Vlagoponlos TP, et al.: Differences in the clinical manifestations of sicca syndrome in the presence and absence of rheumatoid arthritis. Am J Med 66:733, 1979.

Kassan SS, Gardy M: Sjogren's syndrome: an update and overview. Am J Med 64:1037, 1978.

Moutsopoulos HM (moderator): Sjogren's syndrome (Sicca syndrome): current issues. Ann Intern Med 92(Part 1):212, 1980.

Stein HB, Patterson AC, Offer RB, et al.: Adverse effects of D-penicillamine in rheumatoid arthritis. Ann Intern Med 92:24, 1980.

Systemic Lupus Erythematosis

Decker JL, Steinberg SF, Reinertsen JL, Plotz PH, Balow JE, Klippel JH: Systemic lupus erythematosis: evolving concepts. Ann Intern Med 91:587, 1979.

Runyon BA, LaBrecque DR, Anuras L: The spectrum of liver disease in systemic lupus erythematosis: report of 33 histologically proved cases and review of the literature. Am J Med 69:188, 1979.

Klippel JH, Gerber LH, Pollack L, Decker JL: Avascular necrosis in systemic lupus erythematosus. Am J Med 67:83, 1979.

Baker SB, Rovira JR, Campion EW, Mills JA: Late onset systemic lupus erythematosis. Am J Med 66:727, 1979.

Donadio JV Jr, Holley KE, Ferguson RH, Ilstrup DM: Treatment of lupus nephritis with prednisone and combined prednisone and cyclophosphamide. N Engl J Med 299:1151, 1978.

Budman DR, Steinberg AD: Hematologic aspects of systemic lupus erythematosis. Current concepts. Ann Intern Med 86:220, 1977.

Levinski RJ, Cameron JS, Soothill JF: Serum immune complexes and disease activity in lupus nephritis. Lancet 1:564, 1977.

Gladmar DD, Urowitz MB, Keysteon EC: Serologically active clinically quiescent systemic lupus erythematosis. A discordance between clinical and serologic features. Am J Med 66:210, 1979.

Lee SL, Chase PH: Drug-induced systemic lupus erythematosis: a critical review. Semin Arthritis Rheum 5:83, 1975.

Notman DD, Kurata N, Tan EM: Profiles of antinuclear antibodies in systemic rheumatic diseases. Ann Intern Med 83:464, 1975.

Dermatomyositis/Polymyositis

Barnes BE: Dermatomyositis and malignancy: a review of the literature. Ann Intern Med 84:68, 1976.

Schumacher HR, Schimmer B, Gordon GV, et al.: Anticular manifestations of polymyositis and dermatomyositis. Am J Med 67:287, 1979.

Fanci As, Haynes BF, Katz P: The spectrum of vasculitis, clinical, pathologic, immunologic and therapeutic considerations. Ann Intern Med 89:660, 1978.

Huston KA, Hunder GG, Lie JT, Kennedy RH, Elveback LR: Temporal arteritis: a 25-year epidemiologic, clinical, and pathologic study. Ann Intern Med 88:162, 1978.

Goodman BW Jr: Temporal arteritis. Am J Med 67:839, 1979.

Hunninghake GW, Fauci AS: Pulmonary involvement in the collagen vascular diseases. Am Rev Respir Dis 119:471, 1979.

Seronegative Spondyloarthritides

Brewerton Da, Caffrey M, Nicholls A: Reiter's disease HLA B27. Lancet 2:886, 1973.

Butler MJ, Russell AS, Percy JS, Lentle BC: A follow-up study of 48 patients with Reiter's syndrome. Am J Med 67:808, 1979.

Moore SB: HLA. Mayo Clin Proc 54:385, 1979.

Woodrow JC: Histocompatibility antigens and rheumatic diseases. Semim Arthritis Rheum 6:257, 1977.

Calin A, Porta J, Fries JF, Schurman DJ: Clinical history as a screening test for ankylosing spondylitis. JAMA 237:2613, 1977.

Osteomyelitis

Waldvogel FA, Medoff G, Swartz MN: Osteomyelitis: a review of clinical features, therapeutic considerations and unusual aspects. N Engl J Med 282:198-206, 260-266, 316-322, 1970.

Dich VQ, Nelson JD, Hatalein KC: Osteomyelitis in infants and children. Am J Dis Child 129:1273, 1975.

Gout and Pseudogout
Fessel WJ: Renal outcomes of gout and hyperuricemia. Am J Med 67:74, 1979.
Simkin PA: Management of gout. Ann Intern Med 90:812, 1979.
Boss GR, Seegmiller JE: Hyperuricemia and gout: classification, complications, and management. N Engl J Med 300:1459, 1979.
Liang MH, Fries JF: Asymptomatic hyperuricemia: the case for conservative management. Ann Intern Med 88:666, 1978.
McCarthy DJ: Calcium pyrophosphate dihydrate crystal deposition disease (pseudogout syndrome)—clinical aspects. Clin Rheum Dis 3:61, 1977.

Bone Disease
Lutwak L (moderator): Current concepts of bone metabolism. Ann Intern Med 80:630, 1974.
Frame B, Parfitt AM: Osteomalacia: current concepts. Ann Intern Med 89:966, 1978.

Cryoglobulinemia
Gorevic PD, Kassab HJ, Levd Y, et al.: Mixed cryoglobulinemia: clinical aspects and long-term follow-up of 40 patients. Am J Med 69:287, 1980.

Raynaud's Phenomenon
Halperin JL, Coffman JD: Pathophysiology of Raynaud's disease. Arch Intern Med 139:89, 1979.

6
Endocrine System

Derived from the Greek work *krinein,* meaning to secrete, the study of endocrinology is the study of internal secretions. Recent research reveals that the endocrine system is but one part of a vast regulatory network that controls the activity of the working parts of the body. *Endocrine secretions or hormones* are produced by specialized cells and carried to target sites by the circulation; *neurocrine secretions* or neurotransmitters are produced within the nervous system and bridge the short synaptic gap between two neurons; *paracrine secretions* are produced locally and diffuse short distances through the interstitial space to regulate target cells.

The diffuse endocrine system is a network of cells distributed throughout the brain and body that synthesize and release peptide or amine substances. Known as APUD cells (*a*mine *p*recursor *u*ptake and *d*ecarboxylation), their secretions may exert neurocrine, paracrine, or endocrine functions. Cells in the central division of the diffuse endocrine system are located in the pineal body, hypothalamus, and pituitary, and secrete a variety of neurotransmitters, melatonin (pineal origin), posterior pituitary peptides (vasopressin and oxytocin), hypothalamic releasing factors, and pituitary peptide trophic hormones. The peripheral division includes APUD cells located in the pancreas, stomach, intestine, lung, parathyroid, adrenal medulla, sympathetic nervous system, thyroid, and elsewhere. These cells are discussed in other sections, particularly that on gastric secretions.

Secretory products act on other cells by binding to specific receptors; the messenger-receptor combination is a fundamental biologic building block, linking regulatory and working cells. Peptide and amine secretions bind to receptors on the cell surface. These surface receptor-hormone combinations exert their action by producing "second messengers" such as cyclic AMP, cyclic GMP, or calcium within the cell membrane. Once inside the cell, these secondary messengers typically function by converting inactive enzymes to active states.

In contrast, thyroid and steroid hormone receptors are intracellular. Small amounts of free hormone, released from plasma-binding proteins, diffuse into the cell interior and combine with cytoplasmic hormone receptors. Thyroxine, for example, is converted to the active T_3 within the cell itself.

Abnormal function (a recognizable disease state) may result from abnormalities in the hypothalamus, pituitary, classic target organs, cells of the peripheral division of the diffuse endocrine system, membrane receptor abnormalities, or abnormalities in intracellular hormone-binding proteins. Such a complex control network offers many opportunities for malfunction but also provides considerable leverage for therapeutic intervention.

HYPOTHALAMUS AND PITUITARY
Physiology
Bridging the indistinct border between mind and body, the hypothalamus receives afferent information from cortical and subcortical sources and responds with integrated physiologic responses. At one time, the endocrine and nervous systems were believed to be distinct and separate; it is now known that nervous impulses travel from cell to cell by way of neurotransmitters, that neural impulses can cause hormonal release, and that transmitters such as norepinephrine circulate in the bloodstream. The hypothalamus gives rise to cholinergic sympathetic fibers that terminate in preganglionic nuclei located in the spinal cord; it synthes-

izes vasopressin (ADH) and oxytocin; it secretes a group of pituitary-releasing substances that control pituitary function.

The pituitary gland consists of three lobes, each of which differs in embryogenesis and histology. The embryonic pharnyx of Rathke's pouch gives rise to the anterior and intermediate lobes. The posterior lobe is an extension of neural cells and tissues that originate in the hypothalamus. The pituitary gland is the master gland. The anterior pituitary produces seven known polypeptide hormones: growth hormone (GH), prolactin, luteinizing hormone (LH), follicle-stimulating hormone (FSH), thyroid-stimulating hormone (TSH), adrenocorticotropic hormone (ACTH), and melanocyte-stimulating hormone (MSH) or beta-lipoprotein (beta-LPH). The posterior pituitary stores two known hormones: antidiuretic hormone or vasopressin (ADH), and oxytocin.

Anterior pituitary function is controlled by hypothalamic peptides or *releasing factors* and by feedback control from target endocrine organs. Three monamines—*dopamine* (sustantia nigra), *norepinephrine* (locus ceruleus), and *serotonin* (raphe nuclei)—regulate the secretion of releasing factors from the hypothalamus, which then pass through the hypophysial-portal circulation to the anterior pituitary. Releasing factors when characterized chemically are called releasing hormones. Table 6-1 lists releasing and inhibiting factors, neurotransmitters responsible for their secretion, and some agents known to alter their activity.

The destruction of the hypothalamus and interruption of the hypothalamo-hypophysial-portal system (by a craniopharyngioma, for example) may produce a variety of neuroendocrine disorders. Clinical syndromes associated with disturbed hypothalamic neuroendocrine secretions are shown in Table 6-2.

Clinical features of pituitary disease are variable and depend on the type of lesion in the pituitary gland and on whether one or both lobes are involved. Destruction in part or entirely will usually produce hypopituitarism. Enlarging tumors may present with signs attributable to an increased hormonal output or, more commonly, failure of secretion. Some tumors may suppress other

TABLE 6-1—MONOAMINE TRANSMITTERS AND PITUITARY FUNCTION

Hypothalamic Regulator	Neurotransmitter	Stimulates	Inhibits
Corticotropin-releasing factor (CRF)	Serotonin	Serotonin Hypoglycemia	Cyproheptadine Bromocryptine
Prolactin-releasing factor (PRF)	Serotonin	Tryptophan	Tryptophan
Thyrotropin-releasing hormone (TRH)	Norepinephrine		
Luteinizing hormone-releasing hormone (LHRH) (also releases FSH)	Norepinephrine		
Growth hormone-releasing factor (GHRF)	Dopamine Serotonin Norepinephrine	Tryptophan L-Dopa Apomorphine Hypoglycemia	
Prolactin-inhibiting factor (PIF)	Dopamine	L-Dopa Apomorphine Bromocryptine	Phenothiazines Reserpine Morphine
Somatostatin			

TABLE 6-2—HYPOTHALAMIC CAUSES OF CLINICAL SYNDROMES

Hypothalmic Factor	Increased	Decreased
GHRF	Cere' ral giantism Acromegaly (acidophil hyperplasia)	Sexual ateliotic dwarfism (isolated GH deficiency)
TRH	Hypothalamic hyperthyroidism	Isolated TSH deficiency
CRF	Cushing's syndrome Wolff syndrome—tonic ACTH	Isolated ACTH deficiency
LRF	Isosexual precocious	Kallmann's syndrome (olfactory-genital hyperplasia) Psychogenic amenorrhea
PIF		Chiari-Frommel syndrome (nonpubertal galactorrhea); impotence

functions of the gland as a result of hypersecretion of one hormone. Failure of function is often progressive and sequential: the secretion of gonadotropins declines first usually followed by GH, ACTH, and finally TSH.

Evaluation of Hypophyseal-Pituitary-End Organ Control

Physiologic evaluation of end-organ control is based on biochemical observations following: (1) stimulation or inhibition of hypothalamic-releasing hormones, (2) administration of releasing hormones, (3) feedback stimulation or suppression of pituitary trophic hormones, (4) administration of pituitary trophic hormones. Thyroid function, for example, may be studied by administering thyroid-releasing hormone, thyrotropin (TSH), or attempting feedback suppression with thyroid hormone (T_3), which reduces the uptake of radio iodine to below 60% of control in normal individuals. Adrenal function is similarly studied by producing insulin hypoglycemia, which stimulates the secretion of corticotropin-releasing factor, by administering ACTH, by producing feedback suppression of ACTH with dexamethasone, or increasing ACTH secretion with metyrapone, an agent blocking cortisol synthesis. Hypoglycemia also stimulates the production of growth hormone-releasing factor so that the integrity of both ACTH and GH secretion can be evaluated simultaneously. These provocative tests are consistent with the belief that resting physiologic or biochemical values may be within the range of normal early in the natural history of many disease states; stress provocation mirroring everyday activity is necessary for identification of important abnormalities.

Pituitary Hormones and Their Abnormalities
GROWTH HORMONE
Growth hormone begins to affect body growth by the age of 2 and initiates a sharp increase in growth at the beginning of puberty; it appears to act through small peptides (somatomedins) that are produced in the liver and then bind to membrane receptors to stimulate lipolysis and ketogenesis, protein synthesis, and bone and cartilage growth. Pituitary secretion is enhanced by a specific hypothalamic-releasing factor and inhibited by somatostatin (sometimes called somatotropin-release-inhibiting factor). GH raises blood glucose and is considered to be diabetogenic; somatostatin reduces GH secretion as well as the secretion of insulin and glucagon. Somatostatin, which is antidiabetogenic on balance, is also produced by the D cells of the pancreatic islets and by cells in the duodenum and gastric antrum. Hypoglycemia, hyperaminoacidemia, fever, exercise, fasting, and dopaminergic agents such as L-Dopa and apomorphine stimulate the secretion of GH.

Deficiency in growth hormone secretion causes little difficulty after puberty unless it is associated with panhypopituitarism. Before puberty, deficiency leads to dwarfism and delayed puberty; the term sexual ateliotic is frequently applied (ateliotic equals incomplete). The availability of GH assay soon identified proportionate dwarfs with normal GH plasma concentrations (Laron dwarfism). Early postulates suggested that defective somatomedin production in the liver might be responsible, although direct evidence was not available. Most recently, studies on erythroid colonies produced in vitro from bone marrow progenitors harvested from Laron dwarfs have shown cellular resistance to growth hormone. These studies indicate that defective peripheral receptor activity rather than deficiencies in somatomedin synthesis is responsible for some forms of dwarfism. While an important observation in its own right, it demonstrates the variety of abnormalities that may lead to peripheral hormone dysfunction. Obviously, replacement therapy would be useless in these situations. Other conditions producing small stature are infantalism due to starvation or malabsorption, Turner's syndrome, ricketts, achondroplasia, cretinism, renal dwarfism, and juvenile hypothyroidism.

Excess secretion of growth hormone also has varying effects, depending on its relationship to puberty. The classic circus giant is usually an individual with either diffuse hyperplasia of pituitary acidophils or an acidophilic adenoma that develops before puberty. After epiphyseal closure, substantial changes in skeletal length are not possible, but the distal parts of the skeleton enlarge and produce the syndrome of acromegaly.

The cardinal manifestations of acromegaly, frequently obvious when comparing recent and old photographs, are enlargement of hands and feet, coarsening of facial features, muscle aching, easy fatigability, heat intolerance and excessive perspiration, and sexual disturbances due to associated abnormalities in gonadotropins. Hypertension is common, probably due to increased peripheral vascularity and cardiac output, and may lead to congestive heart failure.

The tongue, liver, spleen, kidneys, and other organs are also enlarged. Pressure on the median nerve may cause carpal tunnel syndromes. Hyperglycemia and glucose intolerance are common, demonstrating the diabetogenic action of growth hormone. Type I MEN syndrome (Wermer's syndrome) with pituitary, pancreatic, and parathyroid adenomas (see page 382) may present as acromegaly.

Most acromegalic patients have adenomas, and the presence of visual field defects and bitemporal or frontal headaches frequently assists in the diagnosis. Tomography reveals an enlarged sella turcica, and fasting recumbent GH levels are usually greater than 5 ng/ml. Confirmation of abnormalities in GH secretion may be made by performing a glucose tolerance test. Ingestions of 100 gm of glucose suppresses GH secretion to below 5 ng/ml; suppression does not occur in acromegaly, and the GH level may actually rise. This procedure is obviously the reverse of using hypoglycemia to provoke GH and ACTH secretion.

Treatment is either with radiation (proton beam irradiation) or surgery. Transphenoidal hypophysectomy is becoming the preferred treatment in many centers, particularly if there is suprasellar extension.

THYROID-STIMULATING HORMONES
Thyroid-stimulating hormone (TSH) is a glycoprotein consisting of two subunits, alpha and beta, the former common to LH, FSH, and human chorionic gonadotropin; the normal plasma concentration of TSH is less than 5 μg/ml. In primary thyroid failure, the secretion of TSH is accelerated. Thyroid-releasing factor stimulates the secretion of TSH. Failure to produce thyroid-releasing factor results in isolated TSH deficiency, the most common of the monotropic deficiencies of the anterior pituitary hormones. Administration of synthetic thyroid releasing hormone is useful in the diagnosis of thyroid disorders (see page 335); TRH also stimulates prolactin secretion. Deficiency of TSH often accompanies other anterior pituitary deficient diseases, (Sheehan's syndrome and chromophobe adenoma).

ADRENOCORTICOTROPIC HORMONE (ACTH)
A large glycoprotein prohormone is cleaved to produce ACTH and beta-lipotropin. The latter is a polypeptide containing beta-melanocyte-stimulating hormone and a group of opioid peptides including beta endorphin and enkephalin. The role of beta-MSH is not clear, although excessive ACTH production does appear to increase pigmentation. Corticotropin-releasing factor and ACTH are both controlled by feedback. ACTH concentration varies from 20-60 pg/ml and falls below 10 pg/ml at night.

A total absence of ACTH secretion is incompatible with life. Partial ACTH deficiency occurs in panhypopituitarism and in patients receiving high-dose long-term corticosteroid therapy for nonendocrine diseases. Cushing's syndrome, the result of excessive ACTH secretion, may be caused by hypothalamic abnormalities increasing CRH secretion or pituitary microadenoma. It may also be produced by patients with ACTH-producing pituitary chromophobe adenomas or ectopic ACTH production. There is a loss of circadian rhythm of both ACTH and cortisol secretions and loss of feedback control. Excessive ACTH secretion by a chromophobe adenoma is usually associated with an increased secretion of beta-MSH or beta-LPH, resulting in hyperpigmentation, a common clinical sign of this type of Cushing's syndrome.

GONADOTROPINS

Availability of assays for FSH and LH have permitted analysis of the menstrual cycle. A remarkable midcycle increase in LH (the peak is 6 to 8 times baseline) divides the cycle into follicular and luteal phases. The follicular phase is marked by increasing FSH secretion, granulosa cell proliferation, and increased estrogen production from maturing granulosa cells. The trigger for LH peaking is poorly understood but could be related to falling estrogen levels, which decline at about the same time as LH concentrations increase. FSH also peaks in midcycle, suggesting that both are under negative feedback control from circulating estrogen. Ovulation occurs 12-36 hours after the peaks of LH and FSH; apparently, both trophic hormones are required. The negative feedback of LH and FSH is due to an interdependent action of both progesterone and estrogen; hormonal contraception is based on the administration of these two hormones to inhibit LH and FSH and thus ovulation. LH leads to further maturation of the graafian follicle, which increases its production of progesterone and becomes a corpus luteum. Rising concentrations of progesterone exert negative feedback control on the pituitary, leading to decreases in LH and FSH.

The long-observed relationship between emotions and the menstrual cycle is explained by the importance of a hypothalamic secretion, luteinizing hormone-releasing hormone. FSH-releasing factor may be identical with LHRH, but precise identification has not yet been achieved. Both FSH and LH appear to influence hypothalamic function by a feedback mechanism.

Clomiphene (clomid) binds to hypothalamic estrogen receptor sites and is interpreted by the hypothalamus as reduced circulating estrogen levels. It may be administered to amenorrheic women in an attempt to stimulate an ovulatory cycle by increasing circulating FSH and LH. Failure to respond suggests one of a number of syndromes with either end-organ or pituitary dysfunction. A simpler procedure is to initially administer progesterone, 5 mg/day for 5 consecutive days. Progesterone also acts like clomiphene by binding to hypothalamic estrogen receptors. The increase in LH and FSH secretion apparently leads to sufficient estrogen production that withdrawal bleeding occurs several days after discontinuation of progesterone. About 80% of women who demonstrate a normal axis by withdrawal bleeding will also increase gonadotropins with clomiphene.

PROLACTIN

Unlike the pituitary trophic hormones, the polypeptide hormone prolactin does not regulate a secondary endocrine gland, but acts directly on tissues. The only known function in humans is the initiation and maintenance of lactation. Prolactin secretion is subject to tonic inhibition by prolactin inhibitory factor (PIF), which is under dopaminergic control. Syndromes or diseases associated with altered prolactin secretion in women include Chiari-Frommel (postpartum amenorrhea and galactorrhea), Ahumada-del Castillo (nonpuerperal amenorrhea and galactorrhea), Forbes-Albright (amenorrhea and galactorrhea with a pituitary tumor), and primary hypothyroidism (amenorrhea and galactorrhea). In both men and women, pituitary tumors may produce altered prolactin secretion. Galactorrhea may also be found in men and women as a result of neural stimulation from chest wall surgery, repeated breast stimulation, pituitary stalk section, or during treatment with drugs that inhibit PIF secretion (phenothiazine, reserpine, or methyldopa).

Anterior Pituitary Insufficiency
CHILDHOOD TYPE
In children, anterior pituitary deficiency leads to failure or retardation of growth (pituitary dwarfism). In 35-40% of cases, no discernible cause is found. Approximately another third of children with anterior pituitary insufficiency have craniopharyngiomas that invade the pituitary or interrupt the neural or vascular connection with the hypothalamus. Over half of these children have symptoms before age 15, some of which include diabetes insipidus (posterior pituitary), sexual infantilism, and growth failure.

ADULT TYPE
Anterior pituitary insufficiency in adults (Simmonds's disease) is found in 1 in 1,000 hospital admissions. In adult men, the most common cause of hypopituitarism is a chromophobe adenoma; in adult women, it is caused by postpartum hemorrhage and shock, which produces pituitary infarction and necrosis (Sheehan's syndrome). Spasm of the arterioles of the anterior stalk and lobe is the primary vascular disturbance, although thrombosis due to disseminated intravascular coagulation may play a role. Other causes of anterior pituitary failure in the adult include craniopharyngiomas, certain granulomas, sarcoidosis, xanthomatosis, and metastatic invasion.

Clinically, the features of hypopituitarism depend on the cause, the sex of the patient, and the degree of destruction of the gland. Severe panhypopituitarism is characterized by features of thyroid, gonadal, and adrenocortical insufficiency. Gonadal hormones usually diminish first. Adult men have a loss of libido and potency, with testicular and prostatic atrophy. There is also a loss of axillary and pubic hair, and beard growth is decreased. Adult women experience cessation of menstrual periods, nipples and areolae become depigmented and atrophied, and the skin thins. In Sheehan's syndrome, there is absence of lactation in the postpartum period and failure to resume menses. Thyroid failure is variable, ranging from borderline abnormalities of thyroid function to features of severe primary myxedema.

When adrenocortical failure is present, it is usually limited to diminished androgen and cortisol production. Aldosterone levels are adequate in most patients, because sodium deprivation will induce a rise in aldosterone secretion. Cortisol deficiency produces weakness and fatigue. Hypoglycemia is one of the most serious features of hypopituitarism. Insulin sensitivity is marked, and profound hypoglycemia may lead to death.

PITUITARY TUMORS

Recognized by their effect on function by pressure on adjacent areas, 80% are chromophobe adenomas which produce headache, visual field defects, and may lead to paralysis of the 3rd, 4th, and 6th cranial nerves. The non-functional nature of chromophobe adenomas may be due in part to the difficulty in identifying the glycoprotein hormones (TSH, LH, FSH) since alpha subunits, common to all of these glycoproteins, have been identified in patients with presumably functionless tumors. Increased prolactin concentrations are seen in more than 50% because of interference with prolactin inhibitory factor delivery from the hypothalamus or direct prolactin secretion by the tumor. Large tumors frequently produce pituitary insufficiency; growth hormone deficiency is the most common.

Somewhat more than 10% of pituitary tumors are slow-growing eosinophilic adenomas that are associated with acromegaly or gigantism. Basophilic adenomas are frequently found at autopsy and are usually asymptomatic. Cushing's disease is due to either hypothalamic hyperfunctioning or a chromophobe adenoma that produces ACTH. It is not clear whether Nelson's syndrome results from growth of a preexisting chromophobe adenoma or whether it is actually due to a new chromophobe adenoma that develops after adrenalectomy. Craniopharyngiomas arise from remnants of Rathke's pouch and may present as pituitary tumors. They extend behind and above the sella turcica and may undergo cystic degeneration, becoming suprasellar cysts. Somnolence, delayed sexual maturity, and obesity may occur if they reach the hypothalamus and floor of the third ventricle.

The empty sella syndrome is nonadenomatous enlargement of

the sella turcica due to enlargement of an arachnoid diverticulum that expands below the diaphragm sellae. Individuals with this condition are usually women (90%), obese, and multiparous. Headache is common and leads to skull radiographs. Tomography frequently establishes the diagnosis by demonstrating the characteristic ballooned appearance; visual field changes are rare but may occur.

ECTOPIC HORMONE SYNDROMES
Table 6-3 gives ectopic hormones and associated syndromes.

Disorders of the Posterior Pituitary
Two nonapeptides, differing only by the amino acids at the 3 and 8 positions, are synthesized in the neurons of the supraoptic paraventricular hypothalamic nuclei and transported down the axons of these neurons for storage and subsequent release in the posterior pituitary. Oxytocin has major effects on the uterus; vasopressin or antidiuretic hormone adjusts water excretion by the kidney to water intake. Increases in plasma osmolality, decreases in extracellular volume, and nonspecific stress stimulate vasopressin release, while reduced plasma osmolality, increased extracellular volume, and ethanol administration inhibit its release. Once released, it increases the permeability of the distal nephron, allowing water to pass along an osmotic gradient into the interstitium, resulting in the excretion of a concentrated urine.

VASOPRESSIN EXCESS
Secretion of antidiuretic hormone that is inappropriate to the plasma osmolality is discussed on page 243. This syndrome is characterized by low plasma osmolality, renal sodium wasting, and excretion of concentrated urine. Hyponatremia results from both sodium depletion and vascular volume dilution.

VASOPRESSIN DEFICIENCY: DIABETES INSIPIDUS
Diabetes insipidus results from deficiency in ADH secretion and must be differentiated from other polyuric syndromes such as psychogenic polydipsia or nephrogenic diabetes insipidus (end-

TABLE 6-3—ECTOPIC HORMONE SYNDROMES

Ectopic Hormone	Clinical Syndrome	Type and Site of Usual Tumor
ACTH and/or MSH	Hypokalemic alkalosis, hypertension, edema, pigmentation, hyperglycemia, muscle weakness, wasting	Lung, also pancreas, thymus, thyroid
Parathormone and parathormone-like substance	Elevated calcium, low or normal phosphorus, anorexia, constipation, polyuria, drowsiness, coma	Lung, also kidney, liver
Human chorionic gonadotropin	Precocious puberty, gynecomastia	GI tract, especially pancreas, also lung, breast, teratomas
Antidiuretic hormone	Hyponatremia, increased urinary sodium excretion, lethargy, weakness, confusion, coma	Lung, also pancreas
Calcitonin	None known	Lung, also stomach
Prolactin	Galactorrhea	Lung, kidney
TSH	Signs and symptoms of hyperthyroidism	Lung, kidney

organ failure where renal tubules are unresponsive to vasopressin).

Primary diabetes insipidus may be familial or sporadic. When familial, it is often associated with other congenital defects such as the Laurence-Moon-Biedl syndrome of obesity, hypogenitalism, retinitis pigmentosa, mental deficiency, and polydactyly. Secondary diabetes insipidus is found with metastatic carcinoma of the hypothalamus (most frequent with carcinoma of the lung), following trauma, or in association with Hand-Schuller-Christian disease, histiocytosis, sarcoidosis, other granulomas, or basal meningitis.

Polyuria, excessive thirst (particularly for cold liquids), and polydipsia are characteristic. Patients may excrete 16-24 liters of urine daily, but often urine output is substantially less, and is sometimes in the normal range. Urine osmolality is usually less than plasma osmolality (the opposite, of course, of the situation with inappropriate secretion of ADH). In normal individuals, urine osmolality is below plasma levels until a plasma value of about 285 mOsm/kg is reached; at that point, osmoreceptor stimulation occurs and a concentrated urine is excreted; when osmolality reaches 290, urine osmolality may exceed 800. Water deprivation for 18-24 hours in normals rarely produces a plasma osmolality above 292; plasma ADH at that point is 6-10 μU/ml.

Water deprivation in the patient with diabetes insipidus leads to plasma osmolalities that reach 310; the response is normal in psychologic polydipsia. Administration of vasopressin after dehydration increases urine osmolality and is good evidence of vasopressin deficiency. Failure to respond to vasopressin suggests nephrogenic causes that include the rare inherited form, prolonged hypokalemia, prolonged hypercalcemia, or the chronic ingestion of lithium.

Diabetes insipidus can be treated by nasal spray preparations of 8-lysine vasopressin. Since many patients secrete some vasopressin, chlorpropamide and chlorothiazide may reduce urine output and increase urine osmolality. Atromid and carbamazepine are also useful in some patients. These agents appear to alter the tubular response to vasopressin and may also, in some situations, increase vasopressin secretion.

THYROID GLAND DISORDERS
Thyroid Physiology

The thyroid gland under the stimulus of TSH secretion traps and concentrates iodine from the perfusing blood. The trapped iodine is then bound to tyrosyl residues in thyroglobulin to form monoiodo and diiodo tyrosyl residues, which couple to form three and four iodo residues in thyroglobulin. Proteolytic release from follicular cells liberates thyroxine (T_4) and 3,5,3'-triiodothyronine (T_3) into the circulation. This sequential process may be blocked at several points: (1) thiocyanate and perchlorate block iodine transport, (2) antithyroid drugs inhibit organification, (3) iodide and lithium block release of hormone from thyroglobulin.

Ten times as much thyroxine as T_3 is released from the thyroid, but it has low biologic activity and is probably a prohormone. Approximately 85% of thyroxine is deiodinated to T_3 in kidney, liver, and other peripheral tissues, but not all T_3 is metabolically active. Each molecule has two benzene rings, and each ring has iodine at the 3 and 5 position; the ring most distant from the carboxyl group (outer ring) is designated by the prime mark. About half the time, iodine in the 5' position is lost, producing the active T_3 (3,5,3' triiodothyronine); the remaining 50% of thyroxine destined to lose an iodine is deiodinated at the 5 position, forming the metabolically inactive reverse T_3 (3,3',5' triiodothyronine). In the normal individual, 80% of the T_3 is produced by peripheral deiodination, while in thyrotoxicosis direct thyroid secretion of T_3 accounts for a greater proportion of circulating T_3. In some patients, T_3 is elevated while T_4 is normal. The existence of an active and inactive form of T_3 explains why a reduced T_3 may not mean hypothyroidism. The newborn state, starvation, acute febrile illnesses, cirrhosis, and steroid administration elevate reverse T_3 and reduce the active form. T_3 in comparison to T_4 is loosely bound to plasma proteins, is rapidly cleared from the circulation, and is predominantly intracellular. Many tissues bear membrane receptor sites for both T_4 and T_3; hormone-receptor interaction increases cellular oxygen consumption.

Inorganic iodide has a profound influence on thyroxin biosynthesis. Iodide deficiency (almost unheard of in the United States) leads to increased thyroidal trapping of iodide and to increased T_3 synthesis relative to T_4 synthesis. Excess iodide has the opposite effect on these two functions; it also inhibits release of both T_3 and T_4 from the thyroid and prevents the organification of tyrosyl residues.

Evaluation of Thyroid Function

T_3 and T_4 can be accurately measured in plasma, usually by radioimmunoassay. Normal values for T_4 are 4-12 μg/dl; for T_3 they are 80-160 ng/dl. Since levels of these hormones are influenced by thyroid hormone binding capacity, that capacity should be measured when hormone levels are abnormal.

The T_3 resin uptake (RT$_3$U) is inversely proportional to the numbers of free binding site on the thyroid-binding globulin (TBG). Patient's serum is mixed with radioactive T_3 and a resin; if binding sites are increased, radioactive T_3 will fill them and less will be taken up by the resin (increased TBG and decreased RT$_3$U). If binding sites are decreased, less radioactive T_3 can bind to them and more will be on the resin (decreased TBG, increased RT$_3$U). The normal range is 25-35%. *Therefore, if the RT$_3$U moves in the same direction as the thyroid hormone, the patient has thyroid disease* (increased T_4, increased RT$_3$U in hyperthyroidism, and decreased T_4 and decreased RT$_3$U in hypothyroidism). If the RT$_3$U moves in the opposite direction from thyroid hormones, the patient has an abnormality of binding proteins.

Plasma TSH levels, determined by radioimmunoassay (normal values 0.05-5 μU/ml) are useful in evaluating thyroid function. High values of TSH are characteristic of primary hypothyroidism. Mild elevations occur in clinically euthyroid patients who may be in a prehypothyroid state (Hashimoto's thyroiditis) and in patients who have received RAI therapy for hyperthyroidism. In patients with hyperthyroidism, the levels of serum TSH are usually not detectable.

The response of serum TSH to TRH administration is also helpful. In primary hypothyroidism, the response is exaggerated;

there is no response when it is due to pituitary TSH deficiency and a frequently delayed or prolonged response in hypothyroidism secondary to hypothalamic disease.

Radioactive iodine uptake (RAI) measures the percent of a dose of ^{131}I taken up and bound by the thyroid gland in 24 hours. It is a relatively nonspecific test, since it is markedly affected by the plasma level of inorganic iodide.

Thyroid scanning shows the pattern of distribution of RAI in the thyroid and characterizes the functional activity of nodules ("cold," "warm," or "hot"). It is also used to: (1) distinguish diffuse toxic goiter from toxic nodular goiter, (2) identify ectopic sublingual, metastatic but functional thyroid tissue, and (3) document changes in thyroid function following from subacute thyroiditis, or thyroid size after thyroid-suppressive therapy of nontoxic goiter.

An increased RAI uptake is found in iodine deficiency, thyrotoxicosis (Graves' disease, nodular goiter), TSH excess (early hypothyroidism, defects in thyroid hormone synthesis, and TSH administration), and after administration of antithyroid drugs. Normal RAI uptake values may be found in hypothyroidism, normal subjects, and thyrotoxicosis. Decreased RAI uptake values are found in iodine excess, hypothyroidism, and thyrotoxicosis (factitious thyrotoxicosis, subacute thyroiditis, stroma ovarii, and with massive iodide administration). The RAI uptake obviously cannot always distinguish between hypothyroidism and hyperthyroidism.

Administration of exogenous bovine TSH for 1-3 days will increase RAI uptake as well as T_4 and T_3. A failing thyroid gland will not respond, since it is already functioning maximally (decreased thyroid reserve). This test is used to differentiate primary hypothyroidism (thyroid failure) from hypothyroidism due to deficient endogenous TSH (thyroid intrinsically normal).

The function of the normal thyroid is dependent on TSH. If thyroid hormone is exogenously administered, it will normally suppress endogenous TSH and lead to a decrease in thyroid RAI uptake to 60% or less of the control value, while the hyperthyroid gland is not suppressible.

Intrathyroidal organification of iodide may be measured by

administering perchlorate after a tracer dose of ^{131}I. Further transport of inorganic iodide into the thyroid is inhibited, and any intrathyroidal ^{131}I that has not been organified will diffuse out of the thyroid (normal less than 10-15% discharge). An increased discharge, indicating abnormal organification, is seen in patients taking antithyroid drugs, dyshormonogenetic goiters due to peroxidase deficit, Hashimoto's thyroiditis, and Graves' disease previously treated with radioiodine.

Hyperthyroidism

Hyperthyroidism, five times more common among women than men, has a strong but uncertain familial tendency. There are two major forms of hyperthyroidism: toxic diffuse goiter (Graves' disease) and the less common toxic nodular goiter (Plummer's disease). The manifestations of Plummer's disease are a direct result of increased circulating thyroid hormone, while those of Graves' disease are complicated by immunologic consequences related to its cause. Hyperthyroidism may also be a manifestation of subacute or chronic thyroiditis and may result from excessive ingestion of thyroid hormones.

Graves' disease. The predominant type of hyperthyroidism seen in the U.S., Graves' disease is characterized by hypermetabolism. It is often accompanied by an infiltrative ophthalmopathy with edema, fatty infiltration, deposition of mucopolysaccharides, and lymphocytic infiltration of the ocular muscles and connective tissue, producing venous engorgement, proptosis, and ophthalmoplegia. In addition to this ophthalmopathy, there is also, frequently, dermopathy called myxedema circumscripta, which is a localized mucopolysaccharide infiltration of the skin and subcutaneous tissue. These two manifestations of Graves' disease are pathognomonic but have a course independent of the hyperthyroidism.

A number of observations suggest that both Graves' disease and Hashimoto's thyroiditis may be autoimmune phenomena. Circulating antibodies to thyroid constituents are found in both, and their histologic abnormalities are similar. In addition, patients with Graves' disease have a high frequency of HLA-B8 histocompatibility antigens, and family members may have diseases also thought to be autoimmune, such as Hashimoto's, Addison's, diabetes, or chronic active hepatitis. It is presently believed that one or more immunoglobulins against thyroid tissue act as thyroid stimulators and produce hyperthyroidism. A heritable defect in immune surveillance could lead to emergence of a clone of B lymphocytes that secrete an antibody to thryoid tissue. It is also possible that the antibody might actually be against TSH receptors, so that it could have a stimulator function when bound to specific receptors.

The classic manifestations of hyperthyroidism, directly related to increased circulating thyroid hormone, are goiter, fine tremor, heat intolerance, excessive sweating, emotional lability, weight loss, thirst, diarrhea, and cardiovascular stimulation. Increased cardiac output, due to peripheral vasodilatation and increased oxygen demands, may lead to high output failure. Sinus tachycardia and atrial arrhythmias including atrial fibrillation occur. Patients with preexisting heart disease may show dramatic worsening with the onset of thyrotoxicosis; pure thyrotoxic heart disease in the absence of organic heart disease is rare in the young but may be seen in older individuals, particularly those with toxic nodular goiters.

Two types of eye signs are noted. Spastic changes include the lid retraction and stare (the "frozen terror" of Moebius), failure to converge (Moebius sign). and lid lag (von Graefe sign). Proptosis, ophthalmoplegia, and chemosis are part of the exophthalmic syndromes and are apparently due to immunologic factors not directly related to thyroid hormone. The cardiovascular and spastic eye changes improve dramatically with adrenergic blocking agents, while those of the exopthalmic syndrome do not. In spite of improvement with adrenergic blockade, the precise role of the sympathetic system is not well understood.

Thyrotoxic myopathy is an important consequence, which may be confused with myasthenia gravis or hypokalemic myopathy. Particularly prominent in the pelvic and shoulder musculature, the myopathy responds to control of hyperthyroidism but not to Tensilon.

T_4, T_3, RT_3U, and thyroid RAI uptake are elevated; TRH injection fails to increase serum TSH, and the thyroid RAI uptake is nonsuppressible. Serum cholesterol is often low, while serum calcium, phosphorus and alkaline phosphatase may be high.

Hyperthyroidism Due to Excess Triiodothyronine (T_3 Thyrotoxicosis). Patients are clinically hyperthyroid but have normal levels of total serum T_4; the RT_3U and thyroid RAI uptake may be normal. The hypermetabolism is caused by excess T_3. The incidence of T_3 thyrotoxicosis is probably 4-5% in the United States and has been reported with toxic diffuse goiter, toxic nodular goiter (uninodular and multinodular), and toxic thyroid carcinoma.

Treatment of Graves Disease. Treatment includes antithyroid drugs, surgery, and radioiodine therapy.

The thiocarbamide drugs (propylthiouracil and methimazole) inhibit thyroid organic binding of iodine and thyroid hormone biosynthesis. Therapy for 12-18 months is usually followed by a prolonged remission in 20-50% of patients. The most serious toxic effect of these drugs is agranulocytosis in approximately 0.2% of cases. Rash, fever, and arthralgia occur in about 3% of patients.

Perchlorate and thiocyanate have also been used for the treatment of hyperthyroidism. They reduce iodine transport and so reduce thyroid hormone production but are less well tolerated than the thiocarbamides. When additional iodine is administered, they become less effective, and so cannot be used preoperatively.

Surgery is rarely indicated, and is only undertaken after 3-6 weeks of therapy with the thiocarbamides has rendered the patient euthyroid. Two weeks before surgery, 5 drops of saturated solution of potassium iodide is given three times a day. Complications of subtotal thyroidectomy include hypothyroidism, hypoparathyroidism, vocal cord paralysis, and recurrence of hyperthyroidism. Although surgical therapy is effective in Plummer's disease and reduces the size of the thyroid, it has no real advantage over RAI therapy.

RAI therapy produces a euthyroid state in 10-12 weeks after a single dose. Hypothyroidism, occurring within a few weeks of treatment or developing insidiously after several years, is a major problem. It occurs in approximately 25% of patients treated with radioactive thyroid. In patients over 40, RAI is the treatment of choice, and it is indicated in patients 20-40 years old who have recurrent hyperthyroidism. It is contraindicated in pregnancy and should be used with caution in cases of juvenile hyperthyroidism. Larger doses of RAI are required to treat cases of toxic multinodular goiter.

TREATMENT OF OPHTHALMOPATHY

Noninfiltrative eye changes are corrected when the hyperthyroidism is treated. High doses of steroids (80-120 mg of prednisone a day) are indicated in the treatment of infiltrative ophthalmopathy, especially when there are prominent inflammatory changes or when the disease is progressive. If steroids are ineffective, it may be necessary to surgically decompress the orbit to save vision or ocular integrity. X-ray treatment directed at the orbit is used in some cases of progressive oculopathy. In controlling some cases of malignant exophthalmos, radioablation of all remaining thyroid tissue using ^{131}I has been of some use.

THYROTOXIC CRISIS

A sudden increase in heart rate, body temperature, and all the other manifestations of thyrotoxicosis is called storm or crisis. Precipitated by thyroid surgery in the poorly prepared patient or intercurrent illnesses such as sepsis, the untreated form has a high mortality. Extreme irritability, high fever, tachycardia, diarrhea, and shock are common. One explanation is the possibility of relative adrenal insufficiency. Increased metabolic demands of hyperthyroidism increase corticosteroid requirements, and other stressful situations such as surgery or illness may further increase steroid need so that relative hypoadrenalism occurs. Such an explanation would be particularly important in patients with combined hyperthyroidism and hypoadrenalism.

Treatment includes measures designed to decrease thyroid hormone production, blockade of sympathetic neural activity, and general support measures. A large dose of an antithyroid drug (propylthiuracil, 100-200 mg every 2-6 hours) should be administered to prevent further hormone synthesis, and iodine,

10 mg or more daily, is given to inhibit hormone release. Propranolol (20-80 mg every 4 hours orally or intravenously in some situations) will decrease tachycardia. General supportive measures include adequate fluid replacement, decrease of temperature with cooling blankets, pressor agents for shock, and dexamethasone (1-3 mg every 6 hours depending on severity).

Hypothyroidism

Hypothyroidism is a clinical state resulting from exposure of tissues to an insufficient amount of thyroid hormone. Hypothyroidism dating from birth and resulting in developmental abnormalities is termed *cretinism*. The term *myxedema* is used to describe the severe adult form, characterized by cold intolerance, dry thick skin, constipation, apathy, hoarseness, and retarded speech and movement (see Table 6-4).

Hypothyroidism may develop rapidly (following surgical ablation). Symptoms can evolve in 4-6 weeks and include complaints of myalgias, paresthesias, arthralgias, and emotional disturbance. More commonly, hypothyroidism will develop over 5-10 years

TABLE 6-4—CAUSES OF HYPOTHYROIDISM

DEFICIENCY OF TRH:	Hypothalamic disease
DEFICIENCY OF TSH:	Pituitary tumor (chromophobe adenoma) or infarction (Sheehan's syndrome)
THYROID DESTRUCTION:	Chronic inflammation (Hashimoto's) Surgical ablation Radioactive ablation Irradiation of neck
METABOLIC ABNORMALITY:	Iodine deficiency Iodine excess Antithyroid drugs Biosynthetic defects

(Hashimoto's thyroiditis). Physical examination may reveal a goiter, which should be investigated by laboratory evaluation. Comparing an old photograph with the patient's present appearance may be invaluable in making the diagnosis. When hypothyroidism is due to hypothalamic or pituitary disease, the thyroid gland itself is normal but unstimulated. Hypothyroidism secondary to hypothalamic disorders is less common than that due to pituitary disease.

Laboratory studies may not always correlate easily with clinical states. In the presence of past hypothyroidism, T_4 level is low and TSH is elevated. Serum T_3 and RT_3U, useful in diagnosing hyperthyroidism, are normal in 50% of hypothyroid patients. The cardiac preejection period (PEP) measured noninvasively is prolonged in the hypothyroid state but returns to normal with therapy.

Hormone replacement is very reliable, nonallergenic, nontoxic, and inexpensive. Thyroid hormone replacement, which is indistinguishable from endogenous secretion in its physiologic effect, is obtained with 60-90 mg daily of dessicated thyroid or 100-150 μg of L-thyroxine.

Before instituting therapy, the physician assesses the cardiac status of the patient. In young patients with signficant cardiac disease or in older patients, the initial dose of thyroxine should be lower (25 μg daily for 2-4 weeks) and then increased by gradual increments until a satisfactory therapeutic dose is reached. Measurement of TSH is the best way to determine if hormone replacement is adequate. When TSH is in the normal range, the dose is adequate.

Many patients have been placed on thyroid replacement without any firm laboratory data to prove hypothyroidism. The best way to separate euthyroid from hypothyroid states is discontinuing thyroid replacement. Pituitary-thyroid recovery occurs in 5 weeks, and subsequent measurement of TSH and T_4 should resolve the diagnosis.

MYXEDEMA COMA
Myxedema coma, a rare complication of myxedema usually found in older patients, is characterized by lethargy or coma and hypothermia (temperature 35°C or lower). Hypoventilation with

hypercapnia may occur. The etiology is unknown but patients are usually septic or have been exposed to cold.

Treatment consists of intravenous administration of 250-500 μg L-thyroxine and replacement of fluid volume with special care not to cause hyponatremia. It is important to rule out hypopituitarism as a cause. A plasma cortisol level must be drawn, and 100 mg hydrocortisone hemisuccinate administered every 12 hours intravenously until there is improvement or the cortisol level comes back normal.

THYROIDITIS

Subacute thyroiditis. Presents with fever, pain, and symptoms suggestive of an upper respiratory infection. Painless subacute thyroiditis without goiter and near-normal sedimentation rate has been described, but pain is a usual feature and is located in the anterior neck, throat, or in one or both ears. The thyroid is usually diffusely enlarged, tender with palpation; local adenopathy is not impressive.

There is usually a leukocytosis and an elevated sedimentation rate (50 mm/hour or greater). Thyroid function tests show a combination of elevated T_4 and low radioiodine uptake. The elevated thyroxine level is caused by discharge of stored hormone from ruptured follicles. The radioiodine uptake is suppressed because of the acute inflammation of the gland and the T_4-induced suppression of TSH. Scanning may visualize a "cold spot" during local inflammation. It is important to follow these patients to distinguish them from patients with thyroid neoplasm.

The clinical course of subacute thyroiditis is self-limiting and variable, so treatment must be individualized. The majority of patients respond to salicylates. If they do not, or if they appear more severely ill initially, a month's course of triiodothyronine 25 μg three times daily is indicated. Propranolol may be necessary to offset the side effects (tachycardia, arrhythmias) of triiodothyronine in elderly patients or patients with cardiac disease. For patients refractory to treatment with triiodothyronine, prednisone is indicated.

Subacute thyroiditis does not cause hypothyroidism. The patients should be followed until they are euthyroid and have no symptoms. Neoplasm must be excluded in all patients by repeat scan if the suppression of uptake was unilateral during their clinical course.

Chronic thyroiditis (Hashimoto's disease). A common disorder, occurring most frequently in middle-aged women, this is also the most common cause of sporadic goiter in children. Hashimoto's thyroiditis is a classic example of human autoimmunity. Evidence for this consists of lymphocytic infiltration of the gland and the presence of an increased concentration of serum immunoglobins and antibodies directed against thyroid tissue. Clinically, the most important antibodies are antithyroid antibody, detected by red cell agglutination following coating with thyroglobulin, and antimicrosomal antibody, detected by immunofluorescence or complement fixation. Other pathologic findings in the gland include eosinophilia, follicular rupture, hyperplasia, and fibrosis.

Hashimoto's disease is common with other diseases thought to be autoimmune (pernicious anemia, nontuberculous Addison's disease, myasthenia gravis, Sjögren's syndrome, chronic active hepatitis, rheumatoid arthritis, systemic lupus erythematosus, diabetes, and premature ovarian failure).

Chronic thyroiditis usually presents with hypothyroidism, painless goiter, or both. The most common early state is goiter without hypothyroidism, discovered on routine examination. The goiter is usually diffuse, firm, and involves the pyramidal lobe (a major diagnostic feature). Local lymphadenopathy is unusual, and its presence suggests malignancy.

Hashimoto's thyroiditis, the most common cause of goitrous hypothyroidism in adults, progressively destroys the gland. The thyroid becomes hyperplastic but is eventually unable to produce adequate hormone, so mild to severe hypothyroidism results. Any adult with diffuse goiter should be suspected of having Hashimoto's disease. Thyroid function should be evaluated and repeated at regular intervals, because hypothyroidism can develop insidiously.

Hypothyroid patients should be examined for goiter. Antibody screening is necessary to confirm the underlying disease. In adults, hypothyroidism without goiter is most likely due to a late stage of chronic thyroiditis. High antibody titers will confirm the diagnosis. The term "hashitoxicosis" is used to describe patients with Graves disease (high radioiodine uptake values and frank hyperthyroidism) who have lymphocytic infiltration and high antibody titers. Because the course of Hashimoto thyroiditis is so variable, the best diagnostic approach is careful palpation of the neck, measurement of TSH and T_4 levels, and occasionally needle biopsy if there is a suspicion of malignancy. Treatment consists of thyroxine in therapeutic doses to suppress the goiter or correct hypothyroidism.

Thyroid Enlargements: Nodes, Nodules, and Cancer

Physical findings are often missed in palpating the thyroid. If the gland is diffusely enlarged, the diagnosis of inflammation or hyperplasia is most likely. Neoplasm should be considered if there is irregular, localized, or nodular enlargement of the gland. An irregularly enlarged thyroid gland may be a benign thyroid adenoma, a nodular goiter, or cancer of the thyroid.

Thyroid adenomas. These occur either singly or as part of a benign nodular goiter. They may function as normal thyroid tissue or can even be more active and suppress TSH, leading to hypofunction of the rest of the gland. Hyperfunctioning has been observed only with benign lesions, not in thyroid cancer. A "hot nodule" on diagnostic scanning (the only site of uptake) tends to rule out malignancy.

Nodular goiter. A common disorder, which begins in the fourth decade and is more common in women than men. The etiology is unclear. Clinically, the majority of patients with nodular goiter are euthyroid, but 20-25% have nonsuppressible thyroid function (with exogenous thyroid hormone, the radioiodine uptake values do not fall more than 50%). Hyperthyroidism with nodular goiter usually involves the latter group. Thyroid function should be assessed regularly and the patients watched for development of thyrotoxicosis. Cancer is rare.

Thyroid cancer. Cancer should be considered when a thyroid mass is identified, but it is rare and death from it is even more so. *Papillary carcinoma* of the thyroid occurs in the second and third decades and tends to metastasize to local lymph nodes. It is slow growing both in gland and nodes. Differentiation between benign and malignant lesions requires exacting pathologic study. Invasion of the thyroid capsule or blood vessels indicates malignancy.

Pure *follicular carcinoma*, less common than papillary but as difficult to diagnose histologically, tends to metastasize hematogenously to bone (pelvis, skull, spine) and produce lytic lesions and pathologic fractures. Symptoms arising from bony lesions may be the presenting manifestation.

A mixed *papillary-follicular lesion* is more common than either a pure papillary or pure follicular lesion. The mixed lesion behaves like the papillary lesion (slow growth and local recurrence) but may occasionally metastasize to the lungs. Bone metastasis is less frequent in mixed lesions. The Hürthle cell tumor, the rarest type of tumor, is not well documented but does metastasize locally.

Medullary cancer. A well-differentiated tumor accounting for 3% of thyroid cancers, this arises from parafollicular cells, which secrete thyrocalcitonin. Medullary carcinoma can occur either as a unifocal lesion in elderly patients (75% of cases) or as a bilateral tumor arising from hyperplastic foci in the midportion of the thyroid lobes. The bilateral form is often associated with pheochromacytomas, which tend to be malignant and bilateral. The combination of pheochromocytoma, medullary thyroid carcinoma, and parathyroid hyperplasia is known as *multiple endocrine neoplasia type II* (MEN II), an autosomal dominant disorder. In Men III (also called IIb), mucosal neuromas, and a characteristic facies are present. (See page 382.)

Other clinical syndromes associated with medullary carcinoma include the carcinoid syndrome, intractable diarrhea, elevation of serum calcitonin, amyloidosis (asymptomatic), and Cushing's syndrome secondary to ACTH production by the tumor.

In both types of MEN II, the medullary cancer produces large amounts of thyrocalcitonin. Basal levels can often be determined, but occasionally a provocative test with glucagon, calcium infusion, or pentagastrin is required. Calcitonin assays are important for several reasons: evidence that a nodule in the thyroid is a medullary carcinoma, confirmation of surgical cure, detection of recurrent and residual disease, and study of first-order relatives of affected individuals.

Undifferentiated thyroid cancer. This tends to grow rapidly and often invades locally, with resultant strangulation or esophageal obstruction. Patients present with a neck mass, hoarseness, and stupor. Treatment is a combination of surgery, irradiation, and chemotherapy, but the prognosis is poor.

Favus et al. conducted a series of studies that found a significantly increased incidence of thyroid cancer in patients who had neck irradiation in childhood, usually for benign infections or inflammatory diseases. The study further showed a direct correlation between the dose of radiation given and the occurrence of thyroid neoplasm. The physician must elicit a history of irradiation, and if a node is palpable, the protocol recommended by the American Thyroid Association and National Cancer Institute serves as an excellent clinical guide.

Category I: Patients have a positive history but no palpable nodule in the neck. Scan is recommended, and yearly bimanual palpation is necessary. If a cold area is seen on the scan but no palpable thyroid nodule on repeat exam, surgical studies show that 25-27% of these lesions are malignant. However, it is acceptable to delay surgery until the lesion is clinically detected. Suppression with thyroid is another method of treatment.

Category II: This category includes patients with a history of prior irradiation and one or more palpable nodules. The patients should have a scan. Surgery is indicated if a cold nodule is found.

Category III: This category includes patients with diffuse goiter but no palpable nodules. Required studies include thyroid function tests, antibody titers, and scanning. If there are no nodules, examination for nodules should be repeated in 6 months. If a nodule is found, surgery is indicated.

In patients with no history of irradiation but who have a palpable thyroid nodule, a pertechnetate thyroid scan is recommended. If the nodule is hot and the patient is not hyperthyroid, no further workup is necessary. If the patient is hyperthyroid, surgical or radioiodine ablation of the nodule is the recommended treatment. If the nodule is cold, ^{131}I scanning should be performed since technetium scanning indicates uptake not organification. If the nodule is still cold, ultrasound is indicated to distinguish cystic (no malignant potential) from mixed-solid nodules. To date, there is no definitive noninvasive procedure to distinguish between malignant and benign nodules, and in many centers needle biopsy would be recommended next. If a benign lesion is demonstrated, the internist must be guided by clinical knowledge and expertise and recommend exploratory surgery if necessary.

ADRENAL GLAND DISORDERS
Physiology of Adrenal Cortex
Three principal steroids are produced by the adrenal cortex from cholesterol. *Cortisol*, a glucocorticoid, is hydroxylated at the 11, 17, and 21 positions; *aldosterone*, a mineralocorticoid, is hydroxylated at the 11 and 21 positions; *dehydroepiandrosterone*, an adrenal androgen, has a ketone group at the 17 position. Urine 17-hydroxycorticoids (Porter-Silber chromogens) reflect glucocorticoid excretion, while urine 17-ketosteroids (Zimmermann reaction) reflect adrenal and gonadal production of androgens.

Cortisol is synthesized by both the zona fasciculata and the zona reticularis; most of the 13-20 mg secreted each day is bound to the alpha-globulin transcortin and is biologically inactive. Cortisol and corticotropin are secreted cyclically, with maximum concentrations at 8:00 A.M. and lowest concentrations at midnight.

The synthesis of adrenal androgens takes place in both the zona fasciculata and the zona reticularis. Approximately 10-20 mg of dehydroepiandrosterone sulfate is produced in 24 hours. Small quantities are converted by peripheral tissues (liver and adipose tissue) to a more active androgen—testosterone—and hyperfunction of the hepatic pathway leads to significant masculinization in females. During fetal life and again at puberty, adrenal androgen production increases, reaching a peak in early adulthood and declining to low levels after age 50. The adrenal androgen androstenedione can be converted by the liver and adipose tissue to the estrogen estrone, a major source of estrogen in children and postmenopausal women.

Aldosterone secretion takes place in the zona glomerulosa and is stimulated primarily by angiotensin II, ACTH, and potassium. Approximately 30-150 μg of aldosterone are secreted daily, and

25-50% of the amount is excreted as urinary tetrahydroaldoster-one-3-glucuronide. Aldosterone stimulates the reabsorption of sodium and the secretion of potassium in the distal convoluted tubules and collecting ducts.

Adrenal cortisol and androgen are controlled by ACTH, which is controlled by corticotropin-releasing factor and feedback control. The diurnal variation of cortisol is due to diurnal shifts in ACTH secretion. ACTH production is also triggered by stress, fever, and hypoglycemia.

MEASUREMENT OF ADRENAL HORMONES

Plasma cortisol averages 9-24 μg/dl in the morning and 3-12 μg/dl at night. Estrogens increase, and hepatic disease decreases cortisol-binding protein concentration. Urine 17-hydroxysteroid excretion averages 2-10 mg every 24 hours; usually, more is excreted during the day than at night. Urine 17-ketosteroid excretion averages 7-25 mg every 24 hours for males, 4-15 mg every 24 hours for females. Simultaneous creatinine measurement ensures accuracy of urine collection; adult women excrete about 1000 mg of creatinine daily, adult men about 1800 mg. Fifty to 60% of this occurs in the daytime collection. Resting values of adrenal hormones are of much less clinical importance than values obtained after either stimulation by ACTH or feedback inhibition induced by dexamethasone. ACTH radioimmunoassay can distinguish pituitary hypercorticism from other types.

Adrenocortical Hypofunction (Addison's Disease)

The most common cause in the United States and Western Europe is an autoimmune disorder with lymphocytic and plasma cell invasion of the adrenals and antiadrenal antibodies in the plasma. The only other disease in which these antibodies occur with high prevalence is idiopathic hypoparathyroidism. There is a high incidence of associated endocrine disorders in Addison's disease: premature ovarian failure (24% with primary or secondary amenorrhea), thyroid disease (thyrotoxicosis, primary hypothyroidism, Hashimoto's thyroiditis), diabetes mellitus, and idiopathic hypoparathyroidism. When both adrenal and thyroid deficiencies exist, the term Schmidt's syndrome is applied. The autoimmune disorder is associated with specific HLA antigens, HLA-B8 and Dw3. Other causes of adrenal insufficiency include chronic granulomatous infections (tuberculosis, sarcoidosis, and histoplasmosis), bilateral adrenalectomy, metastatic carcinoma, sepsis, and anticoagulant therapy.

Clinical manifestations are weakness; weight loss; anorexia; hyperpigmentation concentrated over palmar creases, pressure points, and around the areolae of the nipples; hypotension; and hyponatremia. Vitilgo, gastrointestinal symptoms, hypoglycemia, hyperkalemia, and azotemia are helpful diagnostically.

Failure of plasma cortisol to increase more than 8 μg/dl following ACTH stimulation confirms the diagnosis. A useful screening test is the I.M. or I.V. administration of 25 units (0.25 mg) of synthetic ACTH (cosyntropin) with sampling at 30 and 60 minutes. While an adequate increase rules out hypoadrenalism, some normal individuals fail to increase with this dose, and more intense stimulation is necessary. Abnormal results are nonspecific and require further evaluation.

Synthetic ACTH, 40 units in 500 cc normal saline, is infused over an 8-hour period (from 8:00 A.M. to 4:00 P.M.) for two consecutive days with urinary 17-OHS and 17-KS and plasma cortisol measured on a control day and on each day of the infusions. Failure to increase urinary steroids threefold and to absolute levels greater than 12 mg every 24 hours, is strong evidence for hypoadrenalism. Testing should be accompanied by administration of corticosteroids to avoid adrenal collapse during the test. The patient is given dexamethasone 0.5 mg BID and fluorohydrocortisone 0.1 mg daily during testing and until the results are known.

Patients with hypopituitarism causing hypoadrenalism can be distinguished from patients with primary adrenal insufficiency by the presence of other pituitary hormone deficiencies and by the occurrence of a rise in urinary steroids, which is delayed until the third or fourth day of stimulation by ACTH. In some cases, it will be necessary to measure the plasma ACTH to make the distinction. Skull films should be taken to look for an enlarged sella.

If an *acute adrenal crisis* is suspected, blood should be drawn for plasma cortisol levels, and treatment should begin immediately. The therapy for acute adrenal insufficiency is intravenous hydrocortisone hemisuccinate, 100 mg as a bolus and then 50 mg every 4-6 hours during the first 2 days of the crisis. Circulating volume should be restored with plasma expanders, intravenous glucose in saline, and in some cases, blood. When the patient's condition improves, steroid doses can be tapered over 3-5 days to replacement levels.

Since adrenal insufficiency is a lifelong disorder, the clinical response will determine the regimen. The usual replacement therapy for chronic adrenal insufficiency consists of 15-20 mg cortisone on arising in the morning and 10-15 mg cortisone in the late afternoon. The patient also receives fluorohydrocortisone, 0.05-0.1 mg p.o. daily. The effect of the mineralocorticoid is monitored by watching for weight gain and hypokalemia. When the patient with chronic adrenal insufficiency is exposed to major stress, the steroid dosage should be increased.

Secondary Adrenal Insufficiency

Secondary adrenal insufficiency is usually the result of panhypopituitarism. The causes in general include pituitary or hypothalamic tumor, including craniopharyngioma, metastatic tumor to the pituitary or hypothalamus, pituitary infarction (Sheehan's syndrome, diabetes mellitus), surgery or irradiation (therapeutic or unintended ablation), granulomatous disease (histiocytosis, sarcoid), and infection (syphilis, tuberculosis, pyogenic and fungal). Secondary adrenal insufficiency may also be due to glucocorticoid-induced suppression, following either glucocorticoid therapy or surgical removal of an adrenocortical tumor.

With pituitary tumors, ACTH and TSH deficiencies occur relatively late, while other abnormalities such as growth hormone deficiency, gonadotropin deficiency, and prolactin excess occur earlier. Sheehan's syndrome generally produces panhypopituitarism. Except for glucocorticoid-induced suppression, isolated ACTH deficiency is rare.

The clinical manifestations of secondary adrenal insufficiency

are nonspecific and include weakness, fatigability, emotional
lability, and hypoglycemia. Hyperpigmentation is absent because
ACTH and lipotropin concentrations are low. Since aldosterone
production is not control-dependent on ACTH, hyperkalemia is
not seen although hyponatremia results from the water overload
seen with cortisol deficiency. The diagnosis is based on the
evaluation for deficiency or excess of other pituitary hormones.
ACTH reserve may be evaluated by administration of metyrapone, a drug that blocks 11-hydroxylation of cortisol precursors;
3 gm p.o. (70-kg patients) is given with a snack at midnight, and
at 8:00 A.M., plasma for 11-deoxycortisol and cortisol is drawn.
Plasma 11-deoxycortisol of less than 80 μg/dl suggests pituitary
dysfunction.

The block in cortisol stimulates ACTH secretion, which is
recognized by an increase of the nonhydroxylated precursor 11-
deoxycortisol. The increase in plasma cortisol following hypoglycemia has the advantage of testing growth hormone and ACTH
reserve concurrently. Contraindicated in patients with seizure
disorder or cardiac disease, regular insulin 0.1-0.15 units/kg is
administered and blood samples obtained before injection and at
30, 45, 60, 90, and 120 minutes after injection. The normal
response is for blood glucose to fall below 40 μg/dl and the
plasma cortisol to rise by a minimum of 8.0 μg/dl to a value
exceeding 20 μg/dl.

Selective Aldosterone Deficiency

The most common cause of selective aldosterone deficiency in
adults is decreased renin production due to mild or moderate
renal disease (diabetic nephropathy or pyelonephritis). It may
also be due to a defect of aldosterone 18-hydroxylation. Diabetics
have multiple defects, including not only renal disease but a
defective conversion of the inactive renin precursor to renin,
which is manifested as decreased renin activity, enzymatic defects
in aldosterone biosynthesis, and autonomic neuropathy with
decreased catecholamine-induced secretion of renin. Other causes
are chronic heparin administration (decreased aldosterone synthesis) and lead poisoning (decreased renin synthesis).

Clinical manifestations include hyperkalemia and its consequences (muscle weakness, cardiac arrhythmias, and CNS dysfunction). In patients with both insulin-dependent diabetes and aldosterone deficiency, hyperglycemia may induce hyperkalemia. Salt wasting and hyperchloremic acidosis are occasionally seen. Hypoadrenalism, volume depletion, spironolactone or triamterene administration, unrecognized potassium administration, and thrombocytosis must be ruled out as causes of hyperkalemia. The adult hyporeninemic form is diagnosed by measuring plasma renin and aldosterone concentrations following volume depletion and upright posture. The therapy for selective aldosterone deficiency is fludrocortisone (Florinef) 0.05-0.2 mg/day.

Hypothalamic-Pituitary Adrenal (HPA) Suppression Due to Steroid Administration

HPA suppression should be suspected in patients who have received a glucocorticoid in doses equivalent to 20-30 mg of prednisone per day for more than a week. Suppression may not occur for up to 1 month with doses close to but still above the physiologic range. Doses of glucocorticoid equivalent to 5 mg of prednisone daily do not cause suppression if given early in the day. (There have been no documented cases of hypothalamic-pituitary suppression as a result of ACTH administration.)

Recovery from HPA suppression after prolonged exposure to large doses of glucocorticoid is in four phases. During the first month, the pituitary and adrenal are still suppressed. From the second to the fifth month, the pituitary regains normal function but the adrenal remains suppressed. From the sixth to the ninth month, there is partial adrenal recovery, and from the ninth to the twelfth month, full recovery is usually seen. The best test to determine recovery is ACTH stimulation or insulin-induced hypoglycemia.

Alternate-day therapy utilizes short-acting glucocorticoid every 48 hours in the morning. This regimen prevents or ameliorates manifestations of Cushing's syndrome. Alternate-day therapy is associated with normal or nearly normal HPA response to tests and is as effective in controlling a group of diseases as daily therapy in divided doses. The possible exception is in the treatment of giant cell arteritis. Single-dose therapy is indicated for patients who cannot tolerate alternate-day therapy. Single daily-dose therapy produces less HPA suppression than divided daily doses and controls a number of diseases, including giant cell arteritis. However, it does not prevent manifestations of Cushing's syndrome. Caution should be used in withdrawing patients from glucocorticoids. Three possible hazards include adrenocortical insufficiency, steroid withdrawal syndrome, and exacerbation of the underlying disease. Small doses (10-20 mg) of hydrocortisone in the morning may alleviate withdrawal symptoms.

Hyperadrenalism: Cushing's Syndrome

Hyperadrenalism is a relatively uncommon syndrome produced by a variety of causal factors. Clinical presentation depends on the relative secretion rates of glucocorticoids, mineralocorticoids and adrenal androgens.

Excess pituitary ACTH production with bilateral adrenal hyperplasia. This is found in 70% of patients due to either pituitary neoplasm or excess hypothalamic secretion of corticotropin-releasing factor. The onset is gradual; the condition is found mainly in women in the reproductive age group. Early symptoms are menstrual irregularities in women, impotence in men, easy bruising, plethora, and facial rounding. Increased androgen production in women causes hirsutism and balding. Pigmentation reflecting ACTH excess is found in light-skinned people.

Ectopic ACTH production. Found in a group of malignant tumors, most commonly lung, thymus, pancreas, and kidney. Mineralocorticoid effects with weakness, weight loss, and hypokalemic alkalosis predominate. The patient usually does not appear Cushingoid, so that the extremely high cortisol levels contrast with the clinical appearance. An elevated ACTH level indicates excess ACTH production, extremely high levels favoring ectopic production while high concentrations in jugular venous blood suggest pituitary production. The primary tumor must be identified for conclusive differentiation from pituitary excess, since the biochemical studies often overlap.

Excess adrenal cortisol production. Possibly due to adenoma or carcinoma, this occurs in 30% of patients. Benign tumors may be multiple with atrophic surrounding gland and produce a syndrome reflecting intense glucocorticoid secretion. Adrenal carcinoma usually produces hirsutism and defeminization. A palpable mass is present in 50% of patients, and the IVP on the affected side is distorted.

BIOCHEMICAL DIFFERENTIAL DIAGNOSIS OF HYPERADRENALISM

Absence of diurnal variation of plasma ACTH and cortisol levels with evening cortisol levels greater than 10-14 μg/dl suggest the diagnosis. Loss of ACTH suppressibility (lack of negative feedback control) by oral administration of 1 mg dexamethasone at midnight is a useful screening procedure. If the morning cortisol is below 5 μg/dl, indicating negative feedback, hyperadrenalism is very unlikely. Failure to suppress cortisol may indicate hyperadrenalism but may also be a false-positive result, particularly in obese individuals.

A definitive diagnosis is obtained by administering a standard low dose of dexamethasone (0.5 mg q6h for 48 hours). Failure to reduce cortisol to less than 5 μg/dl or 17-hydroxysteroid excretion to less than 3 mg every 24 hours confirms the presence of hyperadrenalism. Free cortisol urinary excretion greater than 100 μg every 24 hours is a useful confirmatory measurement.

High-dose dexamethasone administration (2 mg q6h for 48 hours) allows further separation. Patients with excess pituitary ACTH production will reduce urinary 17-hydroxysteroid excretion to less than half of baseline levels. Patients with either adrenal neoplasm or ectopic ACTH secretion will not suppress with this level of dexamethasone; ACTH concentrations will be normal or low in the former, high in the latter. Metyrapone inhibition of cortisol biosynthesis leads to an increase in 11-deoxycortisol levels in Cushing's disease but not in adrenocortical tumor.

The separation of adenoma from carcinoma is difficult, but carcinoma is suggested if urinary 17-ketosteroids are increased. Usually, 17-hydroxysteroids increase in adenomas but not in carcinomas following ACTH administration. A substantially greater increase in 17-hydroxysteroids compared to 17-ketosteroids is characteristic of adrenal adenomas.

MANAGEMENT OF HYPERADRENALISM

Additional diagnostic information is derived from radiographic and scanning procedures. Ordinary radiographs of the sella turcica are usually normal in individuals with pituitary excess of ACTH, but angiography and tomography frequently reveal microadenomas. Computerized tomography of the abdomen outlines adrenal morphology, assisting in the diagnosis of carcinoma. Differentiation from alcoholism and obesity is occasionally difficult, but neither produces resistance to low-dose dexamethasone suppression.

The treatment of bilateral hyperplasia due to pituitary ACTH excess is controversial. Bromocriptine, a dopamine agonist, and cyproheptadine, a serotonin antagonist, reduce ACTH secretion by inhibiting CRF. Many prefer transsphenoidal microadenomectomy, particularly if the sella is radiographically abnormal. Heavy particle irradiation may be useful in adults, but conventional radiotherapy is ineffective, although it may be useful in children.

Surgical removal is indicated for adrenal carcinoma or adenoma. Either aminoglutethimide or o,p DDD, an analog of DDT, are used for the treatment of metastic disease, since they both inhibit tumor growth and hormone biosynthesis.

Nelson's Syndrome

Approximately 10% of patients with Cushing's syndrome secondary to pituitary ACTH excess develop Nelson's syndrome, whose two main features are hyperpigmentation and chromophobe tumor of the pituitary gland. First described in 1958, the syndrome develops 6 months to 15 years after adrenalectomy. It is therefore imperative that patients who have adrenalectomy for pituitary Cushing's syndrome be followed closely. Hyperpigmentation, sella enlargement, and increased ACTH are diagnostic features. Treatment of Nelson's syndrome includes surgery, heavy-particle irradiation, bromocriptine, and cyproheptadine.

Physiology of Adrenal Medulla

The adrenal medulla, the major source of endogenous epinephrine, consists of chromaffin tissue of neuroectodermal origin. Epinephrine is synthesized from tyrosine through an intermediate compound, dopamine, which is hydroxylated to norepinephrine by the catalytic effect of the enzyme dopamine B-hydroxylase. Norepinephrine is then methylated to epinephrine by catecholamine N-methyltransferase.

Epinephrine has both alpha and beta adrenergic actions, including stimulation of hepatic glycogenolysis and lipolysis with inhibition of hepatic gluconeogenesis and insulin release. Important cardiovascular effects of epinephrine include cardiac stimulation and mixed vasodilator and vasoconstrictor activity.

Pheochromocytoma

Most patients with pheochromocytoma have sustained rather than episodic hypertension. Important additional features include sweating (episodic more often than sustained), episodic palpitations, and hypermetabolism which includes weight loss, myocarditis, focal myocardial necrosis, and mental changes which may include a frank psychosis. Postural hypotension, caused by decreased plasma volume, is a common physical finding. Medullary thyroid carcinoma, a curable form of carcinoma, is a rare disorder associated with pheochromocytomas.

The most frequently used test to detect pheochromocytoma is measurement of urinary vanillylmandelic acid (VMA), one of the principal metabolites of the catecholamines. Eighty-five to 90% are detected by urinary VMA excretion of greater than 9 mg every 24 hours. If this value is normal and clinical suspicion is high, the next step is to determine urinary levels of metanephrines and/or free catecholamines. Pharmacologic testing with phentolamine to lower the blood pressure or with glucagon, histamine, or tyramine to provoke an attack is dangerous, nonspecific, and rarely used.

Preoperatively, patients with pheochromocytomas are prepared by giving an alpha-blocking agent (phenoxybenzamine hydrochloride, 20-40 mg daily in divided doses) to lower blood pressure and increase vascular volume. Alpha blockade is mandatory before invasive diagnostic procedures in order to prevent acute hypertensive crises; beta blockade with propranolol is used to treat severe arrhythmias during surgery.

PARATHYROID GLAND AND
CALCIUM METABOLISM DISORDERS
Physiology

Parathyroid hormone (PTH), calcitonin, and vitamin D act on gut, liver, and kidney to regulate the absorption, distribution, and excretion of calcium, phosphorus, and magnesium. PTH is synthesized in the parathyroid gland and cleaved by kidney and liver into a carboxyl-terminal fragment with long half-life and no biologic activity and an amino-terminal fragment with most of the biologic activity but a short half-life. Commercial radioimmunoassays usually measure the carboxyl-terminal fragment because of its stability.

Reduction in ionized calcium concentration increases PTH secretion, while hypercalcemia inhibits PTH release. PTH increases plasma calcium by (1) increasing bone resorption, (2) promoting renal phosphate excretion and calcium retention, and (3) increasing intestinal calcium absorption by promoting hydroxylation of vitamin D in the kidney to its active form. Renal failure reduces phosphate excretion and leads to PTH secretion by its indirect effect in lowering plasma calcium concentrations. Calcitonin, a polypeptide secreted by the parafollicular cells of the thyroid, exerts negative feedback control by reducing bone resorption when calcium levels become high. Since gastrin and related peptides stimulate calcitonin release, calcitonin may have an effect on calcium absorption from the gut.

Vitamin D_3 (cholecalciferol) from ultraviolet irradiation of skin and the diet is hydroxlated in the liver to $25(OH)D_3$. Feedback control is then afforded by renal conversion to either an active $(1,25(OH)_2\ D_3)$ or inactive $(24,25(OH)_2\ D_3)$ form. Parathyroid hormone, hypocalcemia, and hypophosphatemia stimulate production of the active form, which stimulates the formation of a calcium-binding protein. This protein increases intestinal absorption of calcium, mobilizes calcium from bone, and promotes bone deposition of hydroxyapatite by raising calcium and phosphate levels. Low values of vitamin D (normal value of 25(OH) D, 15-80 ng/ml) occur in vitamin D deficiency, severe liver disease, pregnancy, hyperthyroidism, and with anticonvulsant therapy.

Hypercalcemia

Hypercalcemia, a common problem in medical practice, results from problems in the three organ systems controlling calcium stores: the gut, bone, and kidneys.

Increased GI absorption of calcium occurs in sarcoidosis, the milk alkali syndrome, and hypervitaminosis D. The increased absorption in sarcoid occurs via a poorly understood vitamin D-like mechanism. Other granulomatous diseases such as tuberculosis, berylliosis, and coccidioidomycosis also cause hypercalcemia. Since the milk alkali syndrome is associated with renal insufficiency, alkalosis, and elevated phosphate and calcium levels, it must be distinguished from primary hyperparathyroidism with secondary renal insufficiency; PTH levels will be low in the milk alkali syndrome. Hypervitaminosis D produces renal insufficiency and elevated phosphate in 50% of patients.

Hypercalcemia due to excessive bone resorption is seen with osteolytic malignancies, including hematologic neoplasia and multiple myeloma. It may also be seen in Paget's disease and as a manifestation of hyperthyroidism.

Increased renal reabsorption of calcium is found in patients receiving thiazide diuretics and in adrenal insufficiency.

All three mechanisms account for hypercalcemia in hyperparathyroidism.

TREATMENT

If the serum calcium level is greater than 14 mg/100ml, or 12-14 mg/100 ml and the patient is symptomatic, the situation is an emergency and requires immediate therapy. For most patients, emergency management of hypercalcemia consists of a saline diuresis of 3-4 liters of saline every 24 hours along with 80-160 mg of furosemide. Hypernatremia will be avoided by administering a liter of dextrose for every third or fourth liter of saline. Placement of a central venous line is indicated along with patients with marginal left ventricular function.

In patients with vitamin D intoxication, myeloma, and breast carcinoma with hypercalcemia precipitated by sex steroid therapy, prednisone, 60 mg/day, is a supplemental agent along with the saline diuresis.

Mithramycin, the most potent antihypercalcemic agent, is another therapeutic modality for emergency treatment of severe hypercalcemia. The initial dose is 25 mg/kg, and repeat doses are indicated when the serum calcium begins to rise.

Calcitonin, which works rapidly, is a useful agent when mithramycin is not available. Inorganic phosphate, 1.0-1.5 gm every 24 hours intravenously will temporarily lower serum calcium but should be used with caution, especially if the serum phosphate is elevated because of the risk of extraskeletal calcification.

Hypercalciuria

Hypercalciuria is defined as excretion of 200 mg every 24 hours of urinary calcium on a dietary intake of 400 mg or less. Patients may develop calcium urolithiasis and, except for the stones, are asymptomatic. Hypercalciuria is absorptive, renal, and resorptive. *Absorptive* hypercalciuria is the result of increased gastrointestinal absorption of calcium and suppression of PTH activity. *Renal* calcium excretion is increased because of an increased filtered load and decreased tubular reabsorption of calcium. *Resorptive* hypercalciuria occurs in hyperparathyroidism; urine calcium is increased as a result of increased filtered load.

These three types of hypercalciuria can be distinguished from one another by measuring a fasting serum and urine calcium and then measuring urine calcium after 1 gm of calcium is given by mouth. In absorptive hypercalciuria, fasting calcium levels are normal, but after the calcium load the urine calcium level rises markedly. In primary hyperparathyroidism, fasting serum and urine levels of calcium are high, and the urine calcium does not rise as strikingly after the calcium load. In renal hypercalciuria, fasting serum calcium is normal, and urine calcium is high and rises higher after the calcium load.

It is important to define the mechanisms of hypercalciuria, because treatment depends on distinguishing among the three mechanisms. Parathyroidectomy is indicated for primary hyperparathyroidism. Patients with absorptive hypercalciuria are treated by interfering with gastrointestinal absorption of calcium. Thiazides are indicated in patients with renal hypercalciuria. Adjunctive therapy in all patients includes a high fluid intake and restricted calcium diet.

Primary Hyperparathyroidism
PATHOPHYSIOLOGY
Primary hyperparathyroidism is caused by a single adenoma in 80-90% of patients. Type I patients have large adenomas, a short history, high serum calcium level (10.5 mg/100 ml or greater), and bone involvement or osteitis fibrosa. Type II patients have smaller adenomas, a longer history, moderate hypercalcemia, and renal stones.

The next most frequent cause of primary hyperparathyroidism is chief cell hyperplasia. All four glands are usually involved, and the serum calcium is moderately elevated. This disorder may be the result of some parathyrotrophic substance or a reset of the level of influence of serum calcium on PTH release.

Carcinoma of the parathyroid is the least common cause of hyperparathyroidism, accounting for less than 2%. These lesions grow slowly and metastasize locally or to the liver or bone. Serum calcium values are usually greater than 15 mg/100 ml.

CLINICAL FEATURES
A number of organ systems may be involved in hyperparathyroidism: (1) renal (renal stone disease, nephrocalcinosis, decreased glomerular filtration, thirst, polydipsia, and polyuria), (2) skeletal (bone tenderness and pain and skeletal demineralization, cystic bone lesions, vertebral collapse, and spontaneous fracture), (3) gastrointestinal (abdominal distress, peptic ulcer, acute and chronic pancreatitis, pancreatic calcifications, vomit-

ing, constipation, anorexia and weight loss), (4) neurologic (somnolence, coma, abnormal diffuse EEG findings), (5) mental (fatigue, apathy, depression, psychosis, personality changes), (6) neuromuscular (muscle fatigue, weakness, hypotonia, arthralgias, gout, pseudogout, and periarticular calcifications), and (7) ocular (conjunctivitis, band keratopathy).

Additional manifestations of hyperparathyroidism include tetany in the newborn, hyperparathyroidism among family members, renal transplants, endocrine adenomatosis, and tumors of the upper mediastinum and neck.

Most patients with hyperparathyroidism are discovered by routine multiphasic screening and are found to have hypercalcemia. Other than generalized weakness, physical findings are usually seen in severely ill patients and include pallor, weight loss, and band keratopathy. Vertebral fractures, kyphosis, and pseudoclubbing (which is a result of severe osteitis of the terminal phalanges) are also found in advanced cases.

LABORATORY DIAGNOSES

The most valuable direct test for the diagnosis is measurement of the serum calcium level, which is elevated in 90-95% of patients with primary hyperparathyroidism. If the initial calcium level is normal but clinical evidence is strong, repeat calcium determinations are often valuable because intermittent elevation is common in mild disease. The serum phosphorus level is usually low and the serum chloride value is usually greater than 102 mEq/liter so that the chloride/phosphorus ratio is greater than 30. The elevated chloride and low bicarbonate reflect the influence of excess PTH on renal bicarbonate excretion, producing a hyperchloremic acidosis. Urinary cAMP and PTH are elevated in hyperparathyroidism but not in other hypercalcemic states since hypercalemia suppresses normal PTH secretion. PTH values are less valuable in detecting hyperparathyroidism in patients with mild to intermittent hypercalcemia and in differentiating between primary and ectopic hyperparathyroidism. Patients with severe hyperparathyroidism may have normal calcium levels due to dietary deficiency or malabsorption of calcium or vitamin D, chronic renal insufficiency, magnesium deficiency, or severe hepatic disease. PTH is usually elevated.

Positive radiologic findings include osteitis in the skull, the ends of the clavicles, and the hands. Subperiosteal resorption will be seen in the bones of the hands, particularly in the middle phalanges.

Ectopic Hyperparathyroidism

It is frequently difficult to differentiate between ectopic and primary hyperparathyroidism. The former presents with hypercalcemia and features resembling hyperparathyroidism in association with malignancies of lung, thymus, pancreas, and kidney. The ectopic, or pseudohyperparathyroidism, differs from true parathyroid disease by three features: (1) anemia, (2) serum chloride value less than 102 mEq/liter, and (3) elevated alkaline phosphatase without evidence of parthyroid disease.

TREATMENT OF PRIMARY HYPERPARATHYROIDISM

The treatment of primary hyperparathyroidism is surgical. Patients with mild symptoms, elevated serum calcium, and low phosphorus should have exploration of one side of the neck. If one large parathyroid adenoma and one normal gland are found, the operation may be concluded after resection of the adenoma. Seven-eighths parathyroidectomy is necessary to control the disease and prevent recurrence in patients with hyperplastic involvement of all four glands. If unsure, it is better to expose three glands. If more than one is enlarged and clinically involved, the disease should be treated as hyperplasia. If reoperation is necessary, preoperative studies including arteriography and measurement of PTH in blood aspirated from the veins near the thyroid and parathyroid are necessary to assist in identifying the abnormal tissue. Asymptomatic hyperparathyroid patients with serum calcium under 11 mg/100 ml and no renal impairment or stones may be followed with twice-yearly measurement of serum clacium and alkaline phosphatase, annual hand films, and estimation of creatinine clearance.

Most patients require no special preoperative preparation. However, patients with severe osteitis fibrosa cystica often develop prolonged postoperative hypocalcemia because of "hungry" bones. Preoperative treatment with 12-hydroxyvitamin D_3, 2 mg/day, for 7-10 days will ameliorate the condition. This treatment should be given only to those patients with serum calcium less than 12.5 mg/100 ml and discontinued if severe hypercalcemia develops. Tetany is the principal problem postoperatively. The hypocalcemia may be brief owing to temporary gland injury, more prolonged in patients with osteitis fibrosa cystica and osteomalacia, or permanent owing to permanent damage of the remaining parathyroid tissue. In patients with a single adenoma, a yearly follow-up determination of serum calcium and fasting blood sugar is recommended. If more than one gland is involved, features of the multiple endocrine neoplasia syndrome should be investigated.

Cancer of the Parathyroid
Cancer of the parathyroid is a rare cause of hyperparathyroidism, occurring in 3-5% of cases. The serum calcium level will be high, usually greater than 15 mg/100 ml. On physical examination, a palpable mass that moves with swallowing and is not in the thyroid will often be found. The diagnostic clue at surgery is the adherence of the enlarged parathyroid to the surrounding tissue. En bloc dissection is necessary for successful control of the disease. Chemotherapy and irradiation are of no use.

Secondary Hyperparathyroidism
Secondary hyperparathyroidism results from reactive hyperplasia of the glands in conditions that cause hypocalcemia and osteomalacia, including renal insufficiency, vitamin D deficiency, malabsorption, renal tubular acidosis, and renal tubular defects with phosphate wasting.

In chronic renal insufficiency, diminished formation of $1,25(OH)_2D_3$ leads to decreased absorption of calcium; loss of renal parenchyma leads to hyperphosphatemia. Both hypocalcemia and hyperphosphatemia stimulate parathyroid gland function. In malabsorption secondary to gastrointestinal disease, decreased serum calcium stimulates parathyroid function. When serum calcium is normal in instances where it should be low (malabsorption or renal disease), active parathyroid compensation is probably present.

After diagnosis, the best approach is treatment of the underlying disease with consideration of pharmacologic manipulation. In patients with chronic renal failure, serum phosphorus levels can be controlled with oral phosphate binders or small doses of vitamin D.

Tertiary hyperparathyroidism is found in occasional patients with severe and long-standing secondary hyperparathyroidism. One of the glands becomes autonomous and hyperplastic, which results in continued hypercalcemia and hyperparathyroidism. Some patients who receive a renal transplant for end-stage renal disease occasionally become severely hypercalcemic. The hypercalcemia disappears after 2 or more years. It is presumed that the hyperplastic glandular tissue regressed.

Hypoparathyroidism and Hypocalcemia

Hypoparathyroidism, a deficiency of effective PTH, is due to either a failure of the parathyroids to secrete the hormone or a failure of tissues to respond to hormone (pseudohypoparathyroidism).

PHYSIOLOGY OF HYPOCALCEMIA

One mechanism of hypocalcemia is the absence of PTH resulting from parathyroidectomy or idiopathic parathyroid deficiency, which occurs in three forms. In one form, PTH insufficiency is part of a complex of other endocrine gland deficiencies, especially the thyroid and adrenals. This form is also characterized by mucocutaneous candidiasis and antibodies to endocrine tissues. It is familial, but no specific genetic mechanism has been identified. Parathyroid deficiency occurs in a second form as part of the DiGeorge's syndrome, characterized by lymphocytopenia and aplasia of part of the third brachial arch, including the thymus. In the third form, idiopathic hypoparathyroidism can occur alone. In all forms characterized by the absence of PTH, the assays for PTH are low and for 25-$(OH)D_3$ are normal.

Resistance to PTH action is a second mechanism that leads to hypoparathyroidism. Albright coined the term "pseudohypoparathyroidism" to describe a syndrome in which hypocalcemia, hyperphosphatemia, and parathyroid hyperplasia were associated with obesity, short stature, short metacarpals, and basal ganglia calcification. Assays for PTH are increased, and normal or increased for 25$(OH)D_3$.

There is considerable genetic heterogeneity in some patients with congenital pseudohypoparathyroidism. To describe patients with varying PTH levels and responsiveness, a subclassification has been proposed. The first type includes patients in whom urinary cAMP levels do not rise after an injection of PTH. The second includes patients in whom PTH raises the cAMP level without causing phosphaturia. The third are those patients who secrete an altered biologically ineffective PTH that is recognized by immunoassay.

Acquired resistance to PTH includes impairment of PTH secretion and PTH effect on vitamin D activation. Chronic renal failure, the most common cause of hypocalcemia, presents with elevated phosphorus, creatinine, and BUN levels.

Hypomagnesemia, seen commonly in alcoholics and other malnourished patients, impairs PTH release and results in lowered calcium and phosphorus levels. Correction of the magnesium deficiency will restore PTH secretion, but the response to PTH returns more slowly. Tetany can occur in both magnesium and calcium deficiency, and in this type of hypoparathyroidism the physician must be especially alert.

Patients with small bowel disease may present with malabsorption of both calcium and vitamin D and occasionally with pancreatic deficiency. Small bowel x-ray and stool fat examination may be necessary to provide the diagnosis of malabsorption.

Therapy with phenytoin and other anticonvulsants may cause vitamin D deficiency, but the exact pathogenesis is not known. Patients present with low serum calcium and phosphorus, mildly elevated alkaline phosphatase, and low urinary calcium. All these values are consistent with osteomalacia. Hypocalcemia can aggrevate seizure disorders.

The other causes of hypocalcemia include acute pancreatitis, osteoblastic metastatic disease, and excessive transfusion with citrated blood. The mechanism in blood transfusion is the complexing of calcium with infused citrate, while patients with metastatic disease have extracellular removal of calcium and phosphorus with deposition in osteoblastic lesions.

CLINICAL FEATURES OF HYPOCALCEMIA

The clinical features of hypocalcemia depend on the underlying cause and associated diseases. In patients with acute onset (after thyroidectomy), clinical signs include paresthesias, depression, restlessness, and Chvostek's or Trousseau's sign. Fatigue, cramps, and myalgias are common in patients who develop the disease more gradually. Prolongation of the Q-T interval on the electrocardiogram may be the first sign of hypocalcemia.

Of the three mechanisms responsible for the development of hypocalcemia—GI absorption, bone resorption, or renal resorption—the latter is the least important. If the serum calcium is low—the defect is usually in the gut or bone—and the principal causes are vitamin D deficiency or PTH ineffectiveness. If the mechanism is not apparent, determination of serum vitamin D and PTH assay are indicated.

TREATMENT OF HYPOPARATHYROIDISM

A combination of vitamin D and calcium is used in the treatment of hypocalcemia, since vitamin D mimics the action of PTH.

HYPOCALCEMIA AFTER PARATHYROIDECTOMY

In hyperparathyroid patients with mild osteitis, hypocalcemia after parathyroidectomy is usually transient and may reflect a temporary suppression of the other glands. Temporary calcium replacement is indicated until PTH secretion resumes. The postoperative period for severe osteitis may include several months of osteomalacia, with low calcium and phosphate levels and increased alkaline phosphatase. Vitamin D therapy hastens healing but should be discontinued after 3-6 months. Permanent vitamin

D therapy is necessary for patients who develop tetany after seven-eighths parathyroidectomy.

HYPOCALCEMIA AFTER THYROIDECTOMY

In this clinical setting, acute symptoms can be treated with intravenous calcium gluconate: 10 ml of a 10% solution given slowly provides relief immediately. If more than 7 days of treatment are needed, permanent replacement of 25,000-50,000 units of vitamin D per day are required. Determinations of serum calcium are needed every 2 weeks at the onset and every 6 months when the level is stable, because episodic hypercalcemia is common. The urine calcium in hypoparathyroid patients treated with vitamin D is usually high, and therefore the serum calcium level averages 8.5 mg/100 ml. Periodic checks of urine calcium should be made, and if it is found to be over 250 mg/day, the patient should increase his fluid intake to prevent renal stones.

SYNTHETIC ANALOGUES OF VITAMIN D

Specific analogues are used for treatment of vitamin D deficiency states arising from different causes. $25(OH)D_3$ 50-300 mg/day may be hydroxylated at the 1 position by the kidney and is used in patients with malabsorption or liver disease. $1(OH)D_3$, 2-4 mg/day, is used in patients with renal disease because the liver can hydroxylate at the 25 position. $1,25(OH)_2D_3$, 0.25-1.0 mg/day, raises the serum calcium in patients with hypoparathyroidism. These synthetic agents have a rapid onset and offset so that toxicity disappears when they are discontinued; frequent monitoring of serum calcium is essential.

Calcitonin

PHYSIOLOGY AND DISORDERS

Calcitonin, which was discovered more than 20 years ago, acts to offset sudden hypercalcemia by inhibiting bone resorption either directly or by antagonism of PTH. The absence of calcitonin is not associated with hypercalcemia, and excess amounts, e.g., in medullary carcinoma of the thyroid, do not produce hypocalcemia.

Excess amounts of calcitonin are found in certain diseases, e.g., malignancies of the pancreas, prostate, uterus, lung, bladder, melanoma, and medullary carcinoma of the thyroid. Ectopic calcitonin production is associated with breast cancer, and approximately 20% of patients with breast carcinoma are hypercalcemic.

In Paget's disease, where bone lysis is the basic lesion, calcitonin is valuable in relieving pain, reducing urinary calcium, and antagonizing the hypercalcemia of immobilization. Calcitonin reduces the urinary hydroxyproline and serum alkaline phosphatase levels, which serve as indices of the severity of disease.

DIABETES MELLITUS
Physiology
The beta cells synthesize a polypeptide, *preproinsulin,* which is converted to proinsulin; *proinsulin* is then cleaved to produce equal amounts of *insulin* and C-peptide. Proinsulin may be preferentially secreted in at least one genetic defect; elevated levels are found in 80% of individuals with islet cell tumors and in renal failure.

Glucagon is produced by the alpha cells and maintains glucose concentration during periods of fasting; hyperglycemia decreases its secretion in normal individuals. Glucagon raises glucose by producing glycogenolysis, and gluconeogenesis; it may be important in the development of ketosis. Although pancreatized patients without glucagon do have ketosis, it is less severe. Glucagon stimulates insulin and somatostatin secretion.

Somatostatin inhibits growth hormone (somatotropin), insulin, and glucagon secretion and has been isolated from pituitary, pancreas, and other tissues. It lowers blood glucose concentration in diabetics and reduces the severity of ketoacidosis but has a duration of action too short for clinical use.

Epinephrine has an action opposite to that of insulin. It raises glucose by stimulating glycogenolysis and raises free fatty acids by promoting lipolysis. Elevated glucose tolerance curves in nondiabetic patients may be caused by stress-related epinephrine release.

Diabetes mellitus, hyperglycemia due to a relative or absolute insulin deficiency, is a heterogenous condition of variable genetic determination, most commonly occurring in the fourth decade of life and traditionally divided into juvenile onset/insulin-dependent and maturity onset/insulin independent types. This division has been confirmed by genetic studies, which show a marked difference between the two types of diabetes.

There is a 50% concordance in monozygotic twins for juvenile onset diabetes and a 90% concordance for maturity onset diabetes. This decreased genetic prevalence suggests that environmental factors such as mumps or coxsackie B virus infection may precipitate juvenile onset diabetes in certain predisposed individuals. This is supported by the finding of immunologic abnormalities in these patients that include lymphocytic infiltration of the islets of Langerhans, antibodies to islet cell surfaces or cytoplasm, association with antibodies to thyroid, stomach, and adrenal gland, and an increased frequency of HLA B8, Bw15, Dw3, and Dw4. Maturity onset diabetes, in contrast, is more closely related to genetic determinants.

Insulin levels may be normal or high in maturity onset diabetes but are low relative to blood glucose concentration. Insulin antibodies, humoral insulin antagonists, and a decrease in insulin receptors can lead to hyperglycemia in the presence of normal insulin levels. The number of insulin receptors is related to insulin concentration; the hyperinsulinemia seen in obese patients leads to a decline in receptors, producing hyperglycemia. Weight reduction lowers insulin levels and increases receptor number, thus reducing blood glucose. Growth hormone, cortisol, thyroxine, and glucagon all antagonize insulin. Older women with leukopenia, positive ANA, anti-DNA antibodies, proteinuria, alopecia, and Acanthosis nigricans have hyperglycemia because of an IgG antibody directed against insulin receptors.

INSULIN SECRETION
An elevation of serum glucose level stimulates both the synthesis and the secretion of insulin by the beta cells of the pancreas. This action is significantly greater with oral glucose, suggesting amplification by enteric hormones acting on the pancreatic cells.

Insulin release also occurs following stimulation with sulfonylureas. Insulin secretion is inhibited by catecholamines, somatostatin, beta blockade, diazoxide, and hypokalemia. In early diabetes, there is frequently a sluggish or delayed response in insulin secretion. This may sometimes be responsible for the syndrome of reactive hypoglycemia in early diabetes.

Diagnosis. A random blood glucose over 200 mg/dl or a fasting level over 120 mg/dl (plasma glucose concentration; blood concentrations are 15% lower) raises the suspicion of diabetes. A 2-hour screen (after 50 gm of oral glucose) over 180 mg/dl also suggests diabetes. In borderline cases, an oral glucose tolerance test should be performed with the standard precautions. These include an unrestricted carbohydrate diet during preceding days, an overnight fast, and an abstention from medication known to cause hyperglycemia. The patient should otherwise be in good health and preferably not hospitalized. Many believe the glucose tolerance test is overly sensitive, with many false-positives. In the symptomatic patient with an osmotic diuresis and an elevated blood sugar there is no problem in diagnosis, but in the occasional borderline patient where the 2-hour postprandial blood sugar is below 180 mg/dl but where other, somewhat nonspecific symptoms (such as unexplained neuropathies) are present, an oral glucose tolerance test with strict precautions is justified.

There is considerable agreement that besides the overt clinical diabetic there is a state of "chemical diabetes," with elevation of either fasting or postprandial blood sugars above the accepted norms but without obvious symptomatology. Many such patients show spontaneous recovery and may need no further management except advice on weight reduction where indicated.

Complications of Diabetes

While insulin administration prevents and treats ketoacidosis, the effectiveness of treating diabetes in preventing long-term complications is highly controversial. That good management affords a more comfortable lifestyle and prevents acute complications is not in doubt, but there is considerable debate about the effectiveness of "tight" diabetic control in the prevention of long-term vascular and other complications.

Small and large vessel disease are hallmarks of long-standing diabetes. Most investigators believe that atherosclerosis is no different from that occurring in nondiabetics, except that it occurs at an earlier age. The microvascular lesion unique to diabetes exhibits thickening of capillary basement membranes, endothelial proliferation, and accumulation of PAS-positive material. No definite evidence exists implicating vascular complications to hyperglycemia and inadequate insulin secretion.

At least three causal factors have been suggested.

1. Sorbitol, an alcohol derivative of glucose, may accumulate in vessel walls and produce osmotic changes that alter transmembrane ion fluxes.

2. Diabetic platelets show increased aggregation when exposed to agents like adenosine diphosphate, epinephrine, and arachadonic acid. Aggregation might release thromboxane A_2 or other agents that injure vessel walls.

3. The presence of an abnormal hemoglobin, A1C, has been used to assess control of the diabetic state. Since the abnormality persists for the life of the molecule and produces a greater than normal affinity for oxygen, it is possible that nonenzymatic glycosylation of other proteins would produce vascular disease. The concentration of the enzyme glycosyltransferase has been shown to correlate with glomerular basement proliferation; the activity of the enzyme decreases with insulin therapy. Increased plasma viscosity and decreased pliability of red cells may also contribute to vascular disease, particularly in the eye and the vasavasorum of vessels.

The acute sensory and motor neuropathies may respond to control of hyperglycemia, but chronic abnormalities appear irreversible.

RENAL DISEASE
Renal failure is the most common cause of death in diabetics under 30 years of age. Early renal abnormalities such as micro-

scopic proteinuria, some renal enlargement with increased renal flow, and reduced glomerular filtration rate respond to control of the diabetes. After 2 or 3 years of clinical diabetes, there is frequently some thickening of the capillary basement membrane. Proteinuria usually develops gradually in the younger diabetic, so that after 20 years of diabetes in this age group, about 10% of patients have significant proteinuria. In diabetics presenting in the older age groups, however, the proteinuria may be present at the time of diagnosis or 1-2 years later. Prognosis is related to the level of proteinuria; patients developing nephrotic syndrome do poorly. Coronary artery disease is the leading cause of death in older diabetics.

Diabetic nephropathy is characterized by glomerulosclerosis, pyelonephritis, and renal arteriosclerosis. Medullary necrosis may result in renal pain with hematuria. The classical Kimmelstiel-Wilson syndrome consists of nodular deposits of hyaline material near the periphery of the glomeruli. Renal infection in diabetics tends to be more severe, especially when associated with ischemic necrosis of the renal papillae or necrotizing papillitis. Renal infection should always be suspected and treated vigorously. Patients with significant renal disease may have diminished insulin requirements, partly explained by the fact that the kidney is normally involved in degrading insulin. Diabetics generally tend to do more poorly on renal dialysis programs, but the results from renal transplantation have generally been very promising.

DIABETIC RETINOPATHY

Though most diabetics obviously do not develop blindness, it is the most common cause of legal blindness in the United States and in most Western countries. Increased capillary permeability, identified by injection of fluorescin, was found in 75% of children who had diabetes for more than 1 year. It is traditional to divide diabetic retinopathy into background and proliferative types. In background retinopathy, one sees microaneurysms, dot and blot hemorrhages, hard and soft exudates, and macular edema. Proliferative diabetic retinopathy is characterized by neovascularization. While retinopathy tends to develop sooner in the older onset diabetic, the lesions tend to be more severe when they do occur in the younger patient, where proliferative disease with major hemorrhage into the vitreous and subsequent scar formation with retinal detachment are very serious possibilities. The vast majority of patients who first develop diabetes in childhood or adolescence will go on to develop retinopathy, although patients live for 30 or 40 years with no evidence of eye disease.

Background retinopathy generally does not require treatment unless macular edema develops. Since patients with retinopathy frequently have evidence for increased platelet aggregation, aspirin has been advocated. Improvement of diabetic control and the use of lipid-lowering agents such as clofibrate seem to be of some value in reducing the amount of fatty exudation. Photocoagulation has been quite successful in selected cases, particularly for some proliferative retinopathy, so routine consultation with an ophthalmologist is mandatory. Patients with decreased vision or blindness can be improved by vitrectomy using a needle-like instrument with cutting and aspiration capabilities. Hypophysectomy, once a popular means of treating diabetic retinopathy, has been largely replaced by photocoagulation.

DIABETIC NEUROPATHY

A major cause of morbidity in the diabetic patient, diabetic neuropathy can be acute or chronic, sensory, motor, or autonomic. Clinically, one of the most common presentations of diabetic neuropathy is a loss of vibration sense in the lower limb and of the ankle jerk. Electrophysiologic studies can demonstrate the presence of diminished conduction velocities in sensory and motor nerves long before the development of clinical signs and symptoms. Early neurologic problems in diabetes may be reversible with improved control, but this is not the case in the long-term complications. Many different types of neuropathies may be present in the same patient. Peripheral polyneuropathy may result in pain or paresthesias, with diminution in pinprick and vibration sense. The painful neuropathies are more severe at night and are rather resistant to treatment with analgesics. A trial of phenytoin or carbamazepine should be undertaken. Peripheral sensory loss increases the danger of painless foot ulcers, so the patient should be instructed in foot care with professional help if indicated. Mononeuropathy may occur, particularly of the third, fourth, and sixth cranial nerves. Peripheral mononeuropathy may also occur, resulting in foot or wrist drop. These generally undergo spontaneous recovery within 4 to 6 weeks. Radiculopathy, severe pain occurring over the distribution of a particular spinal nerve, may involve the chest, abdomen, and lateral thigh areas or may mimic the acute abdomen. Prognosis for spontaneous recovery is good. Diabetic amyotrophy is atrophy of the large muscles of the upper leg rather similar to a primary muscle disease. Autonomic neuropathies are frequent and usually permanent. Postural hypotension, disturbances of sweating, nocturnal diarrhea, bladder disturbances, and impotence are the usual manifestations. Impotence is common in the male patient over the age of 40. It is important to rule out nonorganic factors, as the true autonomic impotence has a poor prognosis.

Treatment of diabetic neuropathies is generally unsatisfactory. Fortunately, spontaneous recovery tends to occur in the painful neuropathies and occasionally in some of the autonomic manifestations. Diabetic diarrhea may respond to treatment with anticholinergics, and investigation for evidence of bacterial overgrowth using the C^{14} glycocholate test may be beneficial as these patients respond to antibiotic therapy. Slow gastric emptying may respond to treatment with metoclopramide. Patients should be cautioned against the dangers of postural hypotension. They should be taught to sleep with the head of the bed elevated, to assume the erect posture slowly, and possibly to wear full-length elastic stockings.

DIABETIC CARDIOMYOPATHY
Besides the well-known effect of diabetes in increasing the incidence of coronary artery disease, it also has a primary effect on the cardiac muscle, producing cardiomyopathy. This has been partly explained by the demonstration of glycoproteins and increased collagen deposition in the heart muscle. Diabetics are also prone to cardiorespiratory disorders secondary to diabetic neuropathy. This may result in the so-called silent heart attack,

and also in sudden death where autonomic neuropathy is severe. Both phonocardiography and echocardiography have demonstrated abno malities in patients with microangiopathy.

PERIPHERAL VASCULAR DISEASE

This is most prominent in the lower limbs, where association with neuropathies produces significant morbidity and mortality. Even though diabetes itself is not a contraindication to arterial surgery, the frequent association of microvascular disease diminishes the chances for successful outcome. Lumbar sympathectomy and drugs are of little value in the treatment of intermittent claudication. Prophylaxis and early attention to detail are important.

THE DIABETIC FOOT

The combination of neuropathy with ischemia produces weakness of the intrinsic muscles of the foot with claw toes. Charcot-type radiologic changes may be seen in the midtarsal and ankle joint areas. Foot pulses are absent, and the skin may be plum red when dependent, pale when elevated. Special footwear and appliances may be utilized to correct mobile deformities. Early and careful surgery and drainage of infection may prevent more radical amputation.

KETOACIDOSIS

When it does occur, it is a metabolic emergency of major proportions with a significant mortality of 10%; it may be prevented by good therapy of diabetes, with prompt treatment of infections and other emergencies. The majority of patients respond to prompt and effective management; attention to detail and a rapid response to the changing biochemical profile is critical. While the precise method of treatment (particularly insulin dosage) varies, the single most important element is a flexible and attentive physician who responds promptly to the changing situation.

Ketoacidosis usually results from a severe lack of insulin in the presence of elevated levels of the diabetogenic hormones; it may be secondary to infection, myocardial infarction, or omission of insulin therapy. The hyperglycemia is accompanied by excessive gluconeogenesis, with the accumulation of free fatty acids and their conversion into ketones. The accumulating ketones displace bicarbonate, and the patient develops acidosis with a secondary respiratory alkalosis. Hyperventilation produces hypocapnia and manifests itself as air hunger or Kussmaul respiration. The osmotic diuresis results in a massive loss of water, sodium, and potassium.

Patients are dehydrated and drowsy, may exhibit nausea and vomiting, and may complain of abdominal pain. They are usually hypotensive and have a rapid heart rate. Coma is rare (the most common cause of coma in diabetics is hypoglycemia). Fever is rare and, if present, suggests infection.

Management includes careful fluid and electrolyte replacement, insulin therapy, and the treatment of any underlying condition. An intravenous line should be instituted and blood drawn for glucose, BUN, electrolytes, bicarbonate, and pH determination. An ECG should be done. Vital functions, including urinary output, should be monitored. The first 1-2 liters of fluids should be administered rapidly. Continuing replacement of the fluid deficit must be done gradually, with careful monitoring of the clinical response. A liter of normal saline should be allowed to run in as rapidly as it will go (usually takes approximately 30 minutes). It is generally unwise to add any potassium or other agents to the initial liter of fluid. The potassium level is generally normal or may be elevated at the time of admission, even though there has been a massive loss of potassium from the body. Treatment of ketoacidosis, however, with fluid replacement, institution of insulin therapy, and subsequent correction of the acidosis will invariably produce a fall in the serum potassium. Potassium replacement should therefore be commenced early in therapy, so that more dramatic and dangerous large infusions of potassium are not required later on. Generally 20-40 mEq of KCl or potassium phosphate per liter prevents serious hypokalemia. Because hypernatremia is dangerous and fluid losses exceed salt losses, many advocate the institution of hypotonic saline solutions after the initial 1 or 2 liters. At this stage, fluid should be administered at a rate of 1 liter every 2-3 hours; rapid changes in fluid and electrolyte levels within the body may produce variants of the disequilibrium syndrome. It is important to emphasize that speed is no longer essential.

Bicarbonate therapy is usually not necessary, even though the initial level may be as low at 10 mEq/liter and as long as the pH does not drop below 7.0. Bicarbonate administration has serious disadvantages, including: (1) paradoxically increasing the acidosis of the CSF, (2) increasing the tendency toward hypokalemia, and (3) decreasing the uptake of oxygen by the tissues by shifting the oxyhemoglobin dissociation curve to the left. If sodium bicarbonate is necessary, one or two ampules (44.6 mEq/ 50-ml ampule) should be given in a minimum of 500 ml carrier solution until pH reaches 7.0. Administration of potassium phosphate increases the synthesis of 2-3 diphosphoglycerate (2-3DPG) in red cells and increases the delivery of oxygen to the tissues.

Small doses of insulin by intravenous infusion or hourly I.M. injections have been shown to be highly effective. Generally, the decrease in blood glucose is predictable, and there may be a lower incidence of hypokalemia. Five to 10 units by infusion or 5 units I.M. per hour results in a satisfactory fall in blood sugar levels. (If the intramuscular route is chosen, begin with 10 units I.V.). A close monitoring of the serum glucose and electrolyte levels is important. The patient should not become hypoglycemic; insulin administration by this method is usually discontinued once the blood sugar has fallen to 250 mg/dl. Replacement solutions should then be changed to dextrose and saline; insulin administration is given subcutaneously, 8-12 units at 4-hour intervals. Regular insulin should be continued for 24-36 hours before reinstitution of longer acting insulin preparations. Routine support of therapy and close clinical monitoring must be maintained. Vasopressor agents may be necessary, and a nasogastric tube should be inserted if there appears to be gastric dilatation.

Mucormycosis (phycomycosis) occurs in the immune compromised host and in diabetics, particularly those with ketoacidosis. These aerobic saphrophytic fungi invade from the skin, respiratory, or gastrointestinal tract. Diabetics develop a characteristic rhinocerebral infection that may present with ophthalmoplegia, sinusitis, sudden blindness, or exophthalamos. Crusting, ulcera tion of the palate, and black necrotic debris from infarcted turbinates are valuable clinical signs. Extensive surgical debridement and amphotericin B are necessary.

HYPEROSMOLAR COMA

Profound hyperglycemia without ketosis may be seen in the older and generally milder maturity onset diabetic. The balance of insulin and the diabetogenic hormones appears sufficient to prevent lipolysis but not hyperglycemia; reduced renal function aggravated by dehydration also plays a role by decreasing glucose excretion. It is frequently precipitated by infection, cerebral vascular disease, renal failure, or medications such as steroids, phenytoin, or diuretics. The blood glucose ranges from 800 mg to well over 1000 mg, producing severe dehydration. The absence of ketosis prevents early recognition, since ketosis produces hyperventilation, nausea, and vomiting; these symptoms are generally absent in the hyperosmolar patient. Coma is frequent, and there is a high incidence of other CNS abnormalities. The mortality is well over 50%. Treatment is the same as for ketoacidosis, although fluid deficits are greater and less insulin may be required. Both hypotonic and normal saline infusions are used; potassium levels should be closely monitored, because the absence of acidosis leads to a more rapid decrease in serum potassium. It has been postulated that these patients develop intracellular particles, referred to as idiogenic osmoles, as a protective measure against the hypertonic serum. The rapid delivery of large amounts of hypotonic solutions may precipitate cerebral edema, so normal and hypotonic saline should be alternated. Close monitoring of clinical and biochemical status is necessary.

Management of Diabetes

Following diagnosis, detailed patient instruction is necessary. Most individuals have significant misconceptions about this very prevalent condition, and it is important to encourage as normal a lifestyle as possible while taking maximum precautions and preventive measures to delay or prevent complications. A realistic and sensible diet regimen is the basis of management of all diabetics. The attainment of normal weight is very important, especially in the vast majority of patients who will not require insulin. This may prove to be all that is necessary to remedy the hyperglycemia secondary to obesity. When the patient is receiving insulin, it is important that meals be properly spaced, with the number of calories remaining constant but providing as much variety as possible.

Fat and polysaturates in the diet ought to be modified to protect the diabetic from increased susceptibility to atherosclerosis. The consumption of animal and dairy fat is reduced by replacement with margarines and oils high in polyunsaturates. Highly refined carbohydrates, especially sucrose, are prohibited, and it seems prudent to advise increasing the fiber content of the diet. Carbohydrates normally make up about 50% of the calories in the adult diabetic diet.

ORAL AGENTS

The U.G.D.P. study questions the effectiveness of oral agents in preventing the long-term complications of diabetes. Although the findings of the study remain controversial, they emphasize the importance of dietary management of the mature, overweight diabetic. Oral agents, when used, should be withdrawn at regular intervals to determine whether they are effective.

The oral agents are the sulfonylureas, a group of compounds that stimulate the beta cell of the pancreas to secrete insulin. Their action differs from glucose, since they do not increase synthesis of insulin within the cell. The commonly used agents are tolbutamide (usual dose 0.5 gm t.i.d., maximum 2 gm daily), chlorpropamide given once daily because of its long duration of action (dosage 100-500 mg), and acetohexamide (250-500 mg daily), with a duration of action intermediate between that of tolbutamide and chlorpropamide. Tolazamide is usually given once a day, and the dosage range is between 100 mg and 1 gm. Side effects are not commonly a problem with these agents. Of special interest is the genetically determined body flushing that occurs in some patients and the potentiation of antidiuretic hormone with hyponatremia, which occurs with chlorpropamide.

Hypoglycemia is an important complication, especially in the elderly. When it occurs in patients taking chlorpropamide, they may need observation over a 24-hour period because of the long duration of action of this compound. The oral agents can be potentiated by other medications, particularly oral anticoagulants and some of the anti-inflammatory agents.

INSULIN THERAPY

Short-duration, intermediate-duration, and long-acting insulins are available; regular crystalline and isophane (NPH) insulin suffices for the majority. The intermediate-acting NPH insulin may be required either once or twice daily to achieve optimal control. Individual diabetics exhibit significant variation in response to the various insulins, so that duration of action and peak onset vary widely. When possible, insulin dosage should be modified while the person is ambulatory, because activity and lifestyle influence dosage and frequency of injection. Small doses are tried initially, with sequential increments until optimum control is achieved. The patient should check urine for glucose and ketones before breakfast, lunch, and supper, and before retiring at night. Once good control is achieved, testing could be limited to morning and evenings with the five times per day profile performed once a week. Patient education in this area is extremely important and lends itself to better control of the diabetes.

The Somogyi effect describes the wide fluctuations in blood sugar that occur when hypoglycemia results in secondary hyperglycemia owing to the physiologic response induced in the patient. Hypoglycemia-stimulated secretion of glucagon, catecholamines, corticosteroids, and growth hormone produces compensatory hyperglycemia, and the situation is aggravated if the insulin dose is further increased in response to glycosuria. This problem may be more difficult to diagnose if it occurs during sleep; the presence of morning hypothermia, nightmares, and nocturnal sweating should raise the possibility.

Regular insulin should be used when the patient is being prepared for surgery and in the pregnant diabetic where tight control is critical.

MULTIPLE ENDOCRINE NEOPLASIA

Three multiple endocrine neoplastic syndromes are inherited as an autosomal, dominant trait.

MEN I

Wermer's syndrome includes tumors or hyperplasia of parathyroids, pancreatic islet cells, pituitary, adrenal cortex, and thyroid. The islet cell tumors may produce gastrin and cause the Zollinger-Ellison syndrome, or they may produce insulin and produce hypoglycemia. They may also secrete glucagon, vasoactive inhibitory polypeptide (VIP), prostaglandins, ACTH, ADH, parathormone, or serotonin. Hyperglycemia, weight loss, stomatitis, and necrotizing migratory erythema occur with glucagonomas; watery diarrhea is seen with VIP and prostaglandin-producing tumors.

MEN II

Sipple syndrome includes pheochromotocytoma, medullary thyroid carcinoma, and parathyroid hyperplasia. The first two components arise from the neural crest, and the latter may be due to long-standing calcitonin stimulation. The pheochromocytomas are frequently bilateral, may be extraadrenal, and are often malignant.

MEN III (IIb)

This syndrome includes the endocrine neoplasia of type II but also multiple neuroma involving oral, ocular, upper respiratory, and gastrointestinal mucosa. There may also be generalized hypotonia, kyphoscoliosis, lax joints, and other musculoskeletal abnormalities.

HYPOGLYCEMIA

Hypoglycemia is diagnosed when glucose concentrations of less than 40 mg/dl are accompanied by confusion, agitation, coma, and the signs of sympathetic overactivity (tachycardia diaphoresis).

Both from an etiologic and diagnostic perspective, hypoglycemia is best considered as either: (1) fasting or (2) postprandial.

Fasting hypoglycemia. Usually organic, this can be produced by carefully observing the patient in the fasting state. Important causes are:

1. Insulinoma, or islet cell hyperplasia (may be associated with MEN).
2. Tumors secreting insulin-like substance
3. Underactivity of the hormones that normally oppose the hypoglycemic action of insulin. This includes hypopituitarism, Addison disease (primary or secondary), isolated deficiency of growth hormones, and hypothyroidism.
4. Exogenous insulin, or sulphonylureas.
5. Diffuse liver disease.
6. Glycogen storage disease.
7. Association with alcohol (inhibition of gluconeogenesis by alcohol).
8. Neonatal hypoglycemia in low birth weight infants.

The diagnosis of insulinoma is likely when fasting hypoglycemia is accompanied by levels of insulin higher than expected for the blood glucose concentration. The measurement of C-peptide during hypoglycemia is useful in making the diagnosis of insulinoma, as it is secreted in equimolar quantities to that of insulin. Normally, the levels of C-peptide should fall during hypoglycemia.

Insulinomas are the most common cause of fasting hypoglycemia. They are single in approximately 90%, multiple in the other 10%, and malignant in 10%. They may be associated with the syndrome of multiple endocrine neoplasia (MEN), and a search for other tumors of the pituitary, thyroid, and adrenal glands should be undertaken, particularly if there is a family history of these.

Postprandial hypoglycemia. This form indicates a lack of synchronization between enteric and pancreatic endocrine hormones, glucose absorption from the gut, and utilization and storage by the tissues. It is usually confirmed by 5-hour glucose tolerance test, with appearance of symptoms when glucose concentration falls. Causes include:

1. Reactive hypoglycemia—cause unknown. No definitive hormonal abnormality has been demonstrated. "Eating too fast" in compulsive individuals has been a common clinical impression. There is no consistent abnormality of insulin in these patients.

2. Early mild maturity onset diabetes.

3. Alimentary hypoglycemia—gastric surgery, vagotomy, or rapid gastric emptying from any cause including thyrotoxicosis.

Management of postprandial hypoglycemia involves decreasing the quantity of simple sugars in the diet and substitution of complex carbohydrates, which require longer to digest. The use of small frequent meals and anticholinergic agents to slow gastric emptying has met with limited success. Attainment of ideal body weight and use of hypoglycemic agents to hasten insulin secretion is useful in mild diabetics who present with reactive hypoglycemia.

ANOREXIA NERVOSA

This is a psychoendocrine disorder of teenage girls characterized by severe weight loss, secondary amenorrhea, personality changes, and significant mortality. There is a well-documented disturbance of body image, whereby the patient sees herself as being fatter than she really is. Decreased secretion of gonadotrophin-releasing hormone with decreased pituitary FSH and LH secretion, absent ovarian estrogen production, and amenorrhea are found. This dysfunction is reversible, and recovery occurs with weight gain. Thyroid function is normal. Growth hormone and cortisol levels may be normal or elevated.

Diminution in food intake may occur with fad diets and preoccupation with the caloric content of food. There is a fear of being fat. The patient may induce vomiting and hide food. Personality changes include depression, agitation, obsessive compulsive features, and problems with interpersonal relationships, particularly involving the parents.

Treatment requires hospitalization and a close supervision of eating. A trustful but firm relationship between the patient and her nurses and physician is essential. Supervision is needed to prevent hiding of food and self-induced vomiting. Psychotherapy is important.

The use of medications, especially phenothiazines, is popular but controversial. Tube and parenteral feeding is not useful.

Menstruation returns with weight gain, preceded by the reappearance of gonadotrophins and estrogen secretion. Cyclical hypothalamic pituitary function essential for a normal menstrual cycle is the last function to return. Clomiphene stimulation may bring on menstruation in the presence of pituitary responsiveness.

Abnormalities of Sexual Differentiation and Function

A group of abnormalities may produce changes in external sexual appearance or in gonadal function.

An abnormal number of sexual chromosomes produces disorders of *chromosomal sex*. The presence of two or more X chromosomes in a male produces small testes, infertility, gynecomastia, and elevated levels of urinary gonadotropins because of defective feedback (Klinefelter syndrome). Missing or abnormal X chromosomes in the female causes primary amenorrhea, sexual infantilism, and multiple skeletal abnormalities, which include a low hair line, webbing of the neck, and a small jaw (Turner syndrome). *Gonadal sex* may be abnormal with normal sex chromosomes if the early differentiation and growth of the gonads are abnormal. Some patients with gonadal dysgenesis, for example, have pure sexual dysfunction (amenorrhea, no breast development) but do not have the associated skeletal abnormalities of Turner's syndrome.

Abnormalities in the synthesis of steroid hormones may alter *phenotypic sex* even if chromosomal and gonadal sex is normal. Three adrenal enzymes sequentially convert cholesterol to 17-hydroxyprogesterone, which is the immediate precursor of both glucocorticoids and adrenal androgens. Defects in either of these three enzymes lead to adrenal hyperplasia (because of ACTH feedback stimulation) and defective virilization in the male. Adrenal insufficiency may be severe and life-threatening.

The most common cause of the adrenogenital syndrome is deficiency of the enzyme that converts 17-hydroxyprogesterone to 11-deoxycortisol, 21-hydroxylase. The resultant adrenal hyperplasia from ACTH stimulation causes virilization at birth in the female and precocious sexuality, frequently as early as the second or third year of life, in the male. The level of enzyme deficiency determines plasma cortisol concentrations and the severity of the associated adrenal insufficiency. Deficiency of 11-hydroxylase (the enzyme blocked by the diagnostic agent metyrapone) also produces virilization with the accumulation of deoxycorticosterone, the salt-retaining hormone. Hypertension occurs in some but not all. The adrenogenital syndrome due to 21-hydroxylase deficiency is the most common cause of female pseudohermaphroditism; nonadrenal causes are rare.

Male pseudohermaphroditism occurs from defects in the three enzymes that lead to the synthesis of 17-hydroxyprogesterone or in the two enzymes that lead to testosterone production from 17-hydroxyprogesterone. Defects in the initial three enzymes produce associated hypoadrenalism because of defective cortisol synthesis.

The *Stein-Leventhal syndrome* presents with amenorrhea, sterility, and hirsutism; occasionally virilism is present. Plasma androgen levels are increased, and the pathogenesis may involve abnormalities in the androgen-estrogen conversion pathways. The ovarian cysts appear to result from hypersecretion of LH, which is noncyclical and does not produce ovulation. The value of wedge resection and the antiestrogen compound, clomiphene (clomid), suggests that increased estrogen production from nonovarian sources may initiate the syndrome by interfering with the usual cyclic feedback mechanisms.

ESTROGEN THERAPY

Estrogens are widely prescribed for both premenopausal (contraception and menstrual regularization) and menopausal women. They control vasomotor symptoms and appear to reduce the severity of osteoporosis in the latter group. Recent studies show that the incidence of 11000 cases of endometrial carcinoma in women between the ages of 50-74 is increased 2-20 fold by the use of estrogen. Duration of usage and dosages of more than 0.625 mg per day increase the frequency; the increased frequency declines rapidly when estrogens are withdrawn. Mixed oral contraceptives may actually decrease the incidence of endometrial carcinoma but the use of contraceptives, such as Oracon which contain a predominant estrogenic component, has been shown to increase endometrial carcinoma in younger women.

REFERENCES

Pituitary Gland Disorders

Reichlin S: Regulation of the hypophysiotropic secretions of the brain. Arch Intern Med 135:1350, 1975.

Weitzman ED: Circadian rhythm and episodic hormone secretion in man. Ann Rev Med 27:225, 1976.

Snyder PJ, Jacobs LS, Rabello MM, et al.: Diagnostic value of thyrotrophin-releasing hormone in pituitary and hypothalamic diseases: assessment of thyrotrophin and prolactin secretion in 150 patients. Ann Intern Med 81:751, 1974.

Jenkins JS, Gilbert CJ, Ang V: Hypothalamic-pituitary function in patients with craniopharyngromas. J Clin Endocrinol Metab 43:394, 1976.

Sheehan HL, Stanfield JP: The pathogenesis of post-partum necrosis of the anterior lobe of the pituitary gland. Acta Endocrinol (Kbh)37:479, 1961.

Weisberg LA, Zimmerman EA, Frantz SG: Diagnosis and evaluation of patients with an enlarged sella turcica. Am J Med 61:590, 1976.

Samaan NA, Bakdash MM, Cadaero JB, et al.: Hypopituitarism after external irradiation: evidence for both hypothalamic and pituitary origin. Ann Intern Med 83:771, 1975.

Kurneck JE, Hartman CR, Lufkin EG, et al.: Abnormal sella turcica: a tumor board review of the clinical significance. Arch Intern Med 137:111, 1977.

Ontjes DA, Ney RL: Pituitary tumors. CA 26:330, 1976.

Carmalt MHB, Dalton GA, Fletcher RF, et al.: The treatment of Cushing's disease by transsphenoidal hypophysectomy. Q J Med 46:119, 1977.

Martin JB: Neural regulation of growth hormone secretion. N Engl J Med 288:1384, 1973.

Moses AM, Miller M, Streeter DHP: Pathophysiologic and pharmacologic alterations in the release and action of ADH. Metabolism 25:697, 1976.

Cryer PE, et al.: The diagnosis and therapy of aeromegaly. Arch Intern Med 135:338, 1975.

Sheehan HL, Summer VK: The syndrome of hypopituitarism. Q J Med 18:319, 1949.

Spark RF, Dickstein G: Bromocriptine and endocrine disorders. Ann Intern Med 90:949, 1979.

Golde DW, Bersch N, Kaplan SA, Rimoin DL, Li CH: Peripheral unresponsiveness to human growth hormone in Laron dwarfism. N Engl J Med 303:1156, 1980.

Thyroid Gland Disorders

Vagenakis AG, Braverman LE: Thyroid function tests—which one? Ann Intern Med 84:607, 1976 (editorial).

Brown J (moderator), et al.: Autoimmune thyroid diseases—Graves' and Hashimoto's. Ann Intern Med 88:379, 1979.

Zonszein J, Santangelo RP, Mackin JF, Lee TC, Coffey RJ, Canary JJ: Propranolol therapy in thyrotoxicosis. A review of 84 patients undergoing surgery. Am J Med 66:411, 1979.

Schimmel M, Utiger RD: Thyroidal and peripheral production of thyroid hormones. review of recent findings and their clinical implications. Ann Intern Med 87:760, 1977.

Favus MJ, et al.: Thyroid cancer occurring as a late consequence of head and neck irradiation: evaluation of 1056 patients. N Engl J Med 294:1019, 1976.

Welby ML: Laboratory diagnosis of thyroid disorders. Adv Clin Chem 18:103, 1976.

Larsen PR: Tests of thyroid function. Med Clin North Am 59:1063, 1975.

Evered DC: Endocrine and metabolic diseases. Treatment of thyroid disease. Br Med J 1:264, 1976.

Toft AD, et al.: Thyroid function in the long-term follow-up of patients treated with iodine-131 for thyrotoxicosis. Lancet 2:576, 1975.

Ridgway EC, Maloof F, Federman DD: Rational therapy in hypothyroidism. Ration Drug Thera 10(8):1, 1976.

Sizemore GW, Go VLW: Stimulation tests for diagnosis of medullary thyroid carcinoma. Mayo Clin Proc 50:53, 1975.

The National Cancer Institute: Information for physicians on irradiation-related thyroid cancer. CA 26:150, 1976.

McConahey WM, Hayles AB: Radiation and thyroid neoplasia. Ann Intern Med 84:749, 1976.

Messaris G, Kyrrakoa K, Vasilopoulous P, Tountas C: The single thyroid nodule and carcinoma. Br J Surg 61:943, 1974.

Burman KD, et al.: Clinical observations on the solitary autonomous thyroid nodule. Arch Intern Med 134:915, 1974.

Solomon DH, Kleeman KE: Concepts of pathogenesis of Graves' disease. Adv Intern Med 22:273, 1977.

Irvine WJ, Toft AD: The diagnosis and treatment of thyrotoxicosis. Clin Endocrinol (Oxf) 5:687, 1976.

Stahl TJ: Radioimmunoassay and the hormones of thyroid function. Semin Nucl Med 5:221, 1975.

Mayberry WE: Radioimmunoassay for human TSH. Ann Intern Med 74:471, 1971.

Chopra IJ: A radioimmunoassay for measurement of 3, 3' 5' triiodothyronine (reverse T_3). J Clin Invest 54:583, 1974.

Adrenal Gland Disorders

Spiger M, Jubiz W, Meikle AW, et al.: Single-dose metyrapone test: review of a four-year experience. Arch Intern Med 135:698, 1975.

Tyrnell JB, Brooks RM, Fitzgerald PA, et al.: Cushing's disease. Selective trans-sphenoidal resection of pituitary microadenomas. N Engl J Med 298:753, 1978.

Moore TJ, Dluhy RG, Williams GH, et al.: Nelson's syndrome: frequency, prognosis, and effect of prior pituitary irradiation. Ann Intern Med 85:731, 1976.

Fauci AS, Dale DC, Balow JE: Glucocorticosteroid therapy: mechanisms of action and clinical considerations. Ann Intern Med 84:304, 1976.

Besser GM, Jeffcoate WJ: Endocrine and metabolic disease: adrenal diseases. Br Med J 1:448, 1976.

Gold EM: The Cushing syndromes: changing views of diagnosis and treatment. Ann Intern Med 90:829, 1979.

Weinberger MH, Grim CE, Hollifield JW, Kem DC, et al.: Primary aldosteronism. Diagnosis, localization, and treatment. Ann Intern Med 90:386, 1979.

Mattingly D, Tyler C: Overnight urinary 11-hydroxycorticosteroid estimations in diagnosis of Cushing's syndrome. Br Med J 2:668, 1976.

Axelrod L: Glucocorticoid therapy. Medicine (Baltimore) 55:3955, 1976.

Parathyroid Gland and Calcium Metabolism Disorders

Mazzaferri EL, O'Dorisio TM, LoBuglio AF: Treatment of hypercalcemia associated with malignancy. Semin Oncol 5:141, 1978.

Recker RR, Saville PO, Heaney RP: Effect of estrogens and calcium carbonate on bone loss in post-menopausal women. Ann Intern Med 87:649, 1977.

Sherwood LM, O'Riordan JLH, Auerbach GD, Pott JT Jr: Production of parathyroid hormone by nonparathyroid tumors. J Clin Endocrinol 27:140, 1967.

Schneider AB, Sherwood LM: Calcium homeostasis and the pathogenesis and management of hypercalcemic disorders. Metabolism 23:975, 1974.

Schneider AB, Sherwood LM: Pathogenesis and management of hypoparathyroidism and other hypocalcemic disorders. Metabolism 24:871, 1975.

Patten BM, Heath DA, Doppman JL, Bilezikian JP, Aurbach GD (Moderator): Hyperparathyroidism: recent studies. Ann Intern Med 79:566, 1973.

Mallette LE, Bilezikian JP, Heath DA, Aurbach GD, et al.: Primary hyperparathyroidism: clinical and biochemical features. Medicine 53:127, 1974.

Fogelman I, Bessent RG, Beastall G, Boyle IT: Estimation of skeletal involvement in primary hyperparathyroidism. Use of 24-hour wholebody retention of technetium-99m diphosphonate. Ann Intern Med 92:65, 1980.

Diabetes Mellitus

Boden G, Master RW, Gordon SS, Shuman CR, Owen OE: Monitoring metabolic control in diabetic outpatients with glycosylated hemoglobin. Ann Intern Med 92:357, 1980.

National Diabetes Data Group: Classification and diagnosis of diabetes mellitus and other categories of glucose intolerance. Diabetes 28:1039, 1979.

Koivisto VA, Felig P: Alterations in insulin absorption and in blood glucose control associated with varying insulin injection sites in diabetic patients. Ann Intern Med 92:59, 1980.

Craighead JE: Current views on the etiology of insulin-dependent diabetes mellitus. N Engl J Med 299:1439, 1978.

Kreisberg RA: Diabetic ketoacidosis: new concepts and trends in pathogenesis and treatment. Ann Intern Med 88:681, 1978.

Siperstein MD: The glucose tolerance test. Adv Intern Med 20:297, 1975.

Olesfsky JM: The insulin receptor: its role in insulin resistance of obesity and diabetes. Diabetes 25:1154, 1976.

Cudworth AG, et al.: HLA and diabetes. Diabetes 24:345, 1975; Br Med J 2:846, 1976.

Irvine WJ, et al.: HLA and anti-islet antibodies. Diabetes 26:138, 1977.

Leodrum R, et al.: Anti-islet antibodies in DM. Lancet 1:880, 1975.

Service FJ, Dale AJD, Elvebeck LR, et al.: Insulinoma: clinical and diagnostic features of 60 consecutive cases. Mayo Clin Proc 51:417, 1976.

Seltzer HS: Drug-induced hypoglycemia: a review based on 473 cases. Diabetes 21:9, 1972.

Permutt MA: Postprandial hypoglycemia. Diabetes 25:19, 1976.

Hofeldt FD: Reactive hypoglycemia. Metabolism 24:1193, 1975.

Permutt MA, Keller D, Santiago J: Cholinergic blockade in reactive hypoglycemia. Diabetes 26:121, 1977.

Fajans SS, Floyd JC Jr: Fasting hypoglycemia in adults. N Engl J Med 294:766, 1976.

Multiple Endocrine Abnormalities
Schimke RN: Syndromes with multiple endocrine gland involvement. Prog Med Genet, 1978.

Schimke RN: Multiple endocrine adenomatosis syndromes. Adv Intern Med 21:249, 1976.

Lamers CBHW, Froeling PGAM: Clinical significance of hyperparathyroidism in familial multiple endocrine adenomatosis Type I (MEA I). Am J Med 66:422, 1979.

Estrogen Therapy
Weiss NS, Sayvetz TA: Incidence of endometrial cancer in relation to the use of oral contraceptives. N Engl J Med 302:551, 1980.

Weiss NS, Szekely DR, English DR, Schweid AI: Endometrial cancer in relation to patterns of menopausal estrogen use. JAMA 242:261, 1979.

Acknowledgements
Federman, Daniel, *Scientific American Medicine*, In Rubenstein E, and Federman D, (eds), 1979, Vol 1.

Wilkins RW, Levinsky NG, (eds), *Medicine: Essentials of Clinical Practice*, 2nd ed. Little, Brown, 1978.

The Hematopoietic System

THE ANEMIAS
Biology of Hematopoiesis

Tissue culture and human marker studies confirm earlier speculation that a primitive totipotent stem cell gives rise to pluripotent myeloid and lymphoid colony-forming units or stem cells that mature into erythrocytes, platelets, eosinophils, granulocytes and monocytes, plasma cells, and thymus-derived lymphocytes. A variety of humoral factors regulating proliferation have been described. Abnormalities such as aplastic anemia involving more than one cell line may be understood by considering toxic or immunologic influences operating at a primitive level before final differentiation into specific types.

Anemia is a reduction in the circulating red blood cells and/or hemoglobin caused by decreased production, increased destruction, or both. Tissue oxygenation depends, in addition, on the structural quality of hemoglobin, its ability to acquire and release oxygen appropriately, the metabolic demand of the tissues, and the availability of oxygen to the hemoglobin. The differential diagnosis based on morphology is shown in Table 7-1, and a physiologic classification is presented in Table 7-2.

Hematopoiesis occurs in the sternal, humeral, iliac, and femoral marrow. Approximately 40% of the marrow is hematopoietic;

TABLE 7-1—ANEMIAS: MORPHOLOGIC CLASSIFICATION

Macrocytic
Megaloblastic anemia
Liver disease
Reticulocytosis
Normocytic
Acute blood loss
Hemolytic anemia
Anemia of chronic disease
Microcytic and hypochromic
Iron deficiency
Thalassemia
Sideroblastic anemia

the remainder is composed of fat. Within the marrow, a pluripotential stem cell is capable, with appropriate stimuli, of differentiating into specific stem cells and then to sequentially more mature forms. Erythropoietin, a glycoprotein formed primarily by the kidneys, regulates erythropoiesis and is stimulated by hypoxia and the products of hemolysis; a tenfold increase is possible under certain circumstances. With this stimulus, the committed erythroid stem cell gradually matures and divides through a proerythroblast stage to a reticulocyte in a period of 4-6 days. In the latter portion of this sequence, the nucleus becomes pyknotic and is extruded as the cell enters the bloodstream. The characteristic reticular staining of the reticulocyte is a consequence of the remaining ribosomal RNA; these ribosomes are lost over the next 24 hours, and the cell becomes a mature erythrocyte with a lifespan of 120 days.

If hematopoiesis is abnormal, red blood cells may be destroyed or phagocytosed before entering the circulation (ineffective hematopoiesis). An anemia with few reticulocytes is seen; the bone marrow has increased erythroid cellular elements. Administered radiolabeled iron rapidly enters the erythroid pathways, but only 20-40% appears in the peripheral red cells (normal 70-90%). In addition, ^{14}C-radiolabeled glycine enters the protoporphyrin

TABLE 7-2—ANEMIAS: ETIOLOGIC CLASSIFICATION

I.   Impaired production
A. Disturbances of stem cells
   1. Aplastic anemia
   2. Pure red blood cell aplasia
   3. Anemia of chronic renal failure

B. Disturbances of maturation
   1. Defective DNA synthesis
     a. Vitamin B_{12}
     b. Folic acid
     c. Defects in purine and pyrimidine metabolism
   2. Defective hemoglobin synthesis
     a. Deficient globin synthesis (thalassemia)
     b. Deficient heme synthesis (iron deficiency)
     c. Sideroblastic anemia
   3. Protein malnutrition
   4. Anemia of chronic disease
   5. Myelophthisic anemias

II.   Increased destruction
A. Intrinsic or red blood cell abnormalities
   1. Membrane disorders
   2. Enzyme deficiencies
   3. Hemoglobinopathies

B. Extrinisic or extraerythrocytic abnormalities
   1. Antibody mediated
   2. Physical factors
   3. Chemical or toxic agents
   4. Bacterial or other organisms
   5. Reticuloendothelial sequestration

III. Anemia of blood loss

pathway normally but appears as [14]Carbon monoxide within a few days, compared to the expected 120 days (the lifespan of the normal RBC). Diseases of the bone marrow such as malignant infiltration (myelophithisis) or fibrosis (myelofibrosis) result in compensatory hematopoiesis in extramedullary sites such as the liver and spleen.

Hemoglobin (MW = 65,000) is composed of two pairs of identical polypeptide chains with a heme molecule attached to each pair, so that 97% of the total weight is caused by globin. Balanced synthesis of normal polypeptide chains is necessary; as little as one substitution in an amino acid sequence results in an abnormal hemoglobin. Adults have 97% of hemoglobin A (two alpha and two beta chains, containing 141 and 146 amino acids, respectively), 2% hemoglobin A_2 (two alpha and two delta chains), and 1% fetal hemoglobin (two alpha and two gamma).

The oxyhemoglobin dissociation curve describes the relationship between O_2 and the hemoglobin (Hb) molecule at various partial pressures of oxygen. Any factor—hydrogen ion, carbon dioxide, or 2,3-diphosphoglycerate (2,3-DPG)—that interacts with deoxyhemoglobin to stabilize the reduced state will reduce its affinity for oxygen. The tissue capillary accumulation of acid and carbon dioxide facilitates the release of oxygen from hemoglobin to the tissue, and the intracellular accumulation of 2,3-DPG in chronic anemia or hypoxemia is an adaptive response. Hemoglobin F does not bind 2,3-DPG, and thus its affinity for oxygen is higher and the release to tissues is less.

The erythrocyte has limited metabolic machinery, with a primary purpose of maintaining membrane function and stability. Glucose is the primary nutrient and is metabolized by two pathways: 90% by the Embden-Meyerhof pathway and 10% by the pentose monophosphate pathway (hexose monophosphate shunt).

As the red cell ages during its 120-day life, the cell wall becomes more rigid, leading to sequestration and phagocytosis in the reticuloendothelial system (RES), primarily the spleen. Iron is released and is transported by transferrin, a beta globulin, back to the bone marrow for reutilization. The porphyrin ring is degraded to bilirubin (indirect-reacting), which is conjugated (direct-reacting), in the liver and excreted in the bile. If hemoglobin is freed within plasma, it combines immediately with haptoglobin (an alpha globulin) and is rapidly cleared by the RES and degraded. When the quantity of freed hemoglobin exceeds the availability of haptoglobin, the free hemoglobin is filtered in the urine. Some of the hemoglobin is reabsorbed in the tubule and catabolized, and may then reappear in the urine as hemosiderin.

Anemias Due to Decreased Production
IRON DEFICIENCY ANEMIA

Total body iron is 2-5 gm, and three-fourths of this is contained in hemoglobin of circulating red blood cells; the remainder is in myoglobin, storage forms, and enzymes. Ninety to 95% of the iron from catabolized senescent red blood cells is reused. Normal adults lose approximately 1 mg of iron daily through desquamation (of epithelial cells from the skin and gut) and blood loss (less than 1 mg daily in the stool). Menstruation results in a loss of 30-60 ml of blood each month, thus increasing the daily loss by 0.5-1.0 mg.

The normal daily diet (U.S.) contains 10-20 mg of iron. Usually approximately 10% of the dietary supply is absorbed. Although the entire small intestine has the capacity to absorb iron, the majority of absorption occurs in the duodenum. Except for endogenous reutilization, there is no control mechanism regulating excretion. The small intestinal epithelial cell is capable of increasing absorption up to 20%. Generally, the degree of absorption correlates inversely with the serum and total body iron concentrations; however, certain disorders, such as hemochromatosis, are associated with an inappropriately increased absorption. Metabolic demand may easily exceed availability in such conditions as pregnancy, growth, and acute or chronic blood loss; these conditions may require supplemental iron administration, but the small intestinal mucosa cannot accept more than 100-200 mg daily. Anemia from dietary restriction of iron alone is extremely unusual, although achlorhydria does reduce iron absorption.

Several different proteins are concerned with iron transport and storage.

Transferrin (or siderophilin) is a glycoprotein in the liver. It transports iron in the circulation from sites of absorption, storage, or release from senescent red blood cells to hematopoietic and other areas of utilization. Its half-life is approximately 9 days; half circulates in the plasma, and half is found in extravascular areas. Total iron-binding capacity is an indirect measure of transferrin.

Ferritin. This is a complex macromolecular iron storage protein found principally in the reticuloendothelial elements of the liver and bone marrow. It is also found as an intracellular transport protein in the intestinal epithelium and in normoblasts. Minute amounts circulate in the serum (20-250 μg/liter) and are a useful indicator of body iron stores.

Hemosiderin. An insoluble complex of colloidal iron oxide, it is found primarily in the reticuloendothelial system, and probably represents denatured ferritin.

Iron deficiency is the commonest cause of anemia, and the vast majority of patients have acute or chronic blood loss. In males, blood loss is almost always the cause.

Symptoms correlate with both the degree of anemia and the degree of physiologic adaptation. The general manifestations of anemia include malaise, irritability, difficulty concentrating, pallor, sinus tachycardia, and exertional dyspnea. With severe anemia or compromised blood flow, symptoms of ischemia (particularly cardiac and cerebral) may develop. As the anemia worsens, cardiac flow murmurs may be noted secondary to compensatory increases in both heart rate and contractility; even high-output left ventricular failure may ensue as ventricular filling time lessens and left ventricular end-diastolic pressure rises. Other findings in iron-deficient patients include atrophy of the tongue mucosa (glossitis), koilonychia ("spoon nail"), brittle hair, paresthesias and, rarely, elevated cerebrospinal fluid pressures suggesting pseudotumor cerebri.

Chlorosis. A greenish discoloration of the skin once associated with iron deficiency in young females, this is no longer observed, for unknown reasons. The *Plummer-Vinson syndrome*, the triad of esophageal weblike strictures, iron deficiency anemia, and achlorhydria, is rarely seen in the United States. Gastritis and atrophy of the gastric mucosa are frequently seen in association with iron deficiency anemia. The majority probably represent a secondary phenomenon; a few may have primary achlorhydria, with resultant iron deficiency. Splenomegaly owing to RES phagocytosis of red blood cells may be noted in up to 10% of patients.

When the loss of iron exceeds the metabolic demand, the first stage of iron deficiency ensues. Iron is mobilized from storage forms, first in the liver then in the bone marrow. Although the serum iron remains in the low-normal range, ferritin falls; the bone marrow may show hyperplastic changes. As the tissue stores are depleted, less hemoglobin is made and the red cell is released as a smaller form, giving a microcytic but normochromic appearance on the peripheral smear. Later, the cells become hypochromic as well as microcytic. The diagnosis is supported by a decreased iron saturation. When the total iron-binding capacity (TIBC) is not elevated and iron deficiency is suspected, a low serum ferritin is useful, but the absence of stainable iron in the bone marrow is required for precise diagnosis.

Management must include a thorough search for sites of blood loss; if none are found, intravascular or extravascular hemolysis, defective RBC production, and malabsorption should be excluded, and causes of increased iron requirements should be considered. A complete dietary history should be obtained.

Specific therapy is determined by the quantity and rate of blood loss, the hemoglobin concentration, and the underlying and associated pathology. If the degree of anemia is mild (hemoglobin of 11-13 gm/day), no specific treatment is necessary; the site of loss should be identified and corrected, and adequate dietary iron should be ensured.

Moderate anemia (hemoglobin of 8-11) should generally be treated with iron supplementation. Elemental iron, 200 mg/day orally, allows a maximal hematopoietic response (a daily increase in the hemoglobin of about 0.3 gm/day); more exceeds the absorptive capacity of the small bowel. Ferrous sulfate, 300 mg three times a day, will provide 180 mg of elemental iron. Ten % of patients develop nausea, vomiting, abdominal cramps, or diarrhea. Taking iron on an empty stomach will increase absorption but also increases gastrointestinal side effects. If such side effects occur, the dose should be reduced and/or taken with meals; occasionally other ferrous salts (e.g., gluconate) are better tolerated than the sulfate. Ascorbic acid does not increase absorption to a greater degree than can be accomplished by a small increment in the dose.

Parenteral iron may be administered in the form of iron dextran (Imferon) or iron sorbitex (Jectofer). Indication for parenteral iron is limited to patients with malabsorption syndromes, inflammatory bowel disorders, chronic ongoing losses exceeding the capacity for oral replacement, and noncompliance. The high immediate iron availability achieved with parenteral administration does not significantly increase the rapidity of the erythropoietic response over that achieved with optimal doses of oral iron. Regardless of the route of administration, adequate replacement will result in a reduction of malaise in 2-3 days and an increased reticulocyte count in 5-6 days, which peaks in 12-14 days. Treatment should be continued until stores are replenished.

Severe anemia (hemoglobin less than 8) may often require transfusion. Chronic, severe iron deficiency is often hemodynamically well tolerated. Choice and rapidity of transfusion must be guided by repeated careful assessments of physiologic parameters. Generally, packed red blood cells (PRBCs), rather than whole blood, should be administered to reduce the risk of volume overload.

SIDEROBLASTIC ANEMIAS

The sideroblastic anemias are a group of pathogenetically related iron-loading anemias, all sharing a defect in heme synthesis. Porphyrin synthesis proceeds at the mitochondria through a sequence of enzymatic reactions, beginning with the conversion of glycine and succinic acid to delta-aminolevulinic acid (ALA); defects at any point could result in anemia (Fig. 7-1). Since pyridoxal phosphate is necessary for the synthesis of ALA, a trial of pyridoxine (50-200 mg/daily for 2-4 weeks) is indicated if there is no obvious cause for a sideroblastic anemia. If unsuccessful, parenteral pyridoxal phosphate should be tried.

Most patients have moderate anemia (hemoglobin 7-8 gm/day) with symptoms proportionate to the anemia. The peripheral red cells are normocytic or slightly microcytic and hypochromic. Poikilocytosis and Pappenheimer bodies (iron stippling of the red

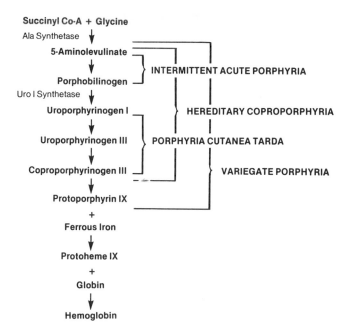

Figure 7-1. Synthesis of erythrocytic heme by a series of porphyrin conversion steps that begin with the production of δ-aminole vulinic acid from glycine and succinic acid.

cell) may be seen. The reticulocyte count is low; platelet and leukocyte counts are normal. The bone marrow shows hypoplasia of the erythroid series, increased iron stores, and ringed sideroblasts on Prussian blue staining. These sideroblasts are normoblasts containing nonheme iron in the perinuclear mitochondrial region of the cell.

Serum iron is normal or elevated; the TIBC is normal. Increased absorption of iron together with inability to incorporate iron because of defective heme synthesis results in systemic iron overload. Transfusions may be necessary and further add to the increase of iron stores. Sometimes, iron-chelating therapy (desferrioxamine) is necessary.

Hereditary sideroblastic anemia is a rare sex-linked recessive syndrome in which a moderate anemia is usually not apparent until the patient is in the mid-20s or early 30s, although a mild undiagnosed anemia is often present earlier. Iron absorption is often even greater in the hereditary form than other sideroblastic anemias and may lead to tissue damage resembling hemochromatosis. A response in some patients to pyridoxine (200 mg daily) suggests a defect in the pyridoxal phosphate-dependent first step; there are usually no symptoms of pyridoxine deficiency. Other patients probably have one of several potential defects.

Thalassemia, a genetic disorder of globin synthesis, may result in a sideroblastic anemia; the inability to incorporate heme into hemoglobin leads to heme accumulation, which inhibits the first step of heme synthesis, resulting in accumulation of perinuclear iron granules. Acquired sideroblastic anemias can be divided into two categories, primary (or idiopathic) and secondary.

Idiopathic sideroblastic anemia is often refractory to any therapy and tends to occur in the elderly. Its occasional association with leukopenia or thrombocytopenia and its infrequent progression to a very refractory acute myelogenous leukemia or erythroleukemia suggests that this form of sideroblastic anemia may be a precursor to, or a part of, the myeloproliferative syndromes.

Secondary causes of sideroblastic anemia include lead poisoning, alcoholism, and several drugs. Lead inhibits the activity of three sulfhydryl enzymes necessary for heme synthesis: delta-aminolevulinic acid synthetase, delta-aminolevulinic acid dehydrase, and heme synthetase. Lead exposure may occur industrially, in children with pica who ingest lead-based paint chips, or by the ingestion of water that has passed through corroded lead pipes. Basophilic stippling of the red cells, gingival lead lines, and increased density of the metaphysis of long bones may suggest the diagnosis of chronic plumbism in older children and young adults. Late chronic exposure in adults may lead only to basophilic stippling (in two-thirds of patients). The diagnosis rests on demonstration of elevated coproporphyrinuria. More severe plumbism is suggested by mental status changes, peripheral neuropathy, ataxia, or seizures. Occasionally, tubular injury results in the Fanconi syndrome of hypophosphatemia, glycosuria, and aminoaciduria. Treatment of lead poisoning requires removal from lead exposure and occasionally chelation therapy when severe.

Alcoholism may produce a sideroblastic anemia by inhibiting the formation of pyridoxal phosphate from pyridoxine. Diagnosis requires the demonstration of a decreased serum pyridoxal phosphate level. Treatment requires cessation of ethanol intake and includes administration of pyridoxal phosphate; the anemia will not respond to pyridoxine therapy.

Two antituberculous antibiotics, isoniazid and cycloserine, metabolically antagonize the action of pyridoxine. Because treatment with pyridoxine does not reduce the antituberculous activity of these agents, prophylactic administration of 10-50 mg of pyridoxine daily is recommended when using these agents.

An unrelated but reversible sideroblastic anemia, which is probably secondary to interference with mitochondrial metabolism, may occasionally be seen with chloramphenicol. This anemia is not related to the aplastic anemias also seen with chloramphenicol.

A wide variety of systemic diseases may be associated with sideroblastic anemia. These include connective tissue diseases (rheumatoid arthritis and systemic lupus erythematosus), viral diseases (infectious mononucleosis), and neoplasia (multiple myeloma). Treatment consists of removal of offending agents and appropriate therapy of the underlying disease.

ANEMIA OF CHRONIC DISEASE

Anemia associated with chronic inflammatory disease is a very common occurrence—perhaps second only to iron deficiency. All treatable causes of anemia must be excluded. The peripheral smear shows slight microcytosis and hypochromia. Although the diagnosis is suggested by a microcytic anemia with a normal or low normal serum iron and a low TIBC (in a patient with malignancy, connective tissue disease, or chronic infection), concurrent iron deficiency can be excluded by examining the bone marrow for stainable iron. A normal serum ferritin also provides firm support that iron deficiency is not present (Table 7-3). Several defects seem to contribute to this anemia: a decreased sensitivity to erythropoietin, a lower elevation in the erythropoietin level than is seen in other anemias, defective mobilization of reticuloendothelial iron (that acquired from catabolism of senescent RBCs) and a slight decrease in red cell survival. The development of this anemia is insidious (2-3 months), and the degree of anemia is usually mild (hemoglobin of 10-13).

Chronic disease may also produce anemia by more obvious mechanisms. Neoplasms may involve the bone marrow or induce blood loss. Iron may be deposited in the inflammatory tissues of connective tissue disease; the treatment of these diseases with nonsteroidal anti-inflammatory agents may produce gastritis or with gold may suppress the bone marrow. Cirrhosis and nephrosis result in increased plasma volume with a resultant lowering of the red cell concentration.

Megaloblastic Anemias

A number of factors may lead to decreased DNA synthesis with delayed cell division, increased nuclear size, and production of the characteristic megaloblast with its decreased nuclear-cytoplasmic ratio. Deficiencies of either B_{12} or folic acid produce megaloblastic anemias, since both are necessary in the initial steps of DNA synthesis (Fig. 7-2). A methyl group is transferred from N^5-methyl tetrahydrofolate to vitamin B_{12} (cobalamin), which acts as a carrier and is converted to methylcobalamin. The nonmethylated tetrahydrofolate is converted to N^5,N^{10}-methylene-tetrahydrofolate, which serves as a cofactor for an initial step of DNA synthesis, the conversion of deoxyuridylate to deoxythymidylate. The methylated form of B_{12} is a cofactor for conversion of homocysteine to methionine. Thus, a lack of B_{12} appears to prevent the transformation of methyl tetrahydrofolate to tetrahydrofolate, explaining why large doses of folic acid can produce a partial hematologic remission in pernicious anemia. Deficiency of another form of B_{12}, adenosylcobalamin, prevents the conversion of methylmalonyl coenzyme A to succinyl coen-

TABLE 7-3—MICROCYTIC-HYPOCHROMIC ANEMIAS

	Iron Deficiency	Sideroblastic	Thalassemia	Anemia of Chronic Disease
FERRITIN	↓	↑	↑	N
FE	↓	N or ↑	↑	N or ↓
TIBC	↑	N or ↓	N or ↓	↓
BONE MARROW IRON	0	↑	↑	N or ↑
SIDEROBLASTS	—	+	+	—
HGB. ELECTRO.	N	N	↑ A$_2$ or F	N

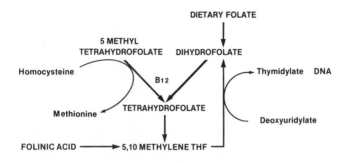

Figure 7-2. Interrelations of dietary folic acid and B_{12} in the synthesis of DNA. Deficiencies of either produce megaloblastic anemias.

zyme A and may be responsible for the neurologic syndrome of vitamin B_{12} deficiency. Increased urinary levels of methylmalonate can be used to identify B_{12} deficiency. Vitamin B_{12} is biochemically similar to heme but has a cobalt atom instead of iron. Intrinsic factor, produced by the stomach, is closely related to two other transportation glycoproteins, the transcobalamins (TC). Following binding of the B_{12}-intrinsic factor complex to the brush border of the terminal ileum, the vitamin is transferred to TC-II in the intestinal capillary bed. Most of the circulating B_{12} is carried by TC-I. TC-I is produced by granules in leukocytes and is markedly elevated in chronic granulocytic leukemia, providing an interesting biochemical marker for that disease.

The bone marrow is highly cellular; 30-50% of the cells are of the erythroid series (normal, 25%), and exceptionally large megaloblasts with fine sievelike nuclear chromatin are found. Peripheral red cells are normochromic and macrocytic. Hypersegmentation of neutrophils is the first hematologic manifestation and is diagnosed when the mean number of lobes exceeds 3.5; other guidelines include seeing one with six lobes, more than 5% with five lobes, or fewer than 20% with two lobes.

The ineffective hematopoiesis and intramarrow hemolysis of

defective precursors often results in elevation of serum bilirubin and lactate dehydrogenase as well as occasional reduction in haptoglobin; serum iron may be elevated.

FOLIC ACID DEFICIENCY ANEMIA

Folic acid is water-soluble, heat labile, and found in a wide variety of foodstuffs: leafy green vegetables, milk, eggs, and most meats. Cooking not only partially destroys the folic acid content but also allows the leaching of the vitamin from the foodstuff into the broth, which is usually thrown away. After ingestion, the polyglutamate must be deconjugated to the monoglutamate at the epithelial brush border of the small intestine before absorption can occur. Absorption occurs primarily in the jejunum. The total body store of folic acid is 4-5 mg, and the daily losses are 40-100 μg; therefore, in the absence of intestinal disease, dietary deficiency results in a very slow development of symptoms. Because enterohepatic cycling accounts for about 100 μg each day, intestinal diseases reducing reabsorption allow the earlier development of symptoms of dietary deficiency.

Clinically, patients present with anemic symptoms proportionate to the degree of anemia, glossitis and diarrhea (and malabsorption) secondary to decreased epithelial cell production (secondary to the decrease in DNA synthesis), and subtle mental status changes (including irritability, forgetfulness, and insomnia). Ten percent of patients are hyperpigmented, 30% have splenomegaly, and many have mild hepatomegaly.

The characteristic smear and bone marrow have already been described. The serum folate and red cell folate levels are low, less than 3 and 150 ng/ml respectively.

As folate deficiency develops (in the absence of blood loss), the serum folate is noted to be low at 1 month, the red cell folate is low at 2 months, hypersegmentation is noted at 3 months, macrocytosis is observed at 4 months and anemia with a megaloblastic marrow is present at 5 months. Therefore, an anemia with a low serum folate level and normal RBC folate level is *not* due to folate deficiency.

While the Schilling test is usually normal, loss of intestinal epithelium with malabsorption of substances such as B_{12} and intrinsic factor may simulate pernicious anemia; reevaluation several weeks after replacement with folate allows correct diagnosis.

Dietary folate deficiency is uncommon and is seen with excess cooking of all foodstuffs or fanatic dieting. A relative dietary deficiency may be noted with increased folate demand from growth (pregnancy and infants), hypermetabolism (malignancy and hyperthyroidism), and compensated chronic hemolytic anemia. Malabsorption and inefficient deconjugation of folate occur in inflammatory and granulomatous small bowel disorders, especially those involving the jejunum. Folate deficiency associated with alcoholism is a combination of dietary deficiency and an alcohol-induced defect in the conversion of folate to its active forms. Estrogens, phenobarbital, phenytoin, and other drugs inhibit intestinal deconjugation of polyglutamate, thus inducing folate deficiency. Methotrexate irreversibly binds and inhibits dihydrofolate reductase.

The normal diet provides approximately 0.5 mg of folate in the polyglutamate form. Treatment of folate deficiency should be directed at correction of the underlying cause. Folic acid (pteroylglutamic acid), the monoglutamate, is readily absorbed in a dose of 1 mg/day orally and will correct the deficiency in *all* the conditions described except that associated with high doses of methotrexate where folinic acid must be administered ("leucovorin rescue").

B$_{12}$ DEFICIENCY ANEMIA

Vitamin B$_{12}$ is heat-stable, water-insoluble, and found in meats and dairy products. The normal diet contains 10-30 μg of B$_{12}$, and the daily requirement is about 5 μg. The vitamin must first combine with intrinsic factor (IF), a glycoprotein secreted by the gastric mucosa, before absorption by the terminal ileum. Diseases of the stomach (such as pernicious anemia and gastric atrophy) or small intestine (such as malabsorption) may result in B$_{12}$ deficiency. After absorption, B$_{12}$ is transported by several plasma proteins; transcobalamin I and III are produced by granulocytes and have a high affinity for B$_{12}$, whereas transcobalamin II is derived from the liver and has a low affinity.

The total body B_{12} content is 4-5 mg; most is found in the liver. As with folate, a prominent enterohepatic cycle is present, so that while dietary reduction has a delayed effect, acute malabsorption may result in relatively rapid changes.

The macrocytic and megaloblastic anemia is associated with serum B_{12} levels below 100 pg/ml. In some situations associated with elevated transcobalamin levels, the total B_{12} level may be normal even though the free (or available) B_{12} is actually low. A measure of the B_{12} binding capacity and percent saturation may be beneficial; in B_{12} deficiency, the saturation is less than 10%.

In addition to the symptoms and signs seen with folate deficiency, patients may develop neurologic abnormalities proportionate to the degree and duration of the B_{12} deficiency. These include paresthesias (numbness, tingling, and burning of the extremities), decreased position sense, and gait disturbances. Distal decreased vibratory sensation involves higher frequencies first. Mental changes may range from irritability and forgetfulness to depression and even paranoia (megaloblastic madness). Combined systems disease (subacute combined degeneration) involves slow progression of the neurologic abnormalities together with degeneration of the dorsolateral columns of the spinal cord, producing upper motor neuron lesions (spasticity and extensor plantar responses) progressing to lower motor neuron lesions (weakness, decreased tendon reflexes, and finally paraplegia). The mental abnormalities may progress to coma and even death.

Dietary deficiency is occasionally seen in strict vegetarians who avoid all dairy products and in hard liquor alcoholics. A relative deficiency secondary to increased need may be found in pregnancy. Absorption of B_{12} will be decreased when there is a lack of intrinsic factor, competitive utilization of B_{12} by intestinal parasites or bacteria, malabsorption and inflammatory diseases of the small intestine, or after surgical resection of the terminal ileum.

Decreased absorption of B_{12} due to gastric atrophy, histamine unresponsive achlorhydria, and decreased intrinsic factor production is termed *pernicious anemia* (PA). The incidence increases with age, and as many as 1 in 200 older people may have PA. More than 60% of patients with PA have circulating antibodies to intrinsic factor, and many have antibodies to gastric parietal cells, suggesting an autoimmune nature.

Gastrectomy may result in B_{12} deficiency owing to the removal of the source of intrinsic factor production; however, because of the large stores and small losses, anemia usually takes several years to develop in the absence of other complicating factors.

The *Schilling test* (Table 7-4) allows the evaluation of the contribution of gastroenterologic abnormalities to a B_{12} deficiency. Radiolabeled B_{12} is given orally, and the urinary excretion of B_{12} over the following 24 hours is measured. Patients with uncorrected B_{12} deficiency should receive parenteral B_{12} (1000 μg) 1 hour after receiving the oral labeled dose so that tissue binding sites are saturated, preventing an artifactual decrease in urinary excretion. In the absence of renal disease, more than 7% of the labeled dose should be excreted into the 24-hour urinary collection. Patients with PA excrete less than 2%. Intermediate levels may be seen in some malabsorption syndromes. A staged Schilling test allows further discrimination as to the etiology. If the standard test is abnormal, it is repeated with concurrent administration of IF; correction of the abnormality suggests gastric disease such as PA. If the second stage is abnormal, the test is repeated after treatment with antibiotics (such as tetracycline)

TABLE 7-4—3-STAGE SCHILLING TEST

	1st No I.F.	2nd With I.F.	3rd After Antibiotics, No I.F.
DIETARY DEFICIENCY	N		
GASTRIC DISEASE (P.A., GASTRECTOMY)	↓↓	N	
BACTERIAL OVERGROWTH (BLIND LOOP SYNDROME)	↓	↓	N
SMALL INTESTINAL DISEASE	↓	↓	↓

but without IF, correction suggests bacterial overgrowth (such as the blind loop syndrome) with competitive utilization of available B_{12}. Abnormalities in all three stages suggest small intestine diseases with malabsorption.

Both folate deficiency and B_{12} deficiency result in mild gastric atrophy and small, intestinal malabsorption, which may lead to misinterpretation of the Schilling test. Therefore, all patients with abnormalities suggesting a primary small-intestinal disease should have the Schilling test repeated several weeks after parenteral replacement with B_{12} or folate. Treatment should be parenteral (I.M.); oral absorption may be unreliable, particularly in the presence of primary or secondary absorptive defects. One hundred μg daily for 5 days followed by monthly injections is adequate. Increased reticulocytes should be noted in 3-5 days, with a peak in 7-10 days. Although many physicians treat patients with secondary neurologic abnormalities with up to 1000 μg, there is no proof of increased efficacy. The neurologic deficits usually respond very slowly (weeks to months), and recovery is often incomplete.

Treatment of patients with chronic pancreatic insufficiency with oral B_{12} may require supplementation with bicarbonate and pancreatic enzymes to allow the endogenous intrinsic factor to work.

Aplastic Anemia

Aplastic anemia is a pancytopenia, associated with a diffuse decrease in all precursor elements in the bone marrow. The incidence in the general population ranges from 1:50,000 to 1:100,000. Although the pathogenesis is unknown, it is probable that the primary defect occurs in the pluripotential stem cell.

A number of causes have been described:

I. Idiopathic
   A. Familial (Fanconi anemia)
   B. Acquired

  II. Associated with a viral illness
     A. Acute
     B. Delayed
 III. Drug-induced
     A. Idiosyncratic (independent of dose)
        1. Chloramphenicol (risk 1:25,000)
        2. Phenylbutazone
        3. Gold
        4. Phenytoin
        5. Sulfonamides
        6. Tolbutamide
     B. Dose-related
        1. Ionizing radiation
        2. Alkylating agents and antimetabolites
        3. Benzene

Predictable reductions in cellularity occur with several of the antineoplastic agents as well as ionizing radiation. Chloramphenicol and phenylbutazone are the classic examples of the idiosyncratic response where aplastic anemia may appear after one or many doses. The risk for this response to chloramphenicol is said to be 1 in 25,000 patients receiving the drug. More often, chloramphenicol produces a dose-related hypocellularity, which involves primarily the red cell line, is reversible, and is characterized by early vacuolization of the red cell precursors on bone marrow examination.

The peripheral smear shows a pancytopenia with a normochromic, normocytic anemia. The reticulocyte count is decreased, and the serum iron is increased.

Thirty percent of patients die in the first year after diagnosis—primarily owing to infections or hemorrhage. Treatment is primarily supportive. All potential etiologic factors should be identified and removed. Occasionally, there will be gradual improvement, particularly with the dose-related agents, that may take weeks to months to normalize. Neither steroids nor splenectomy have been of benefit in reversing the aplasia, although steroids may diminish bleeding due to thrombocytopenia by stabilizing microvascular membranes. Androgens in high doses (oxymetholone at 4 mg/kg/day) may improve the anemia in some patients. At present, bone marrow transplantation from an identical twin or HLA-compatible sibling yields a viable graft in 75% of cases; 50% of these become apparent cures.

A few patients later develop acute myelogenous leukemia, suggesting that aplastic anemia may be a preleukemic state in some patients.

PURE RED CELL APLASIA

Pure red cell aplasia is a rare disease in which red cell precursors are selectively reduced or absent. The causes are similar to those of aplastic anemia; however, the majority of patients have either associated immunologic abnormalities or neoplasia found before or after the diagnosis of pure RBC aplasia. A third to half the patients have a thymoma (usually benign). Some patients have an immunologic inhibitor of erythropoietin. A few patients have lupus or rheumatoid arthritis. These associations suggest an autoimmune etiology, which is further supported by the fact that up to a third of patients with pure RBC aplasia and thymoma improve after thymectomy. Some patients will respond to steroids or immunosuppressive agents. Riboflavin is occasionally effective and should be given to all patients. Folate and B_{12} levels should be determined. If there is no improvement with nutritional adjustment in 1-3 months, the process is not likely to be reversible and immunosuppressive therapy should be considered.

Anemias Caused by Decreased Survival
HEMOGLOBINOPATHIES

Hemoglobin S disease. Hemoglobin S disease is the prototype of the hemoglobinopathies. In these diseases, substitution of a single amino acid in one of the polypeptide chains leads to altered physiochemical properties. The alterations often reduce the molecular solubility under certain environmental conditions, leading to abnormal cell shapes, decreased plasticity of the membrane, and premature destruction of the cell.

Hemoglobin S results from an autosomal genetic substitution of valine for glutamate in the sixth position of the beta chain.

Polymerization of the molecule, resulting in distorted cell shapes (sickled appearance), occurs under conditions of acidosis, hypoxemia, hyperosmolarity, and decreased temperature. Reducing agents such as sodium hyposulfite will produce sickling in vitro.

The heterozygous state (AS), sickle cell trait, is found in about 10% of black Americans and 5% of Americans of Puero Rican origin. Americans with ancestral ties to Mediterranean countries including Italy, Greece, and Syria have a much lower incidence of the trait. On electrophoresis, 25-45% of the hemoglobin is S (Table 7-5). With the trait, unless severely stressed, red cell survival is normal and there is no anemia. Severe physiologic abnormalities, particularly acidosis or hypoxemia, may result in sickling, but generally sickling is not evident. Although survival is normal, many patients will develop renal abnormalities. The medullary conditions of increased osmolarity and decreased oxygen tension and pH result in local sickling, which occludes the medullary microvasculature, resulting in microinfarction. An inability to concentrate the urine occurs, and some patients develop episodic painless microhematuria. The homozygous state (SS), sickle cell disease, is found in approximately 0.2% of all births among black Americans—less than the expected rate because of high fetal wastage. Hemoglobin electrophoresis demonstrates that 70-99% of the hemoglobin is S; the remainder is hemoglobin F. The red cells sickle spontaneously, and thus the RBC lifespan is greatly shortened. Sickled red cells occlude vessels, are easily sheared, and are actively sequestered and destroyed by the reticuloendothelial system. Patients with higher concentrations of fetal hemoglobin have a milder disease.

The peripheral smear demonstrates sickled cells as well as target cells, stippling of the red cell, and Howell-Jolly bodies. Howell-Jolly bodies are remnants of nuclear material, which remain because the spleen cannot "pit" them from the red cell as it normally would. The reticulocyte count is elevated, and the bone marrow demonstrates increased red cell precursors. The hemolysis may result in abnormalities, described below.

Occlusive phenomena produce a variety of clinical presentations, beginning a vicious cycle. Sickling leads to microvascular occlusion; the resultant tissue hypoxia and cellular injury results

TABLE 7-5—HEMOGLOBIN PATTERNS (PERCENT)

Hemoglobin	A $\alpha_2\beta_2$	A2 $\alpha_2\delta_2$	F $\alpha_2\gamma_2$	S 6 Val $\alpha_2\beta_2$	C 6Lys $\alpha_2\beta_2$
STRUCTURE					
NORMALS					
PREMATURE INFANT	10-30		70-90		
BIRTH	15-40		60-85		
4 MONTHS	90-95		0.5-1.0		
ADULT	96-98	1-4			
DISEASE STATES					
SICKLE CELL TRAIT	60-80	1-4	0.5	20-40	—
SICKLE CELL DISEASE	0	1-4	1-40	60-99	—
HEMOGLOBIN C TRAIT	60-80	1-4	0.5	—	20-40
HEMOGLOBIN C DISPOSE	0	1-4	7	—	93
HEMOGLOBIN SC DISEASE	0	1-4	7	40-50	40-50
HETEROZYGOUS BETA THALASSEMIA	85-95	3-8	2-15	—	—
HOMOZYGOUS BETA THALASSEMIA	A2	1-5	40-60	—	—
SICKLE THALASSEMIA	35	1-8	1-25	60-90	—
HBC THALASSEMIA	20	?	1-5	—	65-95

in the release of vasospastic elements; local acidosis, hypoxia, and vasospasm produce further sickling. Fever almost invariably accompanies occlusive crises and must be distinguished from a precipitating infectious illness.

Vasoocclusive phenomena include abdominal crises, hepatic crises, hand-foot syndrome, diffuse pain with fever, pulmonary infarction, and priapism. The white count is usually elevated, with no change or a slight reduction in the red count. Changes compatible with hemolysis include absent haptoglobin, hemoglobinemia, and methemalbuminemia. Fibrinogen is normal or slightly elevated.

Abdominal crises usually present as an acute abdomen with diffuse tenderness and paralytic ileus but without localizing signs. An infectious etiology should always be considered; fever, leukocytosis, and jaundice may be present in both. The leukocyte alkaline phosphatase (LAP) may be helpful; it will usually be elevated more than two and one-half times normal with infections in this setting and normal with an abdominal occlusive crisis. Hepatic crises present with fever, pain, leukocytosis, and laboratory evidence of hepatitis; recovery occurs sooner than the usual course of viral hepatitis, and later cirrhosis is unlikely unless multiple episodes have occurred. The hand-foot syndrome, also known as sickle cell dactylitis, is an occlusive phenomenon occurring in the distal phalanges, producing pain. Painless avascular necrosis may involve the femoral and humeral heads; a similar occurrence in the spine produces vertebral osteoporosis, or a "fish deformity." Diffuse crises manifested as diffuse arthralgias, tenosynovitis, and bone pain are also common.

Occlusion of the pulmonary microvasculature produces a diffuse infarction that resembles pneumonitis; differentiation from pneumonia may be difficult or impossible, and the patient should usually be treated for pneumonia. Priapism may result from sludging of sickled cells in the venous sinusoids of the penis, producing an extremely painful, tense, swollen penis, which may last for days.

The treatment of vasoocclusive crises is symptomatic. Bed rest, hydration, and adequate analgesia and sedation remain the mainstays. Underlying infection must be diagnosed and aggressively treated. Acidosis and hypoxemia should be corrected and underlying causes determined. Vasodilators offer no benefit. Both urea and sodium cyanate reduce sickling in vitro; however, urea has not been of proved benefit in vivo and sodium cyanate must be used in toxic doses. Partial exchange transfusions may help when the crises are life-threatening.

Hematologic crises include aplastic crises and hemolytic crises. Aplastic crisis is an acute reduction in bone marrow production of all elements, which is uncommon, usually lasts several weeks, and is often associated with a viral infection. Hemolytic crises usually occur in association with vasoocclusive crises. A chronic, partially compensated, hemolytic state is common in sickle cell disease. Many patients require supplemental folic acid (0.25-0.5 mg/day).

Other complications include gallstones (caused by the large heme turnover), leg ulcers in older people (due to trauma and decreased microvacularity), and retinal lesions (neovascularization with vitreous hemorrhage and retinal detachment).

Autosplenectomy occurs along with repeated multiple microvascular infarctions with resultant gradual shrinking of size and decrease in function. An increased risk of *Salmonella* and pneumococcal infections is noted, probably owing to ineffective opsonization and reticuloendothelial clearance of these organisms. Up to 50% of osteomyelitis in patients with sickle cell disease is caused by *Salmonella*. Death in the second and third decade due to infection is common, although with better supportive measures, patients with milder forms of the disease are now living longer.

Combination syndromes include sickle thalassemia, in which the concentration of hemoglobin S is higher than that in sickle trait, and sickle C (hemoglobin SC), in which the symptoms and course are intermediate between sickle trait and sickle disease.

There are more than 120 abnormal hemoglobins now known and hemoglobin S is not the only one that sickles. In addition, electrophoresis may not completely separate all forms; when electrophoresis suggests AS or SS but the clinical picture does not fit, a sickle test (sickle preparation) may show no sickling, suggesting that the hemoglobin is actually a variant other than S.

Hemoglobin C disease. The substitution of lysine for glutamine in the sixth position produces hemoglobin C; its solubility is decreased, and precipitation results in attachment to the cell membrane but no sickling. The resultant increased rigidity of the membrane decreases the ability of the cell to traverse capillaries and allows early reticuloendothelial phagocytosis, particularly in the spleen. Individuals with the trait (AC), found in 2% of black Americans, are asymptomatic and not anemic but may have target cells. Homozygous individuals are mildly anemic and have evidence of hemolysis with increased target cells. Abdominal pain and arthralgias may be seen.

Thalassemias. These result from genetically determined repression of either alpha or beta chain synthesis. Beta thalassemia is the most common type. It is found particularly in persons of Mediterranean ancestry. Beta chain production is decreased, alpha chain production is normal or increased, and a partial compensatory increase in gamma (γ) and delta (δ) chain synthesis leads to increased formation of hemoglobins F and A_2 respectively. A hypochromic anemia due to decreased hemoglobin formation is found. Red cell survival is shortened because the excess alpha chains attach to the membrane, decreasing plasticity and allowing phagocytosis. Target cells and stippled red cells may be seen.

Heterozygotes (both thalassemia minors) are mildly anemic but asymptomatic and have normal lifespans. Diagnosis rests on demonstrating a hemoglobin A_2 concentration greater than 5%, with a normal or slightly increased hemoglobin F on electrophoresis.

Beta thalassemia major (Cooley or Mediterranean anemia) is the homozygous state. A severe anemia is noted with poikilocytosis. Electrophoresis demonstrates a normal hemoglobin A_2 level, with hemoglobin F ranging from 20 to 90%. Retarded growth, splenomegaly (from sequestration), and abnormal bones (increased medullary spaces with cortical thinning due to the hyperplastic marrow response) may be seen. Splenectomy may increase red cell survival when there is demonstrable sequestration. Patients in whom ineffective hematopoiesis (hyperplastic marrow with destruction of elements before release into the circulation) predominates will not benefit from splenectomy and will be placed at risk for an increased incidence of infections. Frequent transfusions may result in iron overload and require chelating therapy. Many patients require supplemental folic acid.

Alpha thalassemia is much less common than beta thalassemia. Reductions in alpha chain synthesis reduce formation of hemoglobins A, A_2, and F. The heterozygous state is associated with decreased alpha chain synthesis and a compensatory increase in erythroid activity. Small amounts of hemoglobin B are formed in infancy, and later hemoglobin H (beta-type subunits) is increased. Most patients have only a mild anemia. Intracellular inclusions secondary to precipitated hemoglobin H may be found on the peripheral smear. Homozygous alpha thalassemia is associated with a marked decrease in alpha chain synthesis. Hemoglobin H is increased in the fetus; it is unstable, has a low affinity for oxygen, and usually causes fetal death.

THE HEMOLYTIC ANEMIAS

The hemolytic anemias are a group of disorders characterized by premature destruction of red blood cells, either within the bloodstream (intravascular) or in tissues such as the reticuloendothelial system (extravascular).

Intravascular hemolysis may be further characterized as being caused by factors within the red cell (intracorpuscular) or exogenous intravascular events (extracorpuscular). Intracorpuscular defects include disorders resulting in increased membrane fragility, such as the red cell enzyme deficiencies, the hemoglobinopathies, and the red cell membrane defects. Extracorpuscular disorders resulting in hemolysis include thrombotic states (disseminated intravascular coagulation, thrombotic thrombocytopenic purpura, and hemolytic uremia syndrome), immune mechanisms, toxins (infections, heavy metals, and some drugs), intracellular infections, tortuous endothelial surfaces (cardiac valvular diseases, vasculitis, and vascular tumors), prosthetic surfaces (prosthetic valves and vascular grafts), and exogenous trauma to the red cell within the capillary (march hemoglobinuria).

Hypersplenic states may result in increased reticuloendothelial sequestration and destruction of red blood cells. Liver disease, such as cirrhosis and hepatitis, has been associated with hemolysis. *Zieve syndrome*, once thought to represent hemolysis, is the association of cirrhosis and hypertriglyceridemia with anemia and reticulocytosis seen in some cirrhotic alcoholics after several days of hospitalization. A mild anemia is usually preexistent and worsens with rehydration; the reticulocytosis is thought to be due to improved nutrition and removal of the toxic effects of ethanol.

The peripheral smear in intravascular hemolysis may show poikilocytosis (including schistocytes, helmet cells, spur cells, and spherocytes) and anisocytosis. Depending on the duration and degree of the hemolytic state and the accompanying nutritional status, coexistent deficiencies of iron or folate may be found (owing to the increased utilization of precursors in an attempt to compensate the anemia), thus further altering the morphology. In addition, when the reticulocytosis is brisk, a large proportion of the red cells will be large. Reticulocytosis (usually 3-7%) is always present unless there is marrow failure due to nutritional deficiency or other cause.

The Coombs test may be positive in immune-mediated hemolysis; however, significantly more antibodies are required to give a positive direct Coombs than are required to cause hemolysis. The Coombs test detects the presence of antibody by utilizing an immune serum against human immunoglobulin. The direct Coombs detects antibody attached to the red cell membrane, and the indirect Coombs detects free antibody. The Coombs test may be modified to detect complement by using an antiserum directed against complement. Either complement or immunoglobulin may result in destruction of the red cell by resulting in RES phagocytosis of the coated RBC. The indirect Coombs may be positive in many patients who are not hemolyzing—particularly those with autoimmune phenomena.

Haptoglobin concentrations will be reduced in hemolytic states where hemoglobin is released into the circulation and is proportional to the degree of hemolysis. Once all available haptoglobin is complexed with hemoglobin and rapidly cleared from the serum, hemoglobinemia and hemoglobinuria appear. Moderate to severe hemolysis, regardless of the site, will often be associated with increased serum bilirubin (indirect) and LDH (isoenzymes 3 and 4). Except for the reduction in haptoglobin and the appearance of free hemoglobin, these diagnostic findings are neither specific nor invariably present. A diagnosis of compensated hemolytic anemia might be suggested only by an elevated reticulocyte count. A very mild, well-compensated hemolytic anemia might be detectable only by measuring red cell survival time.

Treatment must be aimed at the underlying cause. Supportive therapy to allow maintenance of compensation includes folate (1 mg/day) and iron (900 mg ferrous sulfate daily). Each transfusion should be preceded by a careful assessment of cross-reacting immune antibodies in states of immune-mediated hemolytic anemia. Splenectomy may occasionally be of benefit, depending on the cause; assessment of the role of the spleen by red cell sequestration studies may determine the expected response to splenectomy.

HEMOLYTIC ANEMIAS DUE TO RED CELL ABNORMALITIES

RED CELL ENZYME DEFICIENCIES

The red blood cell lacks a nucleus and mitochondria and is therefore dependent on glucose for its energy. Ninety percent of the glucose entering the red cell undergoes anaerobic glycolysis (*Embden-Meyerhof pathway*), resulting in the production of adenosine triphosphate (*ATP*), reduced nicotinamide adenine dinucleotide (*NADH*), and 2,3-diphosphoglycerate (*2,3-DPG*). NADH is an essential oxygen receptor in several metabolic steps and helps maintain reduced hemoglobin. ATP is a high-energy compound essential for intracellular metabolic activity, including maintenance of the membrane's sodium pump. 2,3-DPG, by binding to hemoglobin, reduces its affinity for oxygen, allowing easier delivery of oxygen to tissues in the peripheral capillaries.

Pyruvate kinase deficiency. An autosomal recessive abnormality, this is the most common defect of the Embden-Meyerhof pathway (catalyzes conversion of phosphenolpyruvate to pyruvate). Homozygosity leads to deficient anaerobic glycolysis, resulting in decreased cell membrane integrity and hemolytic anemia. Manifestations common to most hereditary abnormalities associated with an inability to maintain membrane integrity include those seen with hemolysis: poikilocytosis and anisocytosis, increased reticulocyte count, splenomegaly, indirect hyperbilirubinemia, scleral icterus, cholelithiasis, and a bone marrow demonstrating erythroid hyperplasia. Demonstration of decreased pyruvate kinase activity establishes the diagnosis; it may be suspected if autohemolysis is corrected by ATP but not glucose. Incubating red cells in vivo for 48 hours depletes energy-storing compounds; glucose, when added, prevents hemolysis when the Embden-Meyerhof pathway is intact. Treatment is primarily symptomatic. Splenectomy may produce a transient improvement in some patients.

The remaining 10% of glucose entering the cell is metabolized aerobically in the *hexose monophosphate shunt* (pentose phosphate pathway), resulting in the production of reduced nicotinamide adenine dinucleotide phosphate (NADP). Reduced NADP is essential in the maintenance of reduced glutathione. Glutathione is an intracellular oxygen scavenger, which protects both hemoglobin and the cell membrane from oxidative degradation.

Glucose-6-phosphatase deficiency. An X-linked recessive trait, this deficiency is the most common defect of the hexose monophosphate shunt (catalyzes conversion of glucose-6-phosphate to glucose). Heterozygous females have approximately half the enzyme activity of males and homozygous females. Either quantitative or qualitative enzyme defects may occur. Approximately 10% of black American males are affected. The measured enzyme activity is about 10% of normal; activity is mildly reduced in young red cells and gradually declines to zero in the senescent red cell. Hemolysis is usually seen only after exposure to oxidizing agents such as quinine derivatives (quinidine and the antimalarials), sulfonamide derivatives (sulfa antibiotics, thiazide diuretics, and sulfonylureas), and aspirin. Acute viral infections may occasionally be associated with hemolysis. Diagnosis rests on demonstrating reduced enzyme activity; when the number of reticulocytes is markedly increased, the activity will appear higher. Heinz bodies (precipitated denatured hemoglobin attached to the red cell membrane) increase cell membrane rigidity and may be observed on the peripheral smear.

A more severe variant is found in persons of Mediterranean ancestry in whom the enzyme activity is less than 5% (often less than 1%). These patients have a chronic hemolytic anemia even in the absence of oxidizing agents. Favism is a state of acute, severe hemolytic anemia precipitated by ingestion of the fava bean or inhalation of the fava pollen.

RED CELL MEMBRANE ABNORMALITIES

Hereditary spherocytosis. An autosomal dominant membrane defect results in increased membrane permeability and rigidity and leads to decreased red cell survival with premature destruction in the spleen. Although present from birth, it may not be diagnosed until adult life.

Hereditary elliptocytosis. An autosomal dominant membrane defect of unknown type occasionally results in hemolysis and decreased red cell survival.

Paroxysmal nocturnal hemoglobinuria (PNH). In this defect, the membrane fixes complement in increased amounts without immunoglobulins. Hemolysis occurs, particularly at night. Twenty to 30% of patients may have gross hemoglobinuria. A few later develop acute stem cell or myelogenous leukemia, suggesting that this may actually be a myeloproliferative disorder.

Immune Hemolytic Anemia

Complement-fixing antibody producing intravascular hemolysis may be producd by exogenous agents such as drugs or be autoimmune. Drug-induced hemolytic anemias may be mediated by at least three different mechanisms:

1. Most drugs have molecular weights that are too low to stimulate antibody formation but can act as haptens with other body constituents. Penicillin in high concentrations, for example, coats the red cell and the red cell-drug complex, then stimulates and binds IgG antibody. The Coombs test with anti-IgG is positive, but negative with anticomplement sera.

2. The drug is not firmly attached to the red cell but stimulates an antibody; the drug-antibody complex activates complement at the red cell surface, producing hemolysis. Since the initial immune reaction does not involve the red cell surface, this reaction is sometimes called an "innocent bystander," although it may be influenced by the red cell itself. Seen with drugs such as sulfonamides, quinidine, chlorpropamide, and chlorpromazine, the Coombs test is negative with anti-IgG but positive with anticomplement sera, since only complement is present on the cells.

3. A third mechanism is the stimulation of an antibody, which cross-reacts with components of the red cell; the drug has actually induced an antibody, which reacts with antigens normally present in the red cell. The Coombs test is positive with anti-IgG, but only a small percentage of those developing antibodies to drugs actually manifest hemolytic anemia. Alpha methyldopa, L-Dopa, procainamide, hydralazine, and phenytoin may induce such "autoantibodies"; actual hemolysis is most common with alpha methyldopa.

Treatment includes removal of the offending agent and general support. With the autoimmune type of hemolysis, hemolysis may decrease with discontinuation of the agent, but the cross-reacting antibody may be produced for several months so that the Coombs test remains positive. Steroid therapy has not been useful.

Autoimmune hemolytic anemias are acquired and fall into three categories:

1. *Hemolytic anemia due to IgG or warm (maximal activity at 37°) antibodies.* These 7-S IgG antibodies are incomplete, since they are less effective than IgM antibodies in fixing complement or causing agglutination. Most have specificity for the Rh antigen. Hemolytic disease of the newborn is a nonautoimmune example of the passive transplacental transfer of maternal antibody (after prior Rh antigen exposure in a Rh-negative mother) directed against the infant's membrane Rh antigen. The spontaneous occurrence of this type of hemolysis as an autoimmune phenomenon is uncommon. Frequently associated with an underlying condition such as connective tissue diseases (systemic lupus erythematosus and rheumatoid arthritis), tumors (ovarian or breast carcinoma), lymphoma or chronic lymphocytic leukemia, or immunodeficiency states (Wiskott-Aldrich syndrome or malignant thymoma), the Coombs test is almost invariably positive. Treatment should be initiated with corticosteroids (1 mg/kg/day of prednisone). If continued high doses are required, immunosuppressive agents such as azathioprine or cyclophosphamide may allow a reduction in steroid dose; however, immunosuppressives tend to only work in steroid-responsive disease, and even then the course does not appear to be shortened. If toxic doses of steroids (with or without immunosuppressives) continue to be necessary after 4 weeks, splenectomy should be performed; two-thirds of patients will improve. None of the above interventions reduce antibody production, so the Coombs test will remain positive.

2. *Hemolytic anemia due to cold-reacting 19S IgM (cryoantibody).* This antibody, which has maximal reactivity at 4°C, is usually directed against the i or I antigens. During the first several months of life, the number of i antigens on the red cell membrane rapidly falls, while the number of I antigens rises. This disorder, known as cold agglutinin disease, is frequently associated with infections such as *Mycoplasma* or infectious mononucleosis or with malignancies such as lymphoma or chronic lymphocytic leukemia. All are antibodies directed against the I antigen, except in infectious mononucleosis where the antibody is against the i antigen. Both infectious varieties tend to have a self-limited course; however, the idiopathic and malignancy-associated varieties may require treatment. Steroids are usually not beneficial; alkylating agents such as chlorambucil may improve the disorder.

3. *Hemolytic anemia mediated by a cold-reacting 7S IgG.* Paroxysmal cold hemoglobinuria is a rare autoimmune disorder in which the antibody is directed against the P antigen on the red cell membrane. This condition may be idiopathic or associated with syphilis. The Donath-Landsteiner test is diagnostic. The idiopathic variety is usually benign and self-limited, and the variety associated with syphilis responds to treatment of the underlying condition.

Methemoglobinemia. Methemoglobin is hemoglobin in which the iron has been oxidized from the ferrous to the ferric state. Normal blood may contain up to 0.25 gm/dl of methemoglobin. Certain oxidant agents such as ferrous sulfate, nitrates and nitrate-producing bacteria, sulfonamides, phenacetin, iodine, and hydrogen peroxide may oxidize hemoglobin to methemoglobin. When the concentration reaches 0.5 gm/dl, cyanosis may be noticed. Symptoms of tissue hypoxia may be noted when about 40% of the hemoglobin is converted to methemoglobin. Concentrations above 70% are lethal. Methylene blue rapidly corrects methemoglobinemia by accelerating the NADP-methemoglobin reductase enzyme.

Sulfhemoglobinemia. This is formed by hydrogen sulfide reacting with oxyhemoglobin to irreversibly alter the polypeptide chain and reduce oxygen affinity while increasing carbon monoxide affinity. Phenacetin, sulfonamides, and *Clostridium welchii* infection may result in the formation of sulfhemoglobin. Marked cyanosis may be noted with as little as 0.5 gm/dl. Concentrations rarely exceed 10% of the hemoglobin content and are invariably asymptomatic.

Carboxyhemoglobin. Carboxyhemoglobin, carbon monoxide hemoglobin, results from exposure of hemoglobin to carbon monoxide. The affinity of hemoglobin for carbon monoxide is more than 200 times its affinity for oxygen; thus, even low concentrations in the ambient air may result in carboxyhemoglobinemia. The high affinity reduces oxygen-carrying capacity and neighboring hemoglobin molecules have increased oxygen affinity. Carboxyhemoglobin imparts a cherry red color that may be seen in the skin or mucous membranes.

With acute carbon monoxide poisoning, symptoms of tissue hypoxia are not usually seen until the carbon monoxide saturation exceeds 25%; however, chronic exposure or children may be symptomatic at much lower concentrations.

POLYCYTHEMIC SYNDROMES
Polycythemia, or erythrocytosis, is an increase in the number of circulating red cells, or more specifically an increase in the total red cell volume.

Relative Polycythemia

Relative polycythemia is actually a reduction in plasma volume disproportionate to any change in the red cell number or volume. Although a direct loss of body fluids as in vomiting and diarrhea is the most common cause, states such as stress or hypertension may be associated with more prolonged reduction in plasma volume, leading to relative polycythemia, and are known as *stress polycythemia* and *Gaisbock's syndrome* (hypertension and polycythemia without splenomegaly) respectively.

Absolute polycythemia is an actual increase in red cell number, volume, or mass. This may be primary or secondary. Secondary polycythemia is a response to tissue hypoxia. Any cause of significant arterial hypoxemia, or more specifically decreased arterial oxygen saturation, may be associated with a secondary polycythemia, apparently due to increased renal production of erythropoietin. Causes include decreased oxygen tension in the air at high altitudes (affecting inhabitants of these areas and producing *Monge's disease*), alveolar hypoventilation (particularly in obese patients in whom the association of hypercapnea and somnolence with hypoxemia and polycythemia is known as the *Pickwickian syndrome*), *pulmonary* (as seen in chronic airway obstruction, actual or effective pulmonary shunts, and diffusion barriers), *heart disease with right-to-left shunts* (particularly cyanotic congenital heart disease), and abnormal hemoglobins (with increased oxygen affinity and inability to "unload" oxygen to the tissues). A mild secondary polycythemia may be noted with elevated corticosteroid levels, as in *Cushing's syndrome* of any cause or with high-dose *androgen administration.* Certain tumors, such as *renal cell carcinoma* and *cerebellar hemangioblastomas,* may produce polycythemia, probably by production of erythropoietin or erythropoietin-like substances; less frequent neoplastic causes include *hepatoma* and *uterine tumors.*

The polycythemic syndromes produce symptoms in direct proportion to the increased hematocrit and viscosity; however, the relationship is curvilinear, and as the hematocrit rises above 60-65, viscosity increases dramatically. Increased viscosity reduces blood flow, thus requiring a compensatory increase in contractility and cardiac output. The decreased flow may result in symptoms of reduced cerebral blood flow (headache, vertigo tinnitus, blurred vision, and syncope) and decreased peripheral blood flow (claudication). Pruritis following a hot bath and a "ruddy" complexion are common with polycythemic vera. Atherosclerosis seems to be accelerated in polycythemia vera, and in combination with increased viscosity favors thrombotic events. Capillary stasis and abnormal platelet function cause bleeding, especially from mucous membranes. Generalized venous engorgement and stasis may lead to thrombophlebitis, hepatic vein thrombosis (*Budd-Chiari syndrome*), and gastrointestinal varices. Duodenal ulcer is common in both polycythemia vera and chronic airway obstruction.

Polycythemia Vera

Polycythemia vera (PV) is also one of the myeloproliferative syndromes. The cause is unknown, hypoxia is not present, and erythropoietin levels are low or absent. More common in Jews of European ancestry and less common in blacks, a familial pattern is occasionally noted. Generally, PV affects persons in the fourth and fifth decades, with a slightly higher incidence noted in males.

The hemoglobin, hematocrit, and red cell mass and number are all elevated. The number of red cells per cubic millimeter generally exceeds 6.5 million and often approaches 10 million with a hematocrit usually over 60. The red cell volume must exceed 36 ml/kg in males and 32 ml/kg in females before the diagnosis can be established. Hypoxia should be ruled out by arterial oxygen saturations consistently greater than 92%. Rarely, nocturnal desaturation due to less apparent pulmonary disease is responsible. The red cells are normochromic and normocytic. The bone marrow demonstrates erythroid hyperplasia, or pan-hyperplasia in the case of PV, and reduced or absent iron stores are commonly noted, probably because of increased use. The reticulocyte count (percentage) is normal, but when corrected it is found to be high. The white blood cell count is elevated in 50-80% of cases, but may be low in up to 20%. Myelocytes and metamyelocytes may be increased in the peripheral blood, and basophils often exceed 6%. Thrombocytosis, noted in 50-60% of patients, frequently exceeds 1 million. Serum B_{12} levels may be elevated in 25-40% of patients; this elevation, due to an increase in B_{12}-binding protein (transcobalamin III), is noted in 60-75%. The leukocyte alkaline phosphatase (LAP) is elevated in 80-90% of cases. Hyperuricemia occurs in 70-80%, although gout is noted in only 5% of cases. A "ruddy" complexion and distended veins are seen with very high red cell concentrations. Splenomegaly is present in more than three-fourths and hepatomegaly in one-third of patients.

The clinical course is widely variable; if untreated, survival averages only 2 years. Patients may die of hemorrhagic or ischemic phenomena. Some patients later develop other myeloproliferative syndromes such as *chronic myelogenous leukemia* or *erythroleukemia*; most, if they live long enough, develop *myelofibrosis* after passing through a phase of myeloid metaplasia in which the hematocrit is normal because even though bone marrow fibrosis is beginning, compensation is maintained by extramedullary sites. At this state, all patients have splenomegaly, half have hepatomegaly, and polychromasia is seen on the peripheral smear.

Treatment is directed at maintaining the hematocrit below 50-60 to avoid the complications of hyperviscosity. Phlebotomy at frequent intervals is the primary treatment for mild disease. If iron deficiency is present, it should *not* be treated because it provides another method of maintaining a lower hematocrit.

Direct myelosuppression may be required in more refractory or severe cases. The choice between radiophosphorus (^{32}P) therapy and myelosuppressive chemotherapeutic agents has not been resolved. ^{32}P is effective and simple to use (single doses at long intervals); however, an increased late incidence of leukemia and possibly an earlier and more severe myelofibrosis have been noted. Many chemotherapeutic agents have been used successfully. Chlorambucil is presently felt to be a better agent; however, when polycythemia is associated with marked thrombocytosis, busulfan may be a better choice.

WHITE BLOOD CELL DISORDERS
Physiology of Polymorphonuclear Leukocytes
Cells of the myelocytic series are derived from the pluripotential stem cell; as myelocytes, they develop specific granules that stain

uniquely with Wright stain and contain lysozymes, alkaline phosphatases, collagenase, histamine, aminopeptidase, and other enzymes. The red-staining granules of eosinophils contain a specific peroxidase; the deep blue granules of basophils are rich in histamine. Neutrophils have 2-5 (average 3.5) nuclear lobules and a circulating life span of 24-48 hours; half circulate, while the remainder are loosely attached to the vascular endothelium and may be mobilized by agents like glucocorticoids, endotoxin, and etiocholanolone, which can double the circulating concentration.

Bacterial products and complement fragments (C_{3a}, C_{5a}, and C_{567}) are chemotactic and attract neutrophils to local areas of inflammation. Coating of foreign material with immunoglobulin or complement (opsonins, C_3 particularly) promotes phagocytosis. Once phagocytosed, the vacuole containing the invader combines with lysosomal granules, destroying the foreign material.

The neutrophil is responsible for phagocytosis and destruction of foreign materials—particularly those coated with opsonins (immunoglobulin and/or complement). Bacteria are destroyed in this fashion. The response to infection or other stresses may be associated with demargination of intravascular neutrophils and increased bone marrow production of neutrophils producing a leukocytosis. Local inflammation results in increased margination in blood vessels in the area. Both bacterial products and complement factors (C_{5a} and C_{567}) are chemotactic and result in enhanced migration of neutrophils into the area. After phagocytosis, the granules (lysosomes) combine with the vacuole containing the organism, resulting in destruction of the organism. An important element in this metabolic sequence is the formation of hydrogen peroxide in the presence of myeloperoxidase, which interacts forming bactericidal free radicals and superoxides.

Disorders of Leukocyte Function

Neutrophil migration is decreased in disorders such as the *lazy leukocyte syndrome* (recurrent fever, stomatitis, and otitis media) and *Job's syndrome* (recurrent staphylococcal abscesses, eczematous dermatitis, and high IgE levels). In addition, deficiencies of components of the complement cascade may result in decreased production of opsonins and chemotactic factors.

The *Chediak-Higashi syndrome* (oculocutaneous albinism with rotary nystagmus, recurrent staphylococcal infection, and lymphadenopathy) is an autosomal recessive defect in which very large granules, which are incapable of degranulating into the phagocytic vacuole, are formed within the neutrophil. *Chronic granulomatous disease* is a syndrome of recurrent and disseminated bacterial infections; it is an X-linked (occasionally autosomal) recessive inability to generate hydrogen peroxide. *Myeloperoxidase deficiency* may occur in an autosomal recessive or sporadically acquired (associated with megaloblastic anemia or myelocytic leukemia) fashion in which recurrent bacterial infections occur.

The Leukopenias

A fall in the circulating count below 5000 per cu mm is termed leukopenia. Neutropenia is a reduction in neutrophils to 2000 per cu mm, while agranulocytosis is their complete absence. The risk of infection rises markedly when the neutrophil count falls below 1,000 and is almost always present below 500. It is best to report absolute cell concentrations by multiplying total leukocyte count and percent of each type.

Neutropenia may be seen with a variety of infections (typhoid fever, brucellosis, tularemia, infectious mononucleosis, infectious hepatitis, measles and rickettsial diseases), folate and B_{12} deficiency, as an early sign of leukemia or aplastic anemia, as heritable or congenital forms that may be cyclic, and with collagen diseases and a large number of drugs. *Felty's syndrome* is splenomegaly with leukopenia, anemia, or thrombocytopenia, and is seen in 10-20% of patients with systemic lupus or rheumatoid arthritis; *Banti's syndrome* is leukopenia due to hypersplenism associated with portal hypertension.

Treatment begins with an exhaustive search for the cause. Patients with a neutrophil count below 500 should be hospitalized, since they may become infected with organisms from their own "normal flora." If infection is suspected, antibiotic coverage should be broad (generally combining a penicillin or cephalosporin with an aminoglycoside, chloramphenicol, or clindamycin if anaerobes are suspected, carbenicillin or ticarcillin for *Pseudomonas*). The choice of agents should be determined by not only the probable organs affected but also by factors that may have altered the normal flora, such as recent antibiotic therapy or hospitalization.

Leukocytosis and Leukemoid Reactions

Leukocytosis (WBC above 10,000 per cu mm) may be seen in response to infection or stress. A persistently elevated count above 25,000 in the absence of infection suggests a leukemoid reaction or leukemia.

Leukemoid reactions are excessive elevations of the white count in response to stimuli that usually produce a simple leukocytosis. Neutrophilic leukemoid reactions are also seen with certain hemolytic anemias and malignancies. Atypical, but not bizarre, cells may be seen in the bone marrow. The leukocyte alkaline phosphatase (LAP) is elevated, and the serum B_{12} is normal in neutrophil leukemoid reactions, whereas the LAP is normal and the B_{12} is elevated in granulocytic (myelocytic) leukemias.

Eosinophilic leukemoid reactions may be seen, particularly in parasitic infestation, but may occasionally be observed in drug allergy or connective tissue diseases (collagen vascular diseases). Eosinophilic leukemia is rare.

Lymphocytic leukemoid reactions may be seen in certain viral infections, particularly infectious mononucleosis, which may occasionally be mistaken for acute lymphocytic leukemia.

Monocytic leukemoid reactions are uncommon and are seen primarily in association with granulomatous diseases or early in the return of bone marrow activity following myelosuppressive chemotherapy.

Differentiation from the leukemias may require examination of the bone marrow. A vigorous search for the underlying cause is essential.

The Leukemias

Leukemia, a neoplastic proliferation of white cell precursors, is one of the myeloproliferative syndromes (Table 7-6). They are considered as acute or chronic, based on a constellation of the clinical presentation, pathologic examination of the peripheral blood and bone marrow, and prognosis. Patients with untreated leukemia have a median survival of 3 months if it is acute and 3-4 years if chronic. In addition, leukemias are generally considered as lymphocytic or myelocytic. The lymphocytic leukemias tend to respond better to treatment and have a less aggressive or stormy course.

The etiology of the leukemias remains unclear. RNA viruses may produce acute leukemias in animals and may even be incorporated into the host's genetic material, producing leukemia in progeny. An RNA-dependent DNA transcriptase is present in all human acute leukemic cells. Evidence for genetic factors is present in the acute leukemias and chronic lymphocytic leukemia. A higher incidence of acute leukemias is noted in multiple syndromes, including *Down's syndrome*, *Fanconi's anemia*, and the *Wiskott-Aldrich syndrome*. Only half of those with acute leukemia have an abnormal karyotype, which becomes normal as the disease is effectively treated. The Philadelphia chromosome (deletion of one of the short arms on chromosome 22) is seen as an acquired defect in 90% of patients with chronic myelogenous leukemia (CML) and less than 5% of those with acute myelogenous leukemia (AML). Ionizing irradiation and benzene may predispose to the development of the acute leukemias and chronic myelogenous leukemia. Immune deficiency may be associated with the development of leukemia.

In all the leukemias, an unregulated proliferation of one (occasionally multiple) cell line gradually develops—probably over several years. Unlike normal precursors, the leukemic cells are released from the bone marrow in various stages of development; often the more premature the cell released, the more aggressive the stage or state of the disease. These cells do not function normally, and since they do not tend to marginate or migrate into tissue, they remain in the circulation much longer than normal cells.

TABLE 7-6—MYELOPROLIFERATIVE SYNDROMES*

	Chronic Myelogenous Leukemia	Myeloid Metaplasia	Polycythemia Vera	Primary Thrombocytosis	Paroxysmal Nocturnal Hemoglobinuria
RED CELL COUNT					
ELEVATED			~100%		
NORMAL				Usually	
DECREASED	Usually slightly	~100%			Usually slightly
WHITE CELL COUNT					
100,000	25%				
ELEVATED	> 95%	Usually	> 50%		
NORMAL	< 5%	Occasionally	40%	Usually	Usually
DECREASED			< 20%		
PLATELET COUNT					
ELEVATED	40%	Often	> 50%	Always	
NORMAL	50%		< 50%		Usually
DECREASED	< 20%	Moderately			
SPLENOMEGALY	~100% (marked)	~100% (marked)	75% (moderate)	~100% (mild)	
HEPATOMEGALY	> 60%	50%	33%		
MARROW FIBROSIS	Mild in 25% at Dx; severe develops 30%	100%			

434

				→
PHILADELPHIA CHROMOSOME	90%			
LEUKOCYTE ALKALINE PHOSPHATASE	↓ 100%	↑ Most	↑ Most	
SERUM B$_{12}$ LEVELS	↑ Most		↑ > 30%	
B$_{12}$ BINDING CAPACITY	↑ Most		↑ < 70%	

* The myeloproliferative syndromes are a group of disorders linked by many similar or overlapping findings probably attributable to closely-linked stem cell abnormalities. Each is discussed separately. The table below gives the page number and the common findings.

Of the leukemias, about half are acute and half are chronic. The overall incidence of acute lymphoblastic leukemia (ALL) and AML are equal; however, in children, 80-90% of all acute leukemias are ALL, whereas in adults only 10-20% are ALL. The chronic leukemias are uncommon in persons less than 35-40 years of age. Chronic lymphocytic leukemia (CLL) is more common (3:2 to 2:1) than CML and after age 70 CLL is five times as common as CML. In children, the sex incidence of leukemias is about equal, but in adults, males are affected more often (3:2) than females. With all leukemias except ALL, the incidence rises with advancing age; the incidence of ALL peaks at ages 2-4 and rapidly falls to a nadir at 15-20, where it remains until the seventh or eighth decade, when it gradually begins to climb again. Leukemia accounts for over half of all childhood neoplasia.

The acute leukemias generally involve proliferation of the very early leukocyte precursors, whereas the chronic leukemias tend to represent proliferation of more mature precursors. In all the leukemias, diminished erythropoiesis and thrombopoiesis are usually noted; this may be due to replacement of the marrow by the leukemic cell line, elaboration of factors that inhibit normal marrow function, or even involvement of the pluripotential stem cell as the site of leukemogenesis. This third mechanism may account for the proliferation of several cell lines in some patients and certainly suggests a common mechanism for the widely varied types of myelogenous leukemia (erythroleukemia, myeloblastic, myelocytic, myelomonocytic, and monocytic).

Symptoms and signs are related to the *reduction in normal hematopoiesis* (erythropoiesis, thrombopoiesis, and leukopoiesis—granulopoiesis and lymphopoiesis), *lack of normal function* of the proliferative cell series (leading to elevations of the counts with increasing viscosity and reduction or absence of normal function), *increased activity of reticuloendothelial system* (clearing the abnormal cells) and *extramedullary hematopoiesis* (both leading to organomegaly, particularly splenomegaly and hepatomegaly), *and infiltration of the leukemic cells* (particularly the blastic cells) in tissues.

Leukocytosis, the "hallmark" of the disease, is not present in everyone with leukemia. One-third of patients with acute leukemia have a white count less than 10,000 per cu mm, 10-15% are over 100,000. Virtually all those with chronic leukemia have white counts above 20,000-30,000, although an occasional patient with CLL will have a normal or low white count; 25% of persons with CML have white counts above 100,000 per cu mm.

The vast majority of patients have abnormal cells in the circulation. In general, these cells comprise the bulk of the circulating white blood cells; normal white cells are absent or present in reduced amounts.

Blast cells are usually found in the circulation of patients with acute leukemia or the "blast phase" of chronic leukemias—particularly in CML in which the frequently preterminal blast phase (occurring in three-fourths) is virtually indistinguishable from AML. Myeloblasts comprise over 25% of the circulating white cells in AML, compared to less than 5% in CML. Lymphoblasts are generally observed in ALL. On Wright stain, myeloblasts may appear similar to lymphoblasts, however, myeloblasts are slightly larger and have more nucleoli; special staining techniques may demonstrate peroxidase-positive granules that are not noted in lymphoblasts. Auer rods, rod-like aggregates of azurophilic granules, are seen in 30-40% of the myeloblasts and promyelocytes of patients with AML.

Increased numbers of promyelocytes and nucleated red cells are generally noted in CML, and the absolute eosinophil and basophil counts are often elevated; an increase in the number of monocytes may be seen. CLL is always associated with a marked increase in the number of lymphocytes; some of these are large and atypical, and "smudge cells" are common.

Neutropenia or pancytopenia may be seen at the time of diagnosis in the myelocytic leukemias, giving rise to the terms preleukemia or aleukemic leukemia.

Anemia is present in most leukemias at the time of diagnosis and is generally mild. The mechanism is bone marrow replacement by leukemic cells in most. Some evidence of bone marrow fibrosis is noted in 25% of patients with CML at the time of diagnosis, and 20-35% will develop myelofibrosis. Twenty percent of patients with CLL develop a Coombs-positive hemolytic anemia during the course of their disease.

Thrombocytopenia of a mild degree is noted in most persons with acute leukemia, although occasionally the platelet count may be normal or even elevated. The platelet count in CLL is often normal at the time of diagnosis, but generally a mild thrombocytopenia ensues. Only 15% of patients with CML are thrombocytopenic; half of the rest (35-50%) have a thrombocytosis.

Twenty percent of patients with CML and up to half with CLL are asymptomatic at the time of diagnosis, with the diagnosis generally being made by noting an abnormal complete blood count. Malaise and easy fatigability are common with all the leukemias and may frequently be unrelated to the degree of anemia; weight loss is seen with chronic leukemia. Fever is common in all the leukemias (particularly the acute leukemias) and, although it may frequently represent a nonspecific expression of the disease process, it should always prompt an aggressive search for an underlying infection.

Infection is the major cause of death in patients with leukemia. Several factors may contribute to the increased incidence, including the degree of neutropenia and/or altered neutrophilic function, altered lymphocytic function with abnormal or decreased immunoglobulin production, and abnormal or reduced reticuloendothelial function. Chemotherapy may further compound these deficiencies, and hospitalization with its attendant invasion reduces natural barriers further and exposes patients to more resistant bacterial strains. Many of these patients are unable to localize neutrophils in an area of an infection, so not only will the classic signs of infection not necessarily be manifested but the infection may not be adequately held in check.

Extramedullary hematopoiesis may result in enlargement of the liver and spleen. Hepatomegaly is very common in the acute leukemias and in CLL; marked hepatomegaly is distinctly uncommon in CML, although a mild enlargement may occur in many. Splenomegaly occurs in over half of patients with AML and in virtually all with other leukemias; it may reach massive proportions in patients with CML. Pathologically, the lymph nodes in CLL are indistinguishable from those of well-differentiated lymphocytic lymphomas.

Arthralgias and bone pain are particularly common in children with acute leukemia and more common in association with ALL than AML.

Hyperuricemia is common in all leukemic patients because of the increased turnover of nucleoproteins; this is particularly evident following chemotherapy. Increased lactate dehydrogenase may also be noted because of increased cell turnover. In CML, the leukocyte alkaline phosphatase (LAP) is characteristically low despite the marked elevation of the white cells. In addition, the serum B_{12} is very elevated in CML due to increased production of the B_{12}-binding protein, transcobalamin I.

The leukemic cells may infiltrate tissues, producing inflammation, defective function of the invaded tissue, or silent lesions. CLL is particularly prone to do this and involves primarily the skin or gastrointestinal mucosa. When leukemic cells infiltrate the pulmonary parenchyma, the signs and radiographic appearance may be indistinguishable from a pneumonia; and antibiotic treatment should usually be instituted until a response occurs or a histologic diagnosis is made.

Infiltration of the CNS is particularly common in ALL, and half of untreated children develop leukemic meningitis.

Infiltration of the gingiva in AML (particularly acute monocytic and myelomonocytic leukemia) produces a characteristic bulging of the interdental papilla. In addition, acute monocytic leukemia may result in renal insufficiency, owing to renal tubular damage induced by a lysozyme released from the leukemic cells.

Acute promyelocytic leukemia may frequently be associated with disseminated intravascular coagulation (DIC) resulting from the release of thromboplastic substances from the leukemic cells.

Patients with CML who do not have the Philadelphia chromosome tend to have a more aggressive form of CML, which is less responsive to therapy.

The bone marrow must be examined in everyone in whom a diagnosis of leukemia is suspected. A needle biopsy must be obtained to avoid mistaking a "packed marrow" for a "dry tap," as might be seen in myelofibrosis. In the acute leukemias, the involved blast cells usually comprise more than 50% of the cellular elements in the bone marrow. In CML, more than 80%

of the marrow cells are mature granulocytic elements; megakaryocyte hyperplasia may be seen. Twenty-five percent of patients with CML have early marrow fibrosis when diagnosed. The bone marrow in early CLL has increased numbers of lymphocytes, which gradually replace the marrow as the course proceeds.

THERAPY
In general, the initial regimen chosen is that which is most likely *to induce remission.* The presence of initial remission and its duration before relapse are important determinants of survival, because subsequent remissions become successively more difficult to achieve. The older the patient, the less likely remission can be obtained, and often the more likely toxic or adverse responses to therapy will occur. For these reasons, a *consolidation cycle* is often added to the regimen early in the course of remission in an attempt to prolong the remission. Remission is usually noted when approximately 99.9% of the leukemic population is killed; unfortunately, the patient at the time of diagnosis has approximately 10^{12} leukemic cells and thus, even though a remission has occurred, as many as 10^9 leukemic cells remain, accounting for the tendency to relapse and the generally poor survival.

Chemotherapy of ALL will induce remissions in more than 90% of children and more than 75% of adults and improves median survival from 3 months if untreated to over 5 years in children and over 3 years in adults.

In AML, more than 60% will obtain a remission lasting about 1 year, and median survival is improved from 2 months if untreated to about 2 years.

CLL is such an indolent disease that chemotherapy may not be necessary. The average survival if untreated is about 6 years. Because CLL is a disease of the elderly, assessing the response (increased survival) to chemotherapy is difficult. Treatment is often reserved for symptomatic patients; 30-50% of these obtain a remission. Survival is probably somewhat improved in treated patients.

Chemotherapy of CML does not significantly improve survival from the $3\frac{1}{2}$ years noted in the untreated patient; however, quality of life is markedly improved. The median survival after the "blast phase" (which occurs in three-fourths of patients) is 2-3 months in untreated patients and improves with treatment in two-thirds of patients to 7-9 months.

Supportive and judicious use of blood products and antibiotics is essential to the management of leukemic patients, particularly after myelosuppressive chemotherapy. The nadir occurs in 2-5 days and lasts for about 10 days before a gradual recovery begins.

Radiotherapy will often improve symptomatic infiltrates, organomegaly, or lymphadenopathy. *Leukopheresis* may be necessary when the white blood count is extremely high because of the dangers of hyperviscosity and sludging.

Immune globulin administration may be required to assist in the control of infections in the hypogammaglobulinemic patient with CLL.

Besides myelo- and immunosuppressive effects, several chemotherapeutic agents have particularly notable adverse effects. Both bleomycin and busulfan are capable of producing similar syndromes of pulmonary fibrosis. The anthracycline antibiotics (adriamycin) may induce a dose-dependent cardiomyopathy. Cyclophosphamide may cause a hemorrhagic cystitis. The vinca alkaloids (vincristine and vinblastine) may produce neurotoxicity, manifested principally as a peripheral neuropathy, and are commonly associated with a thrombocytosis.

Plasma Cell Dyscrasias

The plasma cell dyscrasias are a group of disorders characterized by the abnormal proliferation of a single clone of plasma cells, which produces excess amounts of an abnormal protein. These include (1) multiple myeloma (immunoglobulin G, A, D, or E), (2) Waldenström's macroglobulinemia (immunoglobulin M), (3) heavy-chain disease (alpha, delta, epsilon, gamma, or mu), (4) light chain disease (kappa or lambda), and (5) nonsecretory myeloma (none).

Benign monoclonal gammopathy is a monoclonal paraprotein without plasma cell proliferation. Patients tend to be older, usually have less than 3 gm/day of paraprotein, and have no anemia, bone lesions, or proteinuria. Levels of other immuno-globulins remain normal.

The etiology of each of these is unknown, although antibodies to certain infectious agents (streptococcus and pneumococcus) have been found in some myeloma patients. The etiologic implications of these findings are not clear. Polyclonal gammopathies occur in chronic infections, granulomatous diseases, chronic liver disease, and collagen vascular diseases. Rarely, monoclonal paraproteinemia is associated with carcinoma, leukemia, or polycythemia vera.

MULTIPLE MYELOMA

Multiple myeloma is characterized by bone marrow plasmacyto-sis (more than 15% of the cellularity) and production of a monoclonal paraprotein (IgG in 52%, IgA in 25%) with or without excessive production of light chains (Bence-Jones protein). The peak incidence occurs at the age of 50. As the plasma cells proliferate, they produce *osteoclast activating factor* (OAF), which results in bone resorption. The early lesion is diffuse or regional osteoporosis. Clinical symptoms occur late in the long course of the disease. Osteolytic ("punched out") lesions may be seen in the skull, vertebrae, or pelvis. Painful pathologic fractures of the ribs or vertebrae may occur. Common nonspecific symptoms and findings often include malaise, anemia, or an increased sedimentation rate (ESR). Marked hypercalcemia may be noted.

Stimulation of suppressor cells by the malignant clone leads to inhibition of normal immunoglobulin production, and recurrent infections occur. Patients with Bence-Jones proteinuria develop renal tubular damage from direct toxicity and tubular obstruction, leading to chronic renal insufficiency, the nephrotic syndrome, and occasional progression to chronic renal failure.

When the paraproteinemia is marked, patients develop symptoms of hyperviscosity with its resultant decreased blood flow, sludging, venous engorgement, and diffuse capillary hemorrhages. Symptoms are initially nonspecific (malaise) and progress with developing confusion to frank psychosis, vertigo and tinnitus, congestive heart failure, and peripheral tissue hypoxia.

Tissue deposition of the paraprotein results in amyloidosis in approximately 20%.

Diagnosis rests on finding bone marrow plasmacytosis and a monoclonal paraprotein (M-spike) in the serum (80%) or urine (40%); 98% have the protein in either serum or urine. Rarely, patients with end-stage disease may have diffuse hypogamma-globulinemia with no paraproteinemia.

Treatment with alkylating agents (cyclophosphamide or melphalan) and steroids improves median survival from less than 1 year to more than 4 years. Radiotherapy is useful for localized or symptomatic bone lesions. Hyperuricemia and hypercalcemia should be treated. Symptomatic hyperviscosity may be relieved by plasmapheresis. Renal insufficiency should be treated by avoidance of any degree of dehydration to prevent further tubular precipitation of proteins. Intravenous pyelograms should be avoided.

WALDENSTRÖM'S MACROGLOBULINEMIA

Waldenström's macroglobulinemia is characterized by a macro-globulin (IgM) paraprotein "spike" on serum protein electropho-resis associated with bone marrow proliferation of plasmacytoid lymphocytes. This disorder is seen in older people, and ranges from a slowly progressive form to a widely disseminated lympho-cytic proliferation such as lymphocytic lymphoma or lymphocytic leukemia. In contrast to multiple myeloma, bone lesions are uncommon, and lymphadenopathy, splenomegaly, and hypervis-cosity are common. Other nonspecific phenomena are similar. Tissue biopsy may suggest lymphosarcoma. Choice of treatment depends on the aggressiveness of the disease and varies from no treatment for the benign form to chemotherapy (similar to that used for CLL) for the aggressive form. Symptomatic hyperviscos-ity should be managed with plasmapheresis.

HEAVY CHAIN DISEASE

Heavy chain disease is a distinctly uncommon disorder character-ized by heavy chains of immunoglobulin in serum or urine. Alpha, gamma, and mu chains have been identified in order of decreasing frequency associated with plasma cell proliferation. In alpha heavy chain disease, the proliferation occurs principally in the gastrointestinal tract (Mediterranean lymphoma), resulting in malabsorption and abdominal pain but rarely involves the respi-ratory tract. Gamma heavy chain disease is associated with

recurrent infections, lymphadenopathy (particularly of Wal-
deyer's ring), and hepatosplenomegaly. Mu heavy chain disease
is extremely uncommon and seen in association with chronic
lymphocytic lymphoma.

LIGHT CHAIN DISEASE
Light chain disease may involve either kappa (κ) or lambda (λ)
light chains, appears to be a benign disorder, and is detected by
finding a light chain "spike" on urine (rarely serum) protein
electrophoresis (isolated Bence-Jones proteinuria).

Lymphomas
Lymphocytic leukemia, myeloma, and lymphoma appear to be
caused by excessive production of either T or B lymphocytes.
Ebstein-Barr virus infects B lymphocytes, producing *infectious
mononucleosis* with its characteristic atypical lymphocyte in the
peripheral smear. Failure of T cells to inhibit growth of B cells
may explain the development of *Burkitt's lymphoma*, a neoplastic
lymphoid lesion following Ebstein-Barr infection. *Immunoblastic
lymphadenopathy* (fever, rash, anemia, lymphadenopathy, polyclonal hyperglobulinemia, and Coombs-positive hemolytic anemia) is presently considered to be a non-neoplastic hyperfunction
of the B cell system related to loss of suppressor T-cell control.

Non-Hodgkin's lymphomas are classified into nodular or
diffuse and lymphocytic or histiocytic types. Most are B-cell
proliferations, but T-cell variants have been described. Sezary
syndrome, for example, is a variant of *Mycosis fungoides* with
skin lesions and infiltration of blood and marrow with primitive
T-lymphocytes. Nodular and well-differentiated lymphomas have
the best response to treatment; diffuse histiocytic lymphoma has
been associated with complete remission in about half and the
possibility of "cure" in 40%. Hodgkin's disease accounts for 40%
of all lymphomas and has its peak incidence between 15 and 34.
A second, but lower, peak occurs after the age of 60. The non-
Hodgkin's lymphomas are uncommon below age 40, and the
incidence increases progressively with advancing age.

Presenting symptoms often begin with an enlarging painless
mass in one of the lymph node regions. Local pain or impingement on neurovascular structures may occur. Associated symp-

toms may include fever, night sweats, malaise, weight loss, and pruritus, and are often the first signs of the disease. Intermittent daily fever, which remits to recur days to weeks later, known as the Pel-Ebstein fever, once thought to be a classic symptom of Hodgkin's disease, is actually quite uncommon.

A mild normochromic, normocytic anemia of chronic disease is frequently present. Coomb-positive hemolytic anemia is uncommon. Bone marrow involvement is difficult to assess because of its focal nature. Leukocytosis is common, and leukemoid reactions may suggest leukemia. The leukocyte alkaline phosphatase is elevated. Eosinophilia may occur.

Despite the common anergy to skin tests for delayed hypersensitivity, infections are not more common unless the disease is uncontrolled or resistance has been decreased as a result of therapeutic intervention.

Diagnosis rests on histologic examination; staging is based on extent of disease. Hepatic, splenic, and retroperitoneal involvement may be clinically silent and occur without other evidence of disease. Computed tomography is essential for accurate staging.

For all lymphomas, stage I is disease localized to one group of lymph nodes, stage II for two groups on the same side of the diaphragm, stage III for nodal involvement on both sides of the diaphragm, and stage IV for diffuse disease with one or more extralymphatic organs involved. For the purposes of staging, the spleen is considered as a single lymph node region and the liver is extralymphatic. The suffix A indicates no symptoms, and B indicates systemic symptoms.

The MOPP combination chemotherapy (mechlorethamine, vincristine, prednisone, and procarbazine) alone or with radiation therapy has remarkably extended life expectancy, and many remissions have lasted for more than 10 years. Problems include reduction of rate of relapse, risk of infection due to T-cell lymphocytopenia and B-cell lymphocytosis, and development of acute myelogenous leukemia.

DISORDERS OF HEMOSTASIS
The formation of a platelet plug and the development of a fibrin clot are complementary processes, sometimes known as primary

and secondary hemostasis. Close interrelation of parallel steps permits positive feedback or amplification so that a relatively minor initial stress can produce significant blood coagulation. Vascular injury, activated Hageman factor (factor XII), or epinephrine lead to platelet adherence and aggregation. A small amount of adenosine diphosphate is released, promoting additional aggregation and release of additional ADP, serotonin, platelet phospholipid for platelet factor 3, and thromboxane A_2. Thromboxane A_2 produced by the action of a specific prostaglandin synthetase acting on an endoperoxide (which was produced by the action of cyclooxygenase on arachidonic acid), promotes hemostasis by its intense vasoconstrictor activity and also enhances additional platelet aggregation. Platelets interact with the coagulation cascade by providing binding sites for factors V, VIII, and X_a, by activating factor XI, and by secreting calcium.

Coagulation normally proceeds via one of two pathways (Fig. 7-3), through several sequential steps, ending in the production of a stable fibrin polymer. With the exception of factors III (tissue thromboplastin) and IV (calcium), coagulation factors circulate in an inactive, or procoagulant, form.

Although more complex than is usually presented, the coagulation cascade may be evoked by activation of factor XII (intrinsic pathway) or factor VII (extrinsic pathway). Contact with collagen or foreign surfaces activates factor XII, which in the presence of necessary cofactors sequentially results in activation of XI, IX, VIII, and X. Activated factor X results in completion of the final common pathway with activation of V then II (prothrombin to thrombin) and finally I (fibrinogen to fibrin monomer). Factor XIII allows stabilization of fibrin to occur through polymerization. The extrinsic pathway is activated when factor VII is activated by tissue phospholipid substances known as thromboplastins. Activated factor VII activates factor X, and the ensuing steps are the same as for the intrinsic system. The overall activity of the intrinsic system is tested by measuring the whole blood clotting time or the partial thromboplastin time (PTT). The prothrombin time (protime or PT) measures the activity in the extrinsic system. Defects in the final common pathway will prolong tests of both systems and may be further

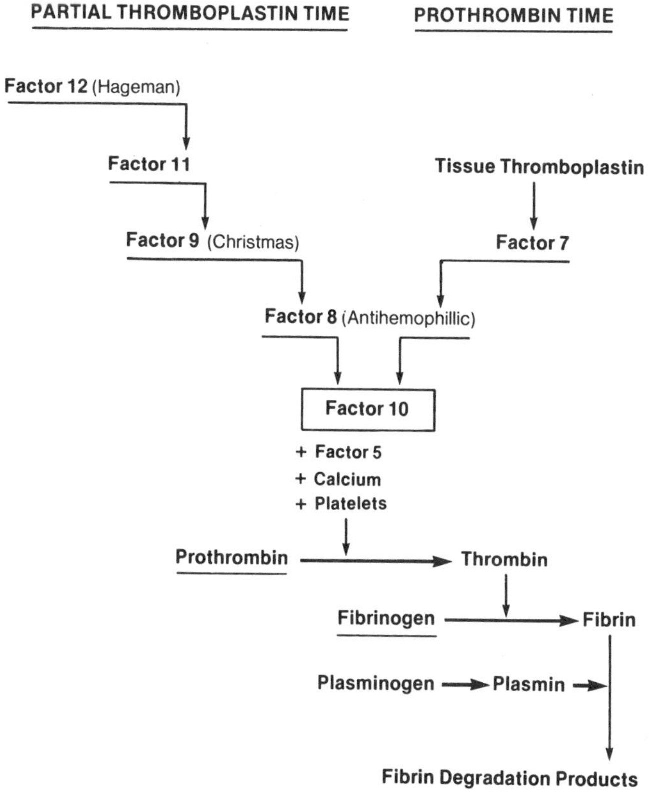

PARTIAL THROMBOPLASTIN TIME   PROTHROMBIN TIME

Figure 7-3. Present understanding of the coagulation sequence includes an intrinsic pathway (left) and an extrinsic or tissue pathway (right) leading to the generation of Factor 10. Factor 8, Factor 5, calcium, platelets, and prothrombin are consumed in the clotting reaction. Fibrin is degraded to its degradation products by plasmin.

evaluated by measuring the thrombin time (TT), which measures the polymerization of fibrinogen when exogenous thrombin is added.

All factors except VIII are synthesized in the liver. Factor VIII is produced by endothelial cells. Synthesis of factors II, VII, IX, and X in the liver depend on vitamin K as a cofactor. The half-lives of the various protein factors range from 5 hours to 5 days.

Excessive or uncontrolled coagulation is prevented by the fibrinolytic system. Plasminogen is an inactive protein, which circulates in plasma and may be deposited during coagulation. A number of factors, including endogenous activated factor XII and exogenous urokinase or streptokinase, may activate plasminogen to plasmin (fibrinolysin). Plasmin proteolytically degrades fibrinogen and fibrin to their respective degradation products.

Thrombocytopenia

Thrombocytopenia is a reduction in the number of platelets below the normal range of 200,000 per cu mm. Bleeding may occur only after trauma with mild thrombocytopenia; but with more severe reductions in the platelet count, spontaneous bleeding from mucosal membranes and the skin are common. The skin lesions may range from petechiae (seen also with increased capillary fragility) to ecchymoses.

The degree of bleeding depends also on platelet function. Younger platelets have a greater potential for adhesion and aggregation, so that the incidence and degree of bleeding is not a linear relationship with reduction of the platelet count. Thrombocytopenias in which a large portion of circulating platelets are young tend to have less bleeding; acute thrombocytopenia has a greater risk of producing bleeding than chronic thrombocytopenia at the same level. In general, unless a qualitative defect is present, an increased bleeding tendency is usually not noted until the platelet count falls below 50,000. Platelet counts below 20,000 are commonly associated with spontaneous bleeding.

Decreased production of platelets may be noted with marrow failure (aplastic anemia) or myelofibrosis. Folate and B_{12} deficiencies may be associated with an ineffective thrombopoiesis in which the megakaryocytes appear normal or increased in number but maturation is incomplete. Certain cases of isolated thrombocytopenia with decreased megakaryocytes may be due to a deficiency of a thrombopoietin.

Thrombocytopenias caused by increased destruction may be immunologic (with intravascular destruction or more commonly splenic phagocytosis of the coated platelet) or nonimmunologic (as mechanical injury, increased utilization, blood loss, and dilution).

Thrombocytopenias due to autoimmune phenomena include idiopathic thrombocytopenic purpura (ITP), the thrombocyto-\enia seen in 10-20% of patients with SLE, posttransfusion urpura, that seen with Coomb-positive hemolytic anemia (Evan's syndrome), in some with lymphoma or chronic lymphocytic leukemia, and in some following certain viral infections (particularly rubella and infectious mononucleosis). In each of these, the primary means of destruction appears to be antibody coating of the platelet followed by reticuloendothelial uptake and destruction, particularly in the spleen.

Idiopathic thrombocytopenic purpura. Autoimmune thrombocytopenic purpura, ITP is the most common of the autoimmune thrombocytopenias. Some patients (particularly children) have had a recent viral infection; however, in general the pathogenesis remains obscure. Although antibodies to platelets are probably present in all patients, they are demonstrable in only 65%. The antibodies are IgG and do not fix complement. Acute ITP, clearing in several weeks, is seen in children; a chronic form of varying severity is seen in young adults (female/male incidence 3-4:1). Diagnosis is generally made by exclusion; a careful drug history is essential.

Lymphadenopathy is not present, and splenomegaly is seen in less than 10% of cases with acute ITP. The bone marrow is unremarkable at the outset, but the megakaryocytes become hyperplastic as the disease continues.

The treatment for the acute phase is primarily supportive. Platelets should be transfused only if the patient is hemorrhaging. Adrenal corticosteroids (0.5-20 mg/kg/day of prednisone) should be used during the acute phase in an attempt to reduce capillary fragility. The platelet count may rise slightly but often does not, and the duration of the thrombocytopenia is not reduced.

Thrombocytopenia persisting longer than 6 months is considered chronic ITP, although patients with thrombocytopenia persisting longer than 4 weeks tend to have a similar prognosis and require similar treatment. Fifteen to 20% of children and most adults with acute ITP develop chronic ITP. Corticosteroids will improve the platelet count in most, although in some the dose required may be toxic.

Exchange transfusions to remove antibodies and replace platelets as well as plasmapheresis to remove immunoglobulin have been beneficial.

Splenectomy should be performed in patients with recurrent or life-threatening hemorrhage unresponsive to repeated platelet transfusion, persistent thrombocytopenia despite adequate steroid therapy, or control requiring toxic doses of corticosteroids. Seventy to 80% of patients will be controlled after splenectomy.

Symptomatic patients unresponsive to splenectomy should receive immunosuppressive therapy with vincristine, azathioprine, or cyclophosphamide. The alkaloids (vincristine and vinblastine) are also associated with an increase in the numbers of megakaryocytes in the bone marrow; other potential mechanisms remain unresolved.

Posttransfusion purpura. This occurs as a result of alloantibody formation in patients following blood or platelet transfusion. It is an uncommon reaction, seen only in patients lacking the PL^{A1} antigen, which is absent in 2% of the normal population. The thrombocytopenia usually occurs several days following transfusion and may be severe. *Neonatal purpura* is a similar phenomenon occurring after transplacental isosensitization of the mother with this or other platelet antigens and transplacental passage of the maternal immunoglobin back to the fetus. See Index for drugs causing thrombocytopenia and page 423 for mechanism.

Nonimmune thrombocytopenia. This results from prosthetic heart valves; *hemangiomas* may produce platelet damage from similar turbulence and shearing. *Viruses* may directly damage platelets, and bacteria may elaborate toxins that injure platelets. In these states, platelet survival may be shortened, but production is usually compensatorily increased and thus thrombocytopenia may be mild or absent.

In *disseminated intravascular coagulation* (DIC), large quantities of platelets aggregate under the stimulus of thrombin.

Microangiopathic processes, particularly when associated with intravascular deposition of fibrin strands, leads to shearing of platelets in addition to deposition of platelets during the process of fibrin formation. The *hemolytic-uremic syndrome* (HUS or Gasser syndrome of microangiopathic hemolytic anemia, thrombocytopenia, and renal failure) and *thrombotic thrombocytopenic purpura* (TTP; microangiopathic hemolytic anemia, thrombocytopenia, and CNS deterioration occasionally with renal disease and fever) are both associated with intravascular deposition of fibrin—HUS is limited to the kidney, but TTP is diffuse. HUS is seen primarily in infants and young children. Both are medical emergencies, and an effective treatment is still unknown. Steroids, heparin, and platelet antiaggregants have been tried, each with a variable degree of success.

Mild thrombocytopenia (50,000-200,000/cu mm) may be found when splenomegaly occurs. In this state, sequestration or pooling of platelets occurs without active destruction. Patients are usually asymptomatic, but if hemorrhage is a problem, splenectomy is indicated (see Banti's and Felty's syndrome, page 431).

Functional Defects of Platelets

Rare disorders of platelet function occur in which platelet numbers may be normal but function is markedly impaired. The disorder must be suspected when a patient presents with a bleeding tendency and is found to have a normal platelet count and tests of the soluble coagulation system. In this disorder, the bleeding time will be prolonged and clot retraction delayed. Aspirin, nonsteroidal antiinflammatory agents, and other drugs may produce bleeding in certain patients by interfering with platelet aggregation.

The "antiaggregant effect" of various agents is the most common functional defect encountered and is discussed in the section on drug-induced blood dyscrasias.

The *Bernard-Soullier syndrome* is a defect in platelet adhesion associated with the presence of bizarre giant platelets. In *von-Willebrand's disease,* there seems to be an absence of serum protein factor necessary for adhesion.

Thrombasthenia (Glanzmann's disease) is a congenital defect in aggregation. *Thrombopathia* is a more common disorder with mild dysfunction of platelets.

Abnormal platelet function may be seen frequently in uremia, myeloproliferative syndromes, and cirrhosis. Other disorders in which abnormalities of platelet function have been reported include several disorders of connective tissue such as osteogenesis imperfecta and Ehlers-Danlos syndrome as well as the Wiskott-Aldrich syndrome.

Thrombocytosis

Thrombocytosis or thrombocythemia is an elevation of the platelet count above 400,000/cu mm. Increased platelet production occurs as a secondary phenomenon in many conditions, including after splenectomy, after stress such as exercise or surgery, in association with severe anemia or iron deficiency, and in some chronic inflammatory states. In addition, it may be associated with carcinoma and the lymphomas.

Essential or primary thrombocythemia is a myeloproliferative disorder in which the platelet count often exceeds 1,000,000. It may precede, follow, or be associated with the other myeloproliferative disorders. The platelets are functionally defective, and bleeding phenomena are common. Thrombotic events may occur. Splenomegaly is almost always found. Treatment includes myelosuppressive agents (particularly busulfan). Heparin may be required during acute thrombotic episodes, and agents that inhibit platelet function may prevent thromboses from occurring.

Vascular Defects in Hemostasis

Bleeding due to defective vessel wall integrity may generally be considered due to defective vascular connective tissue, inflammation of the microvasculature (vasculitis), or ischemia. These broad groups overlap in many disorders; in each bleeding is particularly common from mucous membranes. Skin lesions include petechiae and purpura.

The hereditary connective tissue disorders causing purpura include osteogenesis imperfecta, Ehlers-Danlos syndrome, pseudoxanthoma elasticum, and Morton syndrome. The first three are also associated with defective platelet function. Scurvy (or vitamin C deficiency) and Cushing's syndrome are associated with a not-well-characterized defect in vascular integrity (remember also that steroids in lower doses may protect vascular integrity in certain conditions). Senile purpura is common and probably due to the age-related loss of supporting collagen (of uncertain etiology) and elastic tissues.

Hereditary hemorrhagic telangiectasia (Osler-Weber-Rendu disease) is an autosomal dominant disorder with thin vascular membranes resulting in aneurysms, telangiectasias, and friability. These lesions may produce bleeding from the skin, mucous membranes, lung, and kidney. Up to one-fourth of patients have associated pulmonary arteriovenous fistulas. Active inflammation of the microvasculature (vasculitis) may produce petechiae. Generally, bleeding is much less of a problem than the vascular obstruction. Henoch-Schönlein syndrome (allergic vasculitis, hypersensitivity angiitis, or anaphylactoid purpura) is a hypersensitivity reaction. The disease may affect the small blood vessels of the skin, mucous membranes, and other organs, leading to symptoms of diffuse inflammation including arthralgias, abdominal pain, and in half hematuria (glomerulonephritis); 10% of patients with renal involvement may develop chronic nephritis. Patients with immune vasculitis often benefit from treatment with steroids.

Multiple abnormalities including microvascular defects may be associated with bacteremia (including meningococcemia and gonococcemia), viremia, and circulating endotoxin. The petechial lesions seen in infective endocarditis are probably an immune complex vasculitis as well as an occlusive phenomena from microemboli leading to distal ischemia and increased capillary friability.

Generalized or localized tissue ischemia may result in dimin-

ished capillary integrity and petechial bleeding. It is this phenomenon that is postulated also as a part of the cause of "stress
gastritis." The dysproteinemias such as cryoglobulinemia and
multiple myeloma are often associated with increased viscosity
which may result in capillary ischemia and friability; these
syndromes may also be associated with defective platelet function
attributed to a coating of the platelets by the protein.

INHERITED ABNORMALITIES OF COAGULATION: HEMOPHILIA

Classic hemophilia (or hemophilia A.) This results from the sex-
linked inheritance of reduced or absent activity of factor VIII
(antihemophilic factor). It is the most common of the congenital
disorders of coagulation. Female carriers (heterozygotes) usually
have normal factor VIII coagulant activity. Sporadic occurrences
are relatively frequent. The defect in the intrinsic pathway is
proportionate to the degree of deficiency. Spontaneous bleeding
is uncommon except in severe deficiency. Platelet plugs are
normally formed but not stabilized by fibrin, so that as the
platelet plug is dissolved (hours or days later) bleeding begins.
Minor trauma may result in ecchymoses, muscular hematomas,
or painful hemarthroses. The diagnosis is suspected early in life
and confirmed by finding very low factor VIII procoagulant
activity, usually with normal antigenic activity. The whole blood
clotting time and the PTT are abnormally prolonged, whereas
platelet function and count, PT, thrombin time, and levels of
other factors are all normal. Treatment of bleeding should utilize
factor VIII concentrates, although plasma may be necessary in
emergencies when the concentrate is not available. Infusion of 40
units/kg followed by 20 u/kg every 8 hours for 4-6 doses will
usually produce satisfactory results. The factor VIII procoagulant
activity should be measured and followed when available. Spontaneous bleeding should cease when the level is above 5% and
levels above 25% protect against bleeding from all except major
trauma. For surgery, the level should be maintained above 50%.
No response to therapy or a paradoxical fall in activity may be
the first sign of development of antibodies to factor VIII.
Concurrent administration of cytotoxic agents and factor VIII to

destroy proliferating clones of immunoglobulin-producing cells has brought some success in the 5% of patients in whom this complication occurs.

Von Willebrand's disease. This disorder, transmitted as an autosomal dominant, has three associated defects. The factor VIII coagulant activity is moderately reduced to 30-40%, platelet aggregation in vitro with ristocetin is defective, and factor VIII antigenic activity is reduced (unlike classic hemophilia). Infusion of plasma from a patient with classic hemophilia corrects the abnormalities of patients with vonWillebrand's disease. Treatment of bleeding is with factor VIII concentrate, although in emergencies plasma will be of benefit.

Factor IX deficiency. This disorder, also known as hemophilia B or Christmas factor deficiency, results from sex-linked inheritance of reduced or absent factor IX activity. Clinical manifestations and laboratory abnormalities are identical to classic hemophilia, except factor VIII levels are normal and factor IX is reduced. Treatment is with factor IX concentrate.

Other congenital factor deficiencies. Deficiencies of other factors are uncommon and often mild or asymptomatic. Factor XI deficiency is inherited as an autosomal dominant and, when necessary, is treated with fresh frozen plasma. Factor XII (Hageman factor) deficiency is usually asymptomatic. Factor XIII deficiency is inherited either as an autosomal dominant or a sex-linked trait; symptoms include a moderate bleeding tendency and excessive scar tissue (keloid) formation. Treatment of bleeding is with fresh frozen plasma.

ACQUIRED ABNORMALITIES OF COAGULATION: VITAMIN K DEFICIENCY

The hepatic synthesis of factors II, VII, IX, and X depend on the cofactor role of vitamin K, a fat-soluble essential vitamin. The plasma half-life of these factors ranges from 5 hours for factor VII to 60 hours for factor II (prothrombin). Vitamin K is derived from green leafy vegetables as well as synthesis by the normal intestinal bacterial flora. Reduction in either of these sources may lead to vitamin K deficiency in 10-20 days. Bleeding phenomena similar to those found are noted with hemophilia. The PT is prolonged and reverts to normal several hours following parenteral vitamin K (preferably K_1) administration.

Hepatic disease. Any combination of diminished production of procoagulants, increased plasma proteolytic activity, and mild chronic intravascular coagulation may be noted in acute or chronic liver disease and combine to reduce all factor levels except VIII and result in mild to moderate bleeding. Hemorrhage may be managed with fresh frozen plasma. When intravascular coagulation is a major factor, some improvement may result from heparin infusion (see DIC). Ultimately, prognosis depends on the underlying hepatic disorder.

Anticoagulants. Circulating anticoagulants are immunoglobulins developed against coagulation factors. Any factor can be involved, but the most common is factor VIII. Such antibodies may either develop in patients with congenital deficiency who receive repeated administration of the necessary factor or spontaneously, particularly in association with autoimmune disorders such as SLE (then called the lupus anticoagulant).

Oral anticoagulants such as warfarin and dicumarol competitively inhibit the actions of vitamin K, thus diminishing hemostasis. Hemorrhage may be managed by giving high doses of vitamin K_1 as well as fresh frozen plasma or factor IX concentrate (which is rich in factors II, VII, and X also).

Heparin inhibits coagulation by activating antithrombin III, which combines with (and thus inactivates) factors IX, X, XI, and XII. Its action may be acutely reversed by administering protamine sulfate, which neutralizes heparin, milligram for milligram, by complexing with it.

Urokinase and streptokinase activate plasminogen to plasmin by a proteolytic mechanism. Hemorrhage may be treated by administering epsilon-aminocaproic acid, an inhibitor of plasmin.

Disseminated intravascular coagulation (DIC). DIC results from intravascular activation of the soluble coagulation cascade by products released from cellular or tissue injury. Either or both intrinsic and extrinsic pathways may be activated. Thrombin formed in the process may proteolytically cleave fragments from fibrin and fibrinogen, in addition to the actions of plasmin. These fragments are termed fibrin degradation products (FDP). FDP inhibits both fibrin polymerization and, when deposited, results in a weal and an abnormal fibrin clot. That the action of thrombin is central to the disorder is suggested but not certain. As DIC proceeds, levels of factors V and VIII as well as fibrinogen fall, FDP rises, platelets are consumed, and the prothrombin test is prolonged. These laboratory abnormalities are indices by which the diagnosis is made and the course is followed. Evidence for a central role for thrombin derives from the response to heparin administration. Although the cornerstone of therapy is correction of the underlying disturbance, response may be obtained by administering 5000-7500 units of heparin every 6 hours by intermittent bolus or continuous infusion. With the disordered coagulation profile, monitoring therapy becomes empiric, but gradually the low factor and platelet levels should rise. Acute hemorrhage may respond to plasma administration; however, more FDP will be created, potentially "feeding the fire" and worsening the condition of the patient.

Administration of Blood and Blood Products

Selective therapy with specific blood products, when feasible, is preferable to the use of whole blood. Whole blood carries the risk of volume expansion as well as exposure to various antigens, including the hepatitis virus. The use of whole blood should be limited to uncontrollable acute blood loss. A-B-O and Rh blood group typing and matching should be performed when possible. In emergencies unmatched O-negative whole blood may be used with little risk of incompatibility until cross-matching is completed.

Whole blood and red cells are collected and preserved in an acidic buffer, acid-citrate-dextrose (ACD) or citrate-phosphate-dextrose (CPD), which extends the red cell storage life to 70-75% at 3 weeks, slightly longer with CPD than ACD. Red cell concentrations frozen in glycerol remain viable for years, and such preparation and storage removes many antigens, isoantibodies, and viral contaminants.

Massive transfusion results in administration of acid from the buffer and necessitates therapy with 45 mEq of sodium bicarbonate for every five units of blood administered. In addition, the citrate in the buffer may complex with the patient's serum calcium, and supplementation may be necessary to prevent hypocalcemia. Blood warmers should be used to prevent hypothermia when massive transfusions are given. Supplemental oxygen administration may be necessary because 2,3-DPG is rapidly depleted during storage, resulting in enhanced affinity of hemoglobin for oxygen and resultant decreased delivery to the tissues.

Platelets, granulocytes, and procoagulants have relatively short half-lives during storage. When blood over 1 day old is administered, supplementation with platelets or coagulation cofactors may be necessary to control bleeding and may be accomplished by administering platelet concentrates and fresh frozen plasma.

Leukocyte-poor red cells can be prepared for administration to patients who have been previously sensitized. These leukoagglutinins may cause febrile reactions, which are averted by using leukocyte-poor preparations. Any patient who receives organ transplantation should receive only this type of blood to avoid cross-sensitization.

Granulocytes prepared by leukopheresis from single donors may sustain life in the infected granulocytopenic patient. These white cells survive only several hours after transfusion, and daily administration may be necessary. A close relative with good HLA matching is preferable as the source. Guidelines for granulocyte use are not uniformly accepted, but most agree that the candidate most likely to benefit is the granulocytopenic patient with proven sepsis poorly responsive to antibiotics for 24 or 48 hours.

Platelet concentrates may be viably stored for up to 48 hours, and after administration are effective for 3-5 days. One unit is the amount of platelets obtained from a unit (500 cc) of whole blood. Ten units should raise the platelet count by 20,000-50,000. Spontaneous hemorrhage is common with platelet counts below 10,000 and rare when the count is above 50,000 unless a concomitant disturbance of platelet function is also present. Exogenous platelets may be rapidly consumed in patients with antibodies (such as seen in ITP and SLE) and thus be ineffective.

Albumin is available in a purified preparation in 5% and 25% solutions. It is heat sterilized and free of antigenicity. It is used to provide colloid support of the vasculature, particularly in conditions of acute or subacute plasma or protein loss. Salt-poor albumin is also available when excess sodium administration is to be avoided.

Clotting factors, except for factors V, VIII, and XI, remain stable in refrigerated whole blood or plasma for up to 3 weeks. Factors V, VIII, and XI, when refrigerated, each have a half-life of approximately 1 week. Fresh frozen plasma or concentrates remain stable for over a year. Pooled concentrates, for use with specific deficiencies, carry a high risk of hepatitis. Factor IX concentrate is also rich in factors II, VII, and X.

Pooled immune globulin, collected by plasmapheresis, may be given intramuscularly but not intravenously. Hyperimmune globulins, collected from donors with high concentrations of selected antibodies, are available for Rh(D) antigen and the hepatitis B virus.

Immediate transfusion reactions may be immune-destructive, allergic, febrile (from pyrogens such as leukoagglutin in reactions), contaminant-related (such as bacterial products) or circulatory overload. The typical immune destructive reaction is a hemolytic anemia, but platelets or white cells may be similarly involved. The reaction usually results from antigen exposure in patients with isoantibodies or prior sensitization and is characterized by chills, fever, back pain, and oozing from wounds. Hemoglobinemia and hemoglobinuria may result in acute renal failure. If suspected, DIC should also be evaluated. Treatment should include establishment and maintenance of brisk diuresis with fluid administration and osmotic or loop diuretics.

Allergic responses to antigenic material may include slight fever and rash. These reactions are relatively common and usually not serious. Subcutaneous epinephrine may be administered when necessary. Anaphylaxis is uncommon and acute in onset. This is of particular concern in the infrequent patient with deficient or absent IgA. Manifestations include chest pain, shortness of breath, and hypotension with diaphoresis and cyanosis. Immediate treatment with epinephrine, corticosteroids, and vasopressors is advised.

Febrile reactions develop secondary to pyrogen contaminants or to leukoagglutinin reactions in patients with multiple prior transfusions who become sensitized to specific white cell antigens. Pulmonary infiltrates may transiently appear.

Contaminants such as bacterial endotoxins may evoke immediate reactions seen in patients with gram-negative sepsis such as fever and chills, hypotension, and even DIC. Cultures of donor and patient blood should be obtained to evaluate whether viable organisms are present. Treatment of shock and DIC is as outlined, and appropriate antibiotics may be indicated.

Circulatory overload from excessive volume administration may be minimized by selective use of blood products and should be treated with diuretics and, when indicated, cardiac glycosides.

Later immune destruction may occur in days to weeks secondary to a rise in immune globulin directed against an administered antigen. A Coombs-positive hemolytic anemia or immune thrombocytopenia may develop. Immune thrombocytopenia is particularly common in patients, primarily women, who lack the PI^{A1} antigen and have isoantibodies to it. The degree of the reaction is proportionate to the number of cells transfused, the degree of host immune reactivity, and the extent of cross-reactivity to the host's own cells. Generally the reactions are self-limited.

Late infectious complications of transfusion include posttransfusion hepatitis caused principally by non-A, non-B hepatitis virus. Hepatitis B surface antigen (HBsAg or HAA) screening of donors removes some of the risk of this type of hepatitis; however, commercial unscreened blood, massive transfusion, and use of pooled blood products carry an increased risk of hepatitis. Malaria and syphilis may be transferred by transfusion, and the post-pump syndrome (PPS) occasionally occurs after massive transfusion of fresh whole blood. PPS manifests as fever, lymphadenopathy, hepatosplenomegaly, diffuse maculopapular rash, and atypical lymphocytes in the blood, all very similar to infectious mononucleosis but generally caused by cytomegalovirus infection.

REFERENCES

Anemias

Jacobs A, Wormwood M: Ferritin in serum: clinical and biochemical implications. N Engl J Med 292:951, 1975.

Kagan WA, Ascensao JL, Fialk MA, et al.: Studies on the pathogenesis of aplastic anemia. Am J Med 66:444, 1979.

Najean Y, Pecking A: Prognostic factors in acquired aplastic anemia. A study of 352 cases. Am J Med 67:564, 1979.

Kagan WA, Fialk MA, Coleman M, et al.: Studies on the pathogenesis of refractory anemia. Am J Med 68:381, 1980.

Crosby WH: Current concepts in nutrition: who needs iron? N Engl J Med 297:543, 1977.

Cartwright GE, Deiss A: Sideroblasts, siderocytes and sideroblastic anemia. N Engl J Med 292:185, 1975.

Zucker S, et al.: Bone marrow erythropoiesis in the anemia of infection, inflammation and malignancy. J Clin Invest 53:1132, 1974.

Hemoglobinopathies

Forget BG: Molecular genetics of human hemoglobin synthesis. Ann Intern Med 91:605, 1979.

Dean J, Schechter AN: Sickle cell anemia: molecular and cellular bases of therapeutic approaches. N Engl J Med 299:752-764, 863-870, 1978.

Sears DA: The morbidity of sickle cell trait. Am J Med 64:1021, 1978.

DeFronzo RA, Taufield PA, Black H, et al.: Impaired renal tubular potassium secretion in sickle cell disease. Ann Intern Med 90:310, 1979.

Ballester OF, Warth J: Sickle cell anemia: recurrent splenic pain relieved by splenectomy. Ann Intern Med 90:349, 1979.

Polycythemias

Erslev AJ, Caro J, Kansu E, Miller O, Cobbs E: Plasma erythroprotein in polycythemia. Am J Med 66:243, 1979.

Berlin NI: Diagnosis and classification of the polycythemias. Semin Hematol 12:339, 1975.

Leukopenias

Stuart RK, Braine HG, Lietman PS, et al.: Carbenicillin-trimethoprim/sulfamethoxazole versus carbenicillin-gentamicin as empiric therapy of infection in granulocytopenic patients. A prospective, randomized, double-blind study. Am J Med 68:876, 1980.

Kyle RA: Natural history of chronic idiopathic neutropenia. N Engl J Med 302:908, 1980.

Leukemias

Greenberg PL, Mara B: The preleukemic syndrome. Correlation of in vitro parameters of granulopoiesis with clinical features. Am J Med 66:951, 1979.

Twomey JJ, Lewis VM, Ford R: An inhibitor of thymic hormone activity in serum from patients with lymphoblastic leukemia. Am J Med 68:377, 1980.

Cline MJ, Golde DW, Billing RJ, et al.: Acute leukemia: biology and treatment (UCLA Conference). Ann Intern Med 91:758, 1979.

Blume KG, Beutler E, Bross KJ, et al.: Bone-marrow ablation and allogeneic marrow transplantation in acute leukemia. N Engl J Med 302:1041, 1980.

Lymphomas

Merigan TC, Sikora K, Breeden JH, et al.: Preliminary observations on effect of interferon in non-Hodgkin's lymphoma. N Engl J Med 299:1449, 1978.

DeVita VT Jr, Simon RM, Hubbard SM, et al.: Curability of advanced Hodgkin's disease with chemotherapy. Ann Intern Med 92:587, 1980.

Portlock CS, Rosenberg SA: No initial therapy for stage III and IV non-Hodgkin's lymphomas of favorable histologic types. Ann Intern Med 90:10, 1979.

Fisher RI, DeVita VT, Bostick F, et al.: Persistent immunologic abnormalities in long-term survivors of advanced Hodgkin's disease. Ann Intern Med 92:595, 1980.

Disorders of Hemostasis

Myers TJ, Wakem CJ, Ball ED, et al.: Thrombotic thrombocytopenic purpura: combined treatment with plasmapheresis and antiplatelet agents. Ann Intern Med 92:149, 1980.

DeFino SM, Lachant NA, Kirshner JJ, Gottlieb AJ: Adult idiopathic thrombocytopenic purpura. Clinical findings and response to therapy. Am J Med 69:430, 1980.

Ratnoff OD: Antihemophilic factor (factor VIII). Ann Intern Med 88:403, 1978.

Mant MJ, King EG: Severe acute disseminated intravascular coagulation. A reappraisal of its pathophysiology, clinical significance, and therapy based on 47 patients. Am J Med 67:557, 1979.

Bynum LJ, Wilson JE: Low dose heparin therapy in the long-term management of venous thromboembolism. Am J Med 67:553, 1979.

Brozovic M: Oral anticoagulants in clinical practice. Semin Hematol 15:27, 1978.

Marder VJ: The use of thrombolytic agents: choice of patient, drug administration, laboratory monitoring. Ann Intern Med 90:802, 1979.

Cinas DB, Kaywin P, Bina M, et al.: Heparin associated thrombocytopenia. N Engl J Med 303:788, 1980.

8

The Immune System

O ur rapidly expanding knowledge of the body's immune system emphasizes its critical role not only in host defense against infectious agents, but also in the maintenance of health in numerous physiologic systems and in the pathophysiology of an increasing number of serious illnesses. The singular importance of distinguishing self from nonself is well demonstrated in the autoimmune diseases and in the removal of neoplastic cells.

THE IMMUNE SYSTEM

The body's immune system is located anatomically in the lymphoid tissue of the thymus, spleen, lymph nodes, and bone marrow. Its cellular constituents are the lymphocytes, plasma cells, and macrophages. The basic components of the immune system are: (1) the immunoglobulins derived from B lymphocytes (humoral); (2) the cell-mediated components, and (3) an amplifying system composed of serum complement, the kinin system, and the coagulation-fibrinolytic system. The humoral and cellular components of the immune response are highly specific, whereas the amplifying system is basically nonspecific. An antigenic stimulus is the initiating event in the immune response. An antigen is usually a protein substance whose potential for evoking an immune response is related both to its degree of dissimilarity from host proteins and to genetic host factors. Large polysac-charides (e.g., those of the pneumococcal capsule) can also act as antigens. Haptens are smaller molecules (e.g., penicillin) that require attachment to a larger protein before developing antigenic potential.

Lymphocytes

Lymphocytes are the key cells of immunity. Derived from lymphoid stem cells of the fetal yolk sac, they migrate via the liver to the bone marrow. Peripheral blood lymphocytes can be divided into two distinct categories:

1. T lymphocytes, accounting for 80% of the peripheral blood lymphocytes, are so called because of their dependency on the thymus. They are involved principally in cell-mediated immunity.
2. B lymphocytes, which comprise 20% of normal peripheral blood lymphocytes, are involved in the production of immuno-globulins. The B lymphocytes originally derived their name from the bursa of fabricius in chickens; in humans, these B cells are thought to be marrow-dependent.
3. A portion of peripheral cells do not have the surface criteria for either T cells or B cells. These are referred to as null cells, and are now thought to be B cell precursors. *Thymic-dependent T lymphocytes* are involved in fighting intracellular infections, mycobacteria, fungi, and viral infections; they are also responsible for transplant rejection and are important in preventing neoplastic growth. The T lymphocyte has an extremely varied repertoire following antigenic stimulation. Surface receptors on the T lymphocyte are stimulated by antigen and mutagens, such as phytohemagglutinin, causing a clone of T cells to proliferate and differentiate into cells with varied functions, many of which serve to modify activity of the B lymphocyte. Both suppressor T cells and helper T cells regulate the response of the B lymphocyte to antigens. Further mediators are also elaborated by the stimulated T lymphocytes, the most notable of which is the so-called transfer factor, which is known to be extremely important in the

body's defense against infection. This factor conveys delayed hypersensitivity to specific antigens, particularly important being tuberculosis, diphtheria toxoid, and a number of yeasts. Migration inhibition factor (MIF) released by the T cells inhibits the migration of macrophages. These and other mediators such as interferon all have important effects on macrophage activity at the site of infection. Conversely, it is now known that macrophages can also influence the ability of invading bacteria to antigenically stimulate the T cell.

Another type of T cell developed in response to infection is the cytotoxic T cell, which attaches itself to particular target cells, such as tumor cells, resulting in their destruction. The K or killer cell is another type of T cell, which attacks target cells but only in the presence of and in conjunction with antibody. The cell seems to acquire its target specificity through the antibody and not directly.

Humoral Immunity

The differentiation of B cells into antibody-producing plasma cells occurs after stimulation by antigen. The resulting antibodies are traditionally divided into five classes: IgG, IgA, IgM, IgD, and IgE. These immunoglobulins have a similar basic structure but differ markedly in both functional and physiochemical and electrophoretic activity. Each immunoglobulin is made up of units composed of two light chains and two heavy chains, which come together at the so-called hinge region to form the letter Y. The chains are linked by disulfide bonds. The molecule is traditionally divided into a Fab (fragment antigen binding) portion and Fc (fragment crystallizable) portion. This division is achieved by proteolytic cleavage by papain and pepsin. The arms of the letter Y, the Fab portion, are comprised of both the light chains and the amino terminal halves of heavy chains, while the Fc or stem portion of the Y is comprised of the heavy chains and the carboxy-terminal end of the heavy chains. The variable and highly specific antigen-combining area of the molecule is located in the arms, while the biologic activity and other physiochemical properties are determined by the stem area. The biologic activities located in the Fc part of the molecule determine the effect of the antibody on the complement system, and in the case of IgE, attachment to mast cells and basophils, where it triggers the release of various chemical mediators.

IgM is a macromolecule caused by the polymerization of five of the basic monomeric units. IgA can exist as a monomer or as a dimer.

There are two types of light chains, kappa and lambda, either of which occurs in each immunoglobulin unit; both chains are identical within each monomeric unit.

The antibodies formed in response to infection by specific microorganisms serve their protective function in a number of ways. *Opsonins* are substances which, when bound to an organism, render it more susceptible to phagocytosis. Antibodies such as IgG-1 or IgG-3 act as opsonins because portions of their Fc fragments combine with specific receptors on phagocytes. Other antibodies such as IgM do not possess such fragments but act indirectly by activating complement.

Lysins are antibodies that activate the complement cascade. *Neutralizing* antibodies achieve control of the infective process without either opsonization or lysis of the organism. This action generally occurs against viruses or bacterial toxins and represents the major action of commonly used vaccines.

IgG is the major immunoglobulin in adult serum. It is not produced during fetal life, and any found in the circulation of the newborn is derived from the mother. It is one of the principal antibodies developed in response to infection. It works by opsonization, lysis, and neutralization of the effects of the infecting organism and has a half-life of about 3 weeks.

There are four subclasses of IgG: IgG-1, IgG-2, IgG-3, and IgG-4. These subclasses differ in function and particularly in the ability to bind the first component of complement.

IgA is the predominant immunoglobulin of secretions in the body cavities and externally. It is released by the local plasma cells, usually as a dimer. It is found in high concentrations in respiratory and GI tracts, the genitourinary tract, saliva, tears, and colostrum. It resists autodigestion in areas such as the GI tract by being combined with a polypeptide referred to as the secretory piece, a product of the local epithelial cells. It acts by combining with and neutralizing both bacteria and viruses, thereby lessening the absorption of antigens into the body. It may activate the alternate complement pathway but does not ordinarily bind complement.

IgM is a macromolecule made up of five immunoglobulin monomers linked by disulfide bridges referred to as the J chain. Ultrastructural studies have shown it to resemble the configuration of a star in the human plasma. Although it is found mainly in the serum, it is sometimes found in external secretions. Because of its pentameric form, IgM is highly efficient in both fixing complement and in agglutinating reactions. The iso-hemagglutinins, anti-A and anti-B, are both IgM immuno-globulins, which occur naturally in individuals following cross-reaction with antigens of intestinal bacteria. Cold agglutinins and rheumatoid factor are other examples of IgM immunoglob-ulin.

As already mentioned, the IgM antibody occurs during the acute response to infection and results in the further response of both IgG and IgA antibodies. The IgM-producing cells do not develop antigenic memories, and therefore recurrent infections with the same organism do not result in a higher level of IgM response.

IgD occurs in the serum in small amounts, and its function is generally not known, except that along with IgM it appears on the majority of B cell surfaces. This suggests that it may be an early receptor for antigen.

IgE occurs in very small amounts in the serum, but derives its principal importance from its effect in releasing mediators such as histamine and slow-reacting substance of anaphylaxis from mast cells and basophils. IgE binds to these cells by its Fc portion, and following antigenic stimulation, results in the immediate hypersensitivity reaction with the release of histamine, slow-reacting substance of anaphylaxis (SRS-A) and eosinophil chemotactic factor (ECF-A) of anaphylaxis. SRS-A is a leuko-triene, a newly-characterized substance derived from arachidonic acid. The classic examples of this response are hayfever, extrinsic asthma, and anaphylaxis. IgE levels are elevated in atopic individuals. They are also elevated following infection with worms and other parasites.

Complement

The complement system is composed of at least 20 inactive precursor proteins which, when activated by antigen-antibody combinations, directly by infectious agents, or other nonspecific factors, interact sequentially in an amplifying cascade that results in numerous inflammatory effects. There is release of mediators from mast cells, increased vascular permeability, chemotaxis of neutrophils, monocytes, and eosinophils, and lysis of cell membranes. There is also a direct neutralization of virus and bacterial toxins. Activated complement has a detergent-like nonenzymatic action on cell membranes, resulting in a loss of the integrity of the cell membrane and destruction of the cell by osmotic lysis. This particular capability is peculiar to complement and cannot be achieved by antibodies acting alone.

Both classic and alternate pathways result in the activation and eventual cleavage of C3, bringing about the activation of the terminal sequence C5 through C9 (the "terminal attack unit"). The classic pathway is activated by either a single IgM molecule or two closely placed IgG molecules along with antigen. The alternate pathway (properdin system) is activated by IgA or IgE and also by complex polysaccharides present in cell walls.

Much of our knowledge about the role of complement in human disease comes from measurement of complement levels as well as turnover studies using radiolabeled components. These studies show that complement is important not only for the response to infection but also for maintenance of general health. Deficiency of various complement fractions are associated with disease; SLE is associated with C2 deficiency and glomerulonephritis with C1 deficiency, for example. One of the most common abnormalities of serum complement is its elevation during acute infectious processes. Levels are frequently depressed in patients with immune complex disease. The individual components of complement can be measured immunochemically, one of the most popular measurements being the CH50, a hemolytic assay involving sensitized sheep erythrocytes.

The activity of the complement system is closely controlled by both activators and inhibitors, acting through positive and negative feedback loops. The potent and wide-ranging effects of the complement cascade on vascular permeability, mast cell formation, coagulation, and local inflammation are restrained but poised for action; either excessive activation or inappropriate restraint may produce serious consequences.

GENETIC ASPECTS OF IMMUNITY

Histocompatibility testing before organ transplantation emphasizes the genetic control of immunity. HLA, originally an abbreviation for human leukocyte antigen, is now used to identify all genes controlled by the HLA chromosomal region on human chromosome 6. This area is also referred to as the major histocompatibility complex (MHC). Observations made originally in mice of a correlation of HLA type antigens and susceptibility to various viruses and malignancy raised the possibility of an association between these genes and the body's ability to respond to an antigen. The association of HLA-B27 with ankylosing spondylitis has proved to be the prelude to an increasing number of associations between this and other HLA types and human disease, including Reiter's syndrome, diabetes mellitus, Graves disease, and Addison's disease. The fact that ankylosing spondylitis is over a hundred times more frequent in those with HLA-B27 than in those without it has provided a potent stimulus to further epidemiologic surveys in human disease.

No totally satisfactory explanation has yet been made for the association between HLA factors and increased susceptibility to disease. The favorite explanation is that the HLA genes control the immunologic response to various disease provoking infections. Other theories include similarities between the HLA antigen and the offending agent and an imbalance in the action of the various components of the immunologic system.

HYPERSENSITIVITY

When an immune reaction is harmful rather than helpful to the individual, it is referred to as hypersensitive. The term "allergy," introduced by von Pirquet early in the twentieth century to describe altered immunity following exposure to a foreign antigen, has in current usage become synonymous with hypersensitivity.

Hypersensitivity reactions are generally divided into four types, each with different effector cells.

I. Immediate hypersensitivity
II. Cytotoxic reactions
III. Immune-complex disease
IV. Delayed hypersensitivity

Type I: Immediate Hypersensitivity Reaction

The common clinical manifestations of this hypersensitivity can be either localized or generalized. The localized manifestations include asthma, allergic rhinitis, urticaria, and abdominal cramps. The generalized reaction is that of acute anaphylaxis.

The reaction is mediated on contact of antigen with sensitized IgE (reaginic) antibody bound to mast cells and basophils. The combination of antigen with the antibody results in the release of chemical mediators from the mast cell. These mediators include histamine (SRS-A), prostaglandins, platelet-activating factor (ECF-A), a neutrophil chemotactic factor (NCF), and heparin.

These chemical mediators have potent local and systemic effects. They include increased vascular permeability, contraction of smooth muscle in the bronchi and small blood vessels, and loss of fluid and colloid from the intravascular space. The effects depend to a large extent on the part of the body where they are taking place. The slow-reacting substance of anaphylaxis (leukotrine) is present in both mast cells and basophils. They produce mainly bronchoconstriction and increased vascular permeability. A recently discovered inactivating enzyme in eosinophils, arylsulfatase, may have an important regulatory effect on the reaction.

The reaction can be triggered by other mechanisms besides the classic combination of antigen with the mast cell-attached IgE antibody complex. Certain drugs such as morphine, codeine, hydralazine, and others can cause degranulation of the mast cells directly. Also, antigen-antibody reactions involving IgM or IgA may sometimes trigger the release of these chemical mediators from the mast cells.

The intensity of the immediate hypersensitivity reaction depends on a number of factors, including the actual amount of IgE bound to the mast cells, the presence of blocking IgG antibodies, the level of cyclic AMP in the mast cells, and the presence of inhibiting factors such as arylsulfatase, histaminase, and phospholipase (which acts on the platelet-activating factor).

Treatment of anaphylactic reactions begins with decreasing exposure to responsible antigens and consideration of desensitization with small amounts of antigen, which decreases the production of specific IgE antibody and also produces IgG-blocking antibodies which compete for receptor sites on mast cells. Increasing the intracellular concentration of cyclic AMP by beta adrenergic agonists (isoproterenol or more specific beta-2 agonists) or phosphodiesterase inhibitors (theophylline) decreases the intensity of the response. Beta agonists are also effective bronchodilators. Antihistamines block the effect of histamine on peripheral tissues, and disodium chromoglycolate appears to prevent the release of mediators, including the slow-reacting substance of anaphylaxis. Local or systemic steroids are quite useful. They probably affect the overall immune response, may decrease leukocyte aggregation, and have other important but poorly understood positive effects. Injected epinephrine remains an important agent, in large part by generally increasing cyclic AMP.

Type II: Cytotoxic Reactions

IgG or IgM antibodies can interact directly with a constituent of the cell wall such as a specific receptor, an attached drug, or a viral particle. The resulting reaction frequently ends in the destruction of the cell or tissue via (1) complement-fixing antibody in the case of IgM, or (2) an antigen-antibody reaction in the case of IgG, which can lead to tissue damage without the activation of complement. The IgG attaches to the antigen, with subsequent attraction of and destruction by phagocytic cells. Though cell destruction usually occurs, there is one interesting instance in which stimulation of the cell occurs when long-acting thyroid stimulator (LATS), an IgG, molecule stimulates receptors in the thyroid gland. These receptors are normally acted on by thyroid-stimulating hormone (TSH). The type II cytotoxic reaction is involved in immune hemolytic anemias and thrombocytopenias, Goodpasture's syndrome, and erythroblastosis fetalis. Another example is transfusion reactions where preformed antibodies of the IgG class result in the hemolysis of the transfused cells. In the case of penicillin-induced hemolytic anemia, the penicillin molecule becomes attached to the red blood cell membrane. This results in the production of IgG antibodies, which bind to the penicillin antigen on the red blood cell membrane and lead to its phagocytosis.

Type III: Immune Complex Disease

Circulating antigen-antibody complexes in the circulation may become deposited in tissues, with resultant injury. The release of vasoactive amines results in increased permeability of the blood vessels, with escape of the complexes through the endothelial lining, where they lodge on the basement membranes. Subsequent complement activation provides chemotactic factors, dilatation of the blood vessels, and attraction of neutrophils. These interact with the immune complexes, with resulting inflammation and tissue injury with platelet thrombosis and tissue necrosis. This is the *Arthus phenomonon.*

Immune complex deposition occurs in many diseases; the classic example is serum sickness. Such complexes have also been demonstrated in SLE, bacterial endocarditis, rheumatoid disease, and malignancy. It occurs locally in the lung in extrinsic allergic alveolitis.

Type IV: Delayed Hypersensitivity

In this case, the cell-mediated reactions involve previously sensitized cytotoxic T cells, which kill bacteria or other cells perceived to be "foreign." The tuberculin reaction is a good example of this type of hypersensitivity. It takes 24-48 hours to reach its maximum, as measured by erythema and induration at the site of the tuberculin injection. There is a predominantly mononuclear infiltrate, resulting in the classic induration of the tissue. The foreign antigen is recognized by a number of previously sensitized T cells. These release effector substances (lymphokines), which nonspecifically stimulate lymphocytes and macrophages to attack the antigenic substance. The previously sensitized T cells also stimulate the production of more specifically sensitized T cells. Delayed hypersensitivity is manifested in organ transplant rejection, in the body's defense against malignancy, and in combating intracellular infections, both viral and bacterial. Efforts are sometimes made to augment this activity in patients with malignancy by injecting a bacillus Calmette Guerin (BCG) and other substances designed to stimulate the body's delayed hypersensitivity.

AUTOIMMUNITY

This reflects an impaired tolerance to self with the development of antibodies against the body's own tissues. It encompasses a large number of clinical disorders, increases in frequency with age, and involves both organ-specific and systemic disorders. A number of mechanisms have been proposed.

Genetic predisposition seems well established by the concurrence of various clinical disorders in monozygotic twins and the increased occurrence of disease entities like SLE and rheumatoid arthritis in patients with certain histocompatibility antigens. This may be explained by the close association of histocompatibility antigens with the genes that control the body's immune response. An increase in B cell activity associated with a decrease in suppressor T cells has been noted in a number of autoimmune conditions. There is strong support for the role of viruses in the pathogenesis of some of these disorders. The question remains, however, whether the viral infection produced the abnormality or whether there was a preexisting weakness in the host's defense mechanism. Infective organisms, sometimes acting as haptens, attach themselves to the body's tissues, altering them and provoking an immunologic response that involves the host's own tissues (streptococcal infection and rheumatic carditis). In some cases, self-antigens may have been anatomically sequestered and thus isolated from contact with antibody-producing tissue; when exposed, autoantibodies develop. Antibodies against thyroglobulin that result in autoimmune thryoiditis have been explained by this "forbidden clone" theory. It is not clear whether such antithyroid or antiheart antibodies are cause or effect, since they may be found in individuals without clinical evidence of autoimmune disease.

GRANULOMATOUS DISEASE
In diseases such as tuberculosis, sarcoidosis, and berylliosis, persistence of phagocytized antigens results in the formation of epithelioid cells, which subsequently fuse to form multinucleated giant cells. In the case of sarcoidosis, the antigen has not been identified with certainty. Patients with this condition have impairment of T cell function, hypergammaglobulinemia, and circulating immune complexes. (See Sarcoidosis, page 105.)

THE IMMUNOLOGY OF INFECTION
Besides the three arms of the immunologic system—humoral, complement, and cellular-local defense mechanisms such as an intact skin—the cough and sneeze reflexes and free drainage from body cavities are critically important. Important examples of defects in local defense mechanisms include obstruction in the lower urinary tract caused by prostatic enlargement or urinary calculi, foreign bodies in the anterior nares, and obstructive airways disease.

The mature neutrophil has a primary role in the body's ability to phagocytize invading bacteria. The importance of this line of defense is well exemplified by the patient with neutropenia or in the condition of chronic granulomatous disease of childhood in which there is a qualitative defect of neutrophil function. In the normal individual, products of invading bacteria attract neutrophils to the site of infection. Endotoxin achieves this by activating the alternate pathway of complement. Tissue destruction at the site of infection will also release chemotactic factors. These act on the third and fifth components of complement, and absence of these factors results in an increased susceptibility to infections. Abnormalities of this response also occur in the presence of high doses of steroids, and in certain diseases such as rheumatoid arthritis, diabetes, and uremia.

THE IMMUNOLOGY OF MALIGNANCY

There is increasing evidence for the role of the body's immune system in restraining the spread of mutant neoplastic cells. Cancer is most frequent at the extremes of life when the immune system is least efficient. Immunodeficiency diseases, whether congenital or acquired, are associated with an increased incidence of neoplasia. Where there is loss of cellular immunity, there is a well-documented increase in tumors of lymphoid tissue. It is also well-known, for instance, that the remission of patients with Burkitt's lymphoma is associated with a recovery of cellular immunity. The use of immunosuppressive therapy in patients receiving renal transplantation has resulted in a substantial increase in tumors. There is evidence that the tumor cells themselves can secrete factors that interfere with the host's immune response. These factors can inactivate lymphocytes, complement, and macrophages. The development of suppressor cells results in the suppression of cell-mediated immunity.

If the patient is to react against tumor cells, these cells must change in some way so that they are no longer recognized as self. As evidence, there are numerous cases where *new antigens* have been detected in patients with malignancy. Many of these are only weakly antigenic, so that the resulting immunologic response is not sufficient to cause total rejection of the tumor. Two well-known examples of such antigens, which play an important role in both diagnosis and management, are *alpha-fetoprotein*

(AFP) and *carcinoembryonic antigen* (CEA). Alpha-fetoprotein occurs normally during the first half of prenatal life, disappearing totally in the neonatal period. This has been detected particularly in patients with hepatoma, liver metastases, and malignant teratomas. It may, however, occur in the serum of normal subjects and in those with acute hepatitis, so its chief value is in monitoring the therapy of patients with hepatomas and such tumors rather than in their diagnosis. Carcinoembryonic antigen is elevated in a number of tumors, including those of the gastrointestinal tract, lung, breast, and kidney. Levels are also elevated in cigarette smokers and in patients with a diverse range of clinical conditions including peptic ulcer disease, cirrhosis, and colonic polyps. Its detection is therefore not as useful for diagnosis as in monitoring the effectiveness of treatment and the development of relapse.

There have been numerous reports of the effectiveness of stimulation of the immunologic system in the treatment of patients with malignancy. The nonspecific stimulation of the immune system with BCG, *Corynebacterium parvum,* and other agents has met with some limited success. Since there is general agreement that neoplasia develops when the balance is tipped in favor of the malignancy, and that recovery occurs when the immune system is strengthened, immunotherapy may become an important therapeutic modality.

IMMUNE DEFICIENCY STATES

The most common clinical feature linking patients with this condition is an increased susceptibility to infection. In recent decades, however, the improved ability to treat infections with antibiotics and other modalities has unmasked the other abnormalities of these conditions, principally neoplasia, allergy, and autoimmune disease. Sensitive tests for various limbs of the immune response have resulted in the detection of numerous minor and major defects. Approximately 20 primary immune deficiency diseases (IDD) have now been described. Many of these are genetically determined and inherited by autosomal recessive, autosomal dominant, or X-linked mechanisms.

Selective IgA Deficiency

The most common of the immune deficiency diseases, occurring approximately one in 500 of the population, it generally does not produce significant disease. There is frequently a gross diminution in both serum and secretory IgA to about 5% of normal for serum; serum levels of other immunoglobulins are normal. There has been evidence for suppressor T cells, which block the terminal differentiation of IgA within the plasma cells. Because of the important role of IgA in resistance to mucosal infections and in the maintenance of the mucosal barrier, there is a predictable increase in sinopulmonary infections and IgE-mediated atopic disorders. There is also an increase in IgG antibody to dietary proteins in these patients, which is probably secondary to increased absorption of antigenic material. These patients do not require replacement of their gammaglobulins, since they have normal levels of IgG and IgM. The presence of autoantibodies to human IgA may cause transfusion reactions, as may commercial gammaglobulin, which contains sufficient IgA to produce anaphylactic problems.

Panhypoimmunoglobulinemia (Bruton hypogammaglobulinemia). Caused by a defect in B cell maturation, this is sex linked and usually appears at age 6 months in male subjects when passive resistance to infection wanes. Patients suffer from repeated bacterial infections; respiratory tract infections are common and may cause death. There is also a high incidence of giardiasis and viral hepatitis, as well as enterovirus infections of the CNS. They have a tenfold increase in neoplasia, particularly lymphomas. Replacement therapy with normal plasma or gammaglobulin is of some help, but does not completely eradicate the recurrent infections of the respiratory tract.

Selective T Cell Deficiency (Di George's Syndrome)

Absence of the thymus owing to defective embryogenesis of the third or fourth pharyngeal pouches is associated with defective T cell function. The parathyroids are also absent, with resultant characteristic facies as well as cardiac abnormalities. They have normal immunoglobulin levels and are particularly susceptible to viral and fungal infections. There is also a defect in specific antibody function, exhibiting the interdependence of the T and B cell functions of the immunologic response. Fetal thymus transplants have been successful on occasion.

Combined T Cell and B Cell Deficiency

In this situation, there is a defect in both antibody and T cell-mediated responses. Untreated, the condition is invariably fatal. It may be inherited as either an X-linked or autosomal recessive characteristic. Defects of either the lymphoid stem cell or the enzyme adenine deaminase have been reported in some of these patients. The so called *Swiss-type A gammaglobulinemia* is a well-known example. It is characterized by a severe T and B lymphopenia and is inherited as an autosomal recessive. Varying success has been achieved with transplantations of histocompatible bone marrow from siblings, fetal liver, and thymus transplants.

Ataxia-Telangiectasia

This condition is inherited as an autosomal recessive and is characterized by immunodeficiency together with cerebellar ataxia and telangiectasia. Both lymphomas and chronic pulmonary infections are frequent causes of death. There is poor development of the thymus, with T cell dysfunction and frequently deficiency in serum IgE and IgA (and to a lesser extent IgG). The defect in B lymphocyte function is probably secondary to the T cell dysfunction. A generalized defect involving DNA has been postulated to explain the multiple abnormalities seen in this condition.

Wiskott-Aldrich Syndrome

This is an X-linked disorder probably caused by a basic defect in the B lymphocytes with secondary abnormalities of T cell function. Patients develop eczema, thrombocytopenia, recurrent infection, and lymphoreticular malignancy. It is invariably fatal.

There have been some dramatic responses to transplantations of compatible sibling bone marrow.

Deficiences of Complement

Deficiencies of complement, many of which are related to autosomal recessive inheritance, are associated with recurrent pyogenic infections, autoimmune disease, and in the case of C1 deficiency, hereditary angioedema. Recurrent pyogenic infections are associated with deficiency of C3 and C3$_b$ inhibitor. Recurrent gonococcal septicemia is associated with deficiency of C6, C7, and C8, emphasizing the importance of the terminal attack portion of the complement pathway. SLE and autoimmune nephritis are particularly important complications.

REFERENCES
The Immune System
Reinherz EL, Schlossman SF: Current concepts in immunology: regulation of the immune response-inducer and suppressor T-lymphocyte subsets in human beings. N Engl J Med 303:370, 1980.

Fearon DT, Austen KF: Current concepts in immunology. The alternative pathway of complement—a system for host resistance to microbial infection. N Engl J Med 303:259, 1980.

Parker CW: Control of lymphocyte function. N Engl J Med 295:1180, 1976.

Moretta L, Webb SR, Grossi CE, Lydyard PM, Cooper MD: Functional analysis of two human T-cell subpopulations: help and suppression of B-cell responses by T-cells bearing receptors for IgM or IgG. J Exp Med 146:184, 1977.

Nathan CF, Murray HW, Cohn ZA: Current concepts: the macrophage as an effector cell. N Engl J Med 303:622, 1980.

Genetics and Immunity
Schaller JG, Omenn GS: The histocompatibility system and human disease. J Pediatr 88:913, 1976.

Calin A: HLA-B27 to type or not to type? Ann Intern Med 92:208, 1980.

Dosseter JB, Sinclair NR, Stiller CR: The genetics of HLA. Transplant Proc 10:309, 1978.

Hypersensitivity

Rocklin RE, Sheffer AL, Greineder DK, Melmon KL: Generation of antigen-specific suppressor cells during allergy desensitization. N Engl J Med 302:1213, 1980.

Schur PH: Immune complex assays: the state of the art. N Engl J Med 298:161, 1978.

Daniele RP, Dauber JH, Rossman MD: Immunologic abnormalities in sarcoidosis. Ann Intern Med 92:406, 1980.

Parker CW: Drug allergy. N Engl J Med 292:511-514, 732-736, 957-960, 1975.

Hunt KJ, Valentine MD, Sobotka AK, Lichtenstein LM: Diagnosis of allergy to stinging insects by skin testing with hymenoptera venoms. Ann Intern Med 85:56, 1976.

Dawkins RL, Peter JB: Laboratory tests in clinical immunology: a critique. Am J Med 68:3, 1980.

Autoimmunity

Stuart JM, Postlethwaite AE, Townes AS, Kang AH: Cell-mediated immunity to collagen and collagen a chains in rheumatoid arthritis and other rheumatic diseases. Am J Med 69:13, 1980.

Waldmann Ta, Blaese RM, Broder S, Krakauer RS: Disorders of suppressor immunoregulator cells in the pathogenesis of immunodeficiency and autoimmunity. Ann Intern Med 88:226, 1978.

Williams RC Jr: A second look at rheumatoid factor and other "auto-antibodies." Am J Med 67:179, 1979.

Funderberg HH: Genetically determined immune deficiency as the predisposing cause of "autoimmunity" and lymphoid neoplasia. Am J Med 51:295, 1971.

Rapoport JR, Kozin F, Mackel SE, Jordon RE: Cutaneous vascular immunoflorescence in rheumatoid arthritis: correlation with circulating immune complexes and vasculitis. Am J Med 68:225, 1980.

Brown J, Solomon DH, Beall GN, et al.: Autoimmune thyroid diseases—Graves' and Hashimoto's. Ann Intern Med 88:379, 1978.

Immunology of Infection

Likhite VV: Immunological impairment and susceptibility to infection after splenectomy. JAMA 236:1376, 1976.

Stossel TP: Phagocytosis, clinical disorders of recognition and ingestion. Am J Pathol 88:741, 1977.

Quie PG, Cates KL: Clinical conditions associated with defective polymorphonuclear leukocyte chemotasis. Am J Pathol 88:711, 1977.

Immunology of Malignancy
Go VLW: Carcinoembryonic antigen. Clinical application. Cancer 37(Suppl 1):562, 1976.
Herberman RB: Immunologic tests in the diagnosis of cancer. Am J Clin Pathol 68(Suppl 5):688, 1977.
Whiteside TL, Rowlands DT Jr: T-cell and B-cell identification in the diagnosis of lymphoproliferative disease. A review. Am J Pathol 88:754, 1977.
Hansen HJ, Snyder JJ, Miller E, et al.: Carcinoembryonic antigen (CEA) assay: a laboratory adjunct in the diagnosis and management of cancer. Hum Pathol 5:139, 1974.
Brandstetter RD, Graziano VA, Wade MJ, Saal SD: Carcinoembryonic antigen elevation in renal failure. Ann Intern Med 91:867, 1979.

Immune Deficiency States
Spitler LE: Transfer factor therapy in the Wiskott-Aldrich syndrome and results of long-term follow-up in 32 patients. Am J Med 67:59, 1979.
Agnello V: Association of systemic lupus erythematosus and SLE-like syndromes with hereditary and acquired complement deficiency states. Arthritis Rheum (Suppl)21:S146, 1978.
Abrutyn E: The infancy of immunotoxicity (editorial). Ann Intern Med 90:118, 1979.

9

Infectious Diseases

UNEXPLAINED FEVER

Patients with unexplained fever admitted to community hospitals are frequently found to have viral or bacterial disease, or other conditions such as alcoholic cirrhosis or pulmonary embolization. When a temperature elevation is greater than 101°, persists for 2-3 weeks, and is unexplained despite an intensive laboratory evaluation, the term "fever of unknown origin" is applied. Cost and patient discomfort should be considered in subsequent evaluation, since many fevers remain unexplained or turn out to be protracted viral syndromes. Great effort, however, must be expended to identify potentially fatal but treatable microbial disease.

Studies in university hospital settings have shown the following causes for unexplained fevers lasting more than 2-3 weeks.

Infections are present in 30-50% of patients and include tuberculosis, endocarditis, and localized abscess formation in the abdomen or elsewhere. Extrapulmonary tuberculosis may be difficult to diagnose and may be found in liver, pericardium, peritoneum, bones, hilar nodes, or urinary tract. *Malignant disease* accounts for 15-30%; the most common fever-producing tumors are hypernephroma (the "internist's tumor"), lymphoma, Hodgkin's disease, hepatoma, pancreatic carcinoma, tumors of other abdominal organs, and the leukemias. *Connective tissue*

483

disease occurs in 10-20%. The remainder of patients may have drug fever (usually feel well in spite of the fever), inflammatory bowel disease, sarcoidosis, pulmonary embolization, or thrombophlebitis elsewhere. Factitious fever should always be suspected, particularly in medical personnel.

Detailed and repeated history taking and physical evaluation frequently establish the diagnosis; important historical points include drug exposure, travel, animals in the environment, past medical history, possibility of narcotic addiction, and association with ill patients. The physical examination should emphasize the skin, eyes including the optic fundi (pupillary dilatation is mandatory), oral cavity with special attention to teeth, bones, sternum, and muscles such as trapezius and diaphragm, navel, rectum, testes, heart for evidence of murmurs, abdomen for hepatosplenomegaly, and evidence of lymphadenopathy. Regional lymphadenopathy may be important evidence, but may also reflect unrelated chronic infection, particularly in inguinal, epitrochlear, and axillary areas. *Supraclavicular nodes* are easy to biopsy and have a high yield.

Laboratory evaluation should be systematic, staged, and repeated. Many tests are expensive and should be ordered only as part of a detailed plan. Three blood cultures at 15-minute intervals before institution of antimicrobial treatment and culture of specific body fluids such as cerebrospinal fluid, urine, and ascitic or pleural fluid may give important early information. Three blood cultures should be repeated on the second day.

All medications not necessary should be discontinued. *Eosinophilia* suggests trichinosis, Hodgkin's disease, and periarteritis. *Lymphocytosis* occurs with tuberculosis, syphilis, infectious mononucleosis, toxoplasmosis, and cytomegalic viral disease; *leukopenia* occurs with lymphoma, connective tissue disease, brucellosis, and miliary tuberculosis. Monocytosis suggests tuberculosis, brucellosis, bacterial endocarditis, inflammatory bowel disease, Hodgkin's disease, and malignancy. A normal sedimentation rate makes bacterial endocarditis without congestive failure and connective tissue disease unlikely.

Elevated alkaline phosphatase may suggest hepatic infiltrative disease, elevated uric acid, a lymphoma, and elevated calcium, sarcoidosis. Ten milliliters of serum should be stored in a freezer and labeled "acute phase serum." Later, another "convalescent phase" sample can be analyzed and compared if clinical information suggests specific infectious disease.

Specific scanning, biopsy, or endoscopic procedures may be necessary. Computed tomography is an efficient method for identifying tumor or abscess. Cholecystography, intravenous pyelography, renal or abdominal arteriography, and ultrasonography may be useful, depending on clinical information. Biopsy of skin, pleura, peritoneum, lymph nodes, and liver is frequently useful; adequate tissue for both pathologic and microbiologic examination must be obtained.

Fever in the compromised host is frequently difficult to evaluate because of confusing manifestations due to the underlying disease. Common syndromes include meningitis, encephalitis or brain abscess, pulmonary infiltration, oroesophageal syndromes, and disseminated disease with skin lesions. While bacterial agents such as pneumococci, staphylococci, and gram-negative agents are most common, a variety of unusual microbes may be found:

1. Bacteria—*Listeria, Nocardia, Pseudomonas* and *Mycobacterium tuberculosis.*
2. Fungi—*Cryptococcus neoformans, Aspergillus, Phycomycetes,* and *Candida.*
3. Viruses—*Herpes simplex, varicella-zoster,* and *cytomegalovirus;*
4. Parasites—*Pneumocystis carinii, Toxoplasma gondii,* and *Strongyloides stercoralis.*

Selection of an Antimicrobial Agent

Penicillin and the cephalosporins inhibit synthesis of the microbial cell wall. The aminoglycosides and tetracyclines prevent protein synthesis by binding to the 30S subunit of bacterial ribosomes; chloramphenicol and erythromycin bind to the 50S subunits; and rifampin inhibits bacterial transcription by inhibiting DNA-dependent RNA polymerase. Penicillin, cephalosporins, aminoglycosides, polymixins, and vancomycin are bactericidal, while the tetracyclines, sulfonamides, erythromycin, chloramphenicol, and clindamycin are bacteriostatic. Bactericidal drugs are indicated in indolent infections like endocarditis and in patients with compromised immunity.

Penicillin G remains the agent of choice for most cocci with the exception of enterococci (where an aminoglycoside is added in combination), staphylococci, and rare strains of gonococci and pneumococci. Penicillinase-producing gonococci are rare in the United States, so that penicillin G is the appropriate first drug; resistant pneumococci have been isolated, particularly in countries such as South Africa, but are almost unheard of in the U.S. at the present time. A phenoxy side chain leads to a semisynthetic penicillin (penicillin V) that is resistant to acid digestion in the stomach.

Methicillin (methoxy groups at positions 2 and 6 in benzene ring) is resistant to staphylococcal penicillinase; *oxacillin* and *dicloxacillin* are both acid-resistant and resistant to penicillinase. Recently, methicillin-resistant strains of *S. aureus* have been identified; up to 40% of *S. epidermidis* are resistant to methicillin. There is almost always cross-resistance to other penicillins, but resistant strains of *S. epidermidis* are frequently sensitive to the cephalosporins.

Vancomycin has been improved so that phlebitis, drug fever, and nephrotoxicity have been almost completely eliminated. It is useful in the treatment of methicillin-resistant staphylococci, endocarditis in the penicillin-allergic individual, penicillin-resistant pneumococci, bacteremia with *Corynebacterium* in the compromised host, and for treatment of the toxogenic strains of *Clostridia* that are believed to cause clindamycin-associated colitis.

Tetracyclines are active against many gram-positive and gram-negative organisms, although resistance is frequent. More than 50% of staphylococci, 5-20% of pneumococci, and 20-40% of group A streptococci are resistant. The gonococcus remains sensitive. The tetracyclines are also effective against *Chlamydia, Mycoplasma, Legionella, Brucella,* and *Pasteurella tularensis.*

Doxycycline and minocycline are two newer tetracyclines with similar activity but with long half-lives, so that they may be administered twice daily. The tetracyclines are usually not the drug of choice for most infections.

Cephalosporins are versatile, expensive, and have been used indiscriminately because of their wide spectrum. Cephalothin (Keflin), cephapirin (Cefadyl), and cephradine (Velosef) have similar pharmacodynamic properties; cefazolin (Ancef, Kefzol) produces substantially higher blood levels. Cephalexin (Keflex) is active orally. All are active against cocci, including staphylococci-producing penicillinase, and against many gram-negative rods. Enterococci, *H. influenzae, P. aeruginosa,* and *B. fragilis* are not sensitive. Excellent activity against *Klebsiella pneumoniae* makes them useful for treatment of bacterial pneumonias of uncertain etiology or in the penicillin-sensitive individual.

Two newer cephalosporins have a broader spectrum. Cefamandole (Mandol) is active against *H. influenzae;* both this agent and cefoxitin (Mefoxin) are effective agents for treating infection with *Enterobacter,* indole-positive *Proteus,* and *B. fragilis.* The other cephalosporins, like penicillin, are active against most anaerobes with the exception of *B. fragilis.*

A "third generation" of cephalosporins, noted for their broad spectrum and long half-life will be shortly available. Active against gram-negative and gram-positive bacteria, they are limited for parenteral use at present. Cefotaxamine was released in May, 1981, and cefoperazone, an agent quite effective against pseudomonas, is expected within months. The group appears active against anaerobes including *B. fragilis.* Contrasted to aminoglycosides they are remarkably non-toxic although change in intestinal flora may produce vitamin K deficiency.

The *aminoglycosides* remain effective agents for the treatment of severe gram-negative infections; they are also active against *S. aureus* but ineffective against most other cocci. Gentamicin, tobramycin, and amikacin have similar ototoxicity and nephrotoxicity and have the same efficacy when used for treatment of sensitive organisms. Amikacin, however, appears more resistant to enzymes that inactivate the other two aminoglycosides and has been extremely useful for organisms insensitive to gentamicin or tobramycin.

Two semisynthetic penicillins, *carbenicillin* and *ticarcillin,* have expanded activity against gram-negative organisms and are particularly useful for *Pseudomonas* infections. They appear to be synergistic with the aminoglycosides for that organism.

Selection of agents is facilitated by dividing gram-negative bacteria into enteric and nonenteric varieties. *Nonenteric rods* such as *H. influenzae, L. monocytogenes, Actinomyces, Clostridia,* and *Bacteroides* species with the exception of *B. fragilis* are sensitive to penicillin. *H. influenzae* is sensitive to both penicillin and ampicillin, although a few strains have developed beta lactamase activity and are resistant to both drugs. It is resistant to the older cephalosporins but sensitive to cefamandole.

Enteric bacteria are much less sensitive to penicillin, although ampicillin is effective against *P. mirabilis, E. coli,* and *Salmonella.* Aminoglycosides or semisynthetic penicillins such as carbenicillin or ticarcillin are generally indicated. Most cephalosporins are active against *K. pneumoniae.*

Clindamycin inhibits most gram-positive cocci but is most commonly used for anaerobic infections below the diaphragm where *B. fragilis* is a potential agent.

Rifampin, derived from a *Streptomyces* species, is extremely active against most cocci as well as enjoying clinical usage for tuberculosis and leprosy. Group A streptococci, pneumococci, staphylococci, meningococci, gonococci, and anaerobic streptococci are relatively sensitive; enterococci are less sensitive, but the agent may be useful together with an aminoglycoside in the treatment of enterococcal endocarditis in individuals allergic to penicillin. Acquired resistance to rifampin will probably become a problem; the drug should be used only in specific situations when other agents are not appropriate for sensitive organisms, but should be remembered for difficult coccal problems, particularly in the penicillin-allergic patient.

Treatment of Unexplained Fever or Bacterial Disease Due to Unidentified Agents

The vigor of therapy in the absence of diagnosis depends on the severity of illness. An unexplained fever in a moderately ill patient may be subjected to therapeutic trial with a single agent for diagnostic purposes after cultures have been obtained. In contrast is the intensive antimicrobial therapy to critically ill patients when life is at stake but the microbial agent unknown. Broad-spectrum therapy should include agents active against gram-positive cocci including resistant staphylococci, gram-negative rods, and anaerobic organisms. Oxacillin, ampicillin, and aminoglycoside is one combination that is broad, but not effective for *B. fragilis.* Vancomycin or clindamycin could be substituted for the penicillins in the penicillin-allergic patient; both clindamycin and the aminoglycoside could be expected to have antistaphylococcal activity. Third generation cephalosporins will certainly play an important role in these patients.

Considerable experience has developed with granulocytopenic patients with fever where delay may be disastrous. Usually, an aminoglycoside (for gram-negative coverage) and a semisynthetic penicillin (for gram-positive and staphylococcal coverage) is used. There is evidence that carbenicillin and ticarcillin are synergistic with aminoglycosides for *Pseudomonas,* so that triple therapy with these two agents and a cephalosporin or other semisynthetic penicillin such as methicillin is begun. One study showed that mortality in leukopenic patients varied in the following manner: synergistic combination, 18%; additive but not synergistic, 44%; single agent, 71%; inappropriate therapy, 100%.

Local Collections of Pus

Abscess in various locations can present as pain and fever, or as either manifestation without the other. Frequently silent on conventional diagnostic study, their presentation is altered by intermittent antibiotic therapy, and they may not produce evidence of systemic infection such as leukocytosis or elevation of the erythrocyte sedimentation rate. Abscesses may be due to a single organism or contain mixed flora. Gram-negative and positive organisms are common, depending on the abscess location. These organisms lower oxygen concentration and provide an environment for the growth of anaerobic agents. Usually, anaerobes above the diaphragm are sensitive to penicillin, while

B. fragilis, an agent resistant to penicillin, is common in abscesses below the diaphragm.

Brain abscess. This presents with headache (75% of patients), focal neurologic signs (40%), seizures (30%), and evidence of increased intracranial pressure. Direct extension from paranasal sinuses, ears, and mastoids or hematogenous spread from other septic foci is frequently demonstrable and may be a clue to diagnosis. The cerebrospinal fluid commonly shows increased pressure, lymphocytosis, normal glucose, and increased protein content. *Lumbar puncture may be dangerous;* in one series, 25% of patients developed evidence of brainstem compression following lumbar puncture. Computed tomography has revolutionized diagnosis and should be performed before lumbar puncture unless meningitis is strongly suspected as the primary problem. Technetium scanning, which detects an abnormality in the blood-brain barrier, has also been useful. Brain abscess may be confused with epidural abscess, subdural empyema, and cerebral thrombophlebitis.

Abdominal abscesses. Symptoms are produced depending on location. *Subphrenic abscesses* are frequently postoperative and should be suspected in patients with unexplained postoperative fever. They may also arise from trauma, perforation of peptic ulcer, cholecystitis, or pancreatitis. Sixty percent are on the right, 25% on the left, and the rest are bilateral. Pleural effusions and diaphragmatic elevation are common. *Intrahepatic abscess* may be amebic, result from purulent infection in contiguous organs, or occur with bacteremia.

Pancreatic abscesses. Abdominal pain, fever, and leukocytosis are noted 10-21 days after an episode of pancreatitis. A mass is present in 50%, but serum amylase may be normal. *Diverticular* and *appendiceal abscesses* present as abdominal pain or low-grade fever. Distal *rectal abscesses* are easy to identify on rectal examination, but those located higher may produce vague rectal discomfort and be mistaken for disease of adjacent organs. Rectal abscesses are particularly common in the compromised host. Abdominal abscesses contain gram-negative aerobic rods, aerobic streptococci, and anaerobic bacteria. *B. fragilis* is the most common anaerobe cultured and is resistant to many antibiotics but sensitive to clindamycin, chloramphenicol, carbenicillin, and ticarcillin.

Perinephric abscesses. These usually contain *E. coli, Proteus,* or other gram-negative bacteria, since they result from pyelonephritis, microabscess formation, and perinephric rupture. They are common in the diabetic, occur frequently in patients with hydronephrosis or urinary calculi, and may present without fever, pyuria, or bacteriuria. Perinephric abscess may suggest pyelonephritis that is poorly responsive to antibiotic therapy but also presents as unexplained fever, pyuria, or back pain.

Vertebral osteomyelitis and paravertebral abscess. These may produce back pain, be confused with spinal epidural abscess, subdural abscess, disc space infection, neoplasm or degenerative joint disease, and develop from direct or hematogenous spread. Presentation may be acute with chills and fever or chronic with pain of long duration, absent fever, and vague constitutional symptoms. Tuberculous disease may occur with negative chest radiographs; other organisms include staphylococci, fungi, and organisms such as *Salmonella* or *Brucella.*

Computed tomography or ultrasonography has been of great value in identifying local abscess formation. The former is useful in patients with substantial body fat, since periorgan fat collections allow separation of one intra-abdominal organ from another; the latter is more useful in slender patients. Computed tomographic direct needle aspiration for diagnosis and drainage is frequently effective. While antibiotic selection is important in the critically ill patient, percutaneous or operative drainage is almost always necessary in patients with abscesses.

SEXUALLY TRANSMITTED DISEASES
Gonococcal Infections
Neisseria gonorrhoeae is extremely prevalent in young individuals of any socioeconomic group. Syndromes include gonococcal urethritis, epididymitis, anorectal and pharyngeal infection in homosexuals, pelvic inflammatory disease, Bartholin gland infection, and gonococcal perihepatitis with right upper quadrant or bilateral upper abdominal pain (Fitz-Hugh-Curtis syndrome).

Disseminated gonococcal infection with gonococcemia may produce an immune complex disease with fever, polyarthralgias, and a skin rash that may be papular, petechial, hemorrhagic, pustular, or necrotic. Tenosynovitis of wrists, fingers, knees, and ankles is frequent.

Demonstration of intracellular gram-negative diplococci is simple and reliable. Culture requires Thayer-Martin medium in an atmosphere of 3-10% carbon dioxide supplemented by chocolate agar cultures. Standard broth medium for blood culture with 3-10% carbon dioxide is used for culturing blood and synovial fluid. Immunofluorescent staining may increase the yield when used together with Gram staining.

The uniquely penicillin-sensitive gonococcus became progressively resistant in Southeast Asia and Africa in the early 1960s. Strains isolated in the United States about that time required higher concentrations of penicillin, owing in part to disease contracted in Vietnam. In 1976, beta lactamase-producing strains were found in the U.S. but have not become widespread. These were insensitive to penicillin and ampicillin. At present, the recommended treatment for uncomplicated gonococcal infection is aqueous procaine penicillin G, 4.8 million units injected I.M. at two sites with probenecid 1 gm by mouth. Alternatively, tetracycline, 0.5 gm q.i.d. for 5 days may be administered.

Chlamydial Infections

An organism formerly considered to be viral and closely related to that producing psittacosis, *C. trachomatis*, may produce urethritis, cervicitis, salpingitis, and other manifestations similar to those produced by the gonococcus. Three immunotypes (L1, L2, and L3) cause lymphogranuloma venereum. A primary genital lesion is associated with purulent inguinal lymphadenopathy with fever and occasionally meningitis. Hemorrhagic proctocolitis is found in women. It is the most common cause of nongonococcal urethritis and of epididymitis in those under the age of 35. The agent must be isolated by tissue cell culture, and the diagnosis is usually assumed if nongonococcal urethritis is documented. It is insensitive to penicillin, and treatment is tetracycline 500 mg q.i.d. for 7 days.

Another cause of nongonococcal urethritis is *Ureaplasma urealyticum*, a strain of *Mycoplasma*. It responds to tetracycline and, unlike *Chlamydia*, to spectinomycin.

Herpes Infections

Eighty percent of genital herpetic lesions are due to herpes virus type 2. Note the aphorism, type 2 below the diaphragm, type 1 above (oral mucosa). Following an incubation period of 4 days, a painful vesicular genital lesion appears that persists for several weeks; infectivity occurs during the first few days. The virus migrates to sacral neural cell bodies, where it remains quiescent and may recur following nonspecific stimulation. There is no known treatment. Ether is painful and not useful.

Syphilis

The infection caused by *Treponema pallidum* has three stages: *a primary lesion* with regional lymphadenopathy 3 weeks after infection, *a secondary bacteremic stage* with widely distributed maculopapular, pustular, and necrotic lesions that involve the palms, soles, face, and scalp and may last for several months, and *tertiary* involvement of aorta, CNS, skin, and muscles.

Syphilitic infection is identified by tests for either nonspecific reaginic or specific antitreponemal antibody. Purified cardiolipin antigens react with an IgG-IgM antibody. The rapid plasma reagin (RPR) can be automated, and the VDRL is a slide flocculation test that allows determination of titer. Twenty to 40% of positive VDRL tests are false-positive owing to recent infections, connective tissue disorders, or drug addiction, but the titer is usually less than 1:8. The titer rises fourfold or more in primary syphilis and falls with adequate treatment. True false-positive results are rare with specific antitreponemal antibody tests like the FTA-ABS. In early primary syphilis, the FTA-ABS is positive while the VDRL is negative. In later primary and in tertiary syphilis, both tests are positive. One-third of patients with late disease have a negative VDRL, but the FTA-ABS is generally positive. One percent of those patients with secondary syphilis have a negative VDRL with undiluted serum which becomes positive with serum dilution (prozone phenomenon).

Primary, secondary, or early latent syphilis is treated with 1.2 million units of benzathine penicillin G in each hip or 600,000 units of aqueous procaine penicillin G for 8 days. Erythromycin 500 mg q.i.d. or tetracycline 500 mg q.i.d. for 15 days is recommended for individuals with penicillin allergy. Late neurosyphilis is treated with aqueous procaine penicillin G, 600,000 units daily for 14 days, and late cardiovascular with benzathine penicillin G, 2.4 million units weekly for 3 weeks.

Trichomonas Infections
Found in about 25% of the sexually active population, *Trichomonas vaginalis* may cause a persistent vaginitis with itching and profuse creamy yellow, frothy discharge. In the male, it may be asymptomatic or produce urethritis. Oral metronidazole (Flagyl) is administered, 250 mg t.i.d. for 7 days or in a single 2-gm dose. There is evidence that it is carcinogenic in rodents and should probably not be used unless significant symptomatology is present. It has an antabuse-like action, and alcohol is contraindicated during therapy.

FEVER WITH LYMPHADENOPATHY
Fever lasting for 10 days-2 weeks with generalized lymphadenopathy suggests the following diagnostic possibilities:

1. *Infectious*—Ebstein-Barr (EB) or cytomegoloviruses (CMV), tuberculosis, atypical mycobacteria, syphilis, tularemia, brucellosis, toxoplasmosis, lymphogranuloma venereum.
2. *Neoplastic*—-Hodgkin's and non-Hodgkin's lymphoma, angioimmunoblastic lymphoma.
3. *Connective tissue*—rheumatoid arthritis, juvenile rheumatoid arthritis (JRA), Sjögren's syndrome, SLE, mixed connective tissue disease.
4. *Drug-induced*—phenytoin, para-amino salicylic acid.
5. *Granulomatous diseases*—sarcoidosis, Whipple's, catscratch fever.

These conditions may present with protracted fever, weight loss, general weakness, hepatosplenomegaly, and normal WBC count; lymphocytosis and virocytes are noted in some.

Brucellosis. This is a disease of meat packers, farmers, veterinarians, and livestock producers; *B. abortus* is acquired from cow's milk, *B. suis* from hogs and contact with pork products, *B. melitensis* from goat milk and cheese. Infection may be from ingestion, dermal contact, or inhalation. 7S and 19S antibodies appear during the second or third week of illness and may be identified by an agglutination test. Agglutinins may persist after infection, but a titer greater than 1:100 or presence of 7S globulins suggest activity. *Brucella* may be cultured from blood. The intradermal test indicates past or present infection (like the PPD) and may confuse the diagnosis by stimulating production of 7S globulins. The disease is usually self-limited, but the course is shortened and complications prevented by tetracycline 500 mg q.i.d for 3 weeks.

Tularemia. Hunters, butchers, housewives, and others in rural areas who are exposed to animal carcasses, particularly the wild cottontail rabbit (also squirrels, woodchucks, skunks and other animals), contract this disease. It is transmitted by direct contact or by insect vectors such as ticks. A mucocutaneous primary lesion with regional lymphadenopathy is characteristic. Oculoglandular, gastrointestinal, and typhoidal forms also occur and relate to the portal of entry. Agglutinins appear in the second week but may cross-react with *Brucella;* the organism may be cultured from blood, nodes, or lesions. Treatment requires streptomycin, 0.5-1 gm q12h for 10 days.

Toxoplasmosis. This is transmitted by oocysts from *Toxoplasma gondii,* which is found in many mammals, birds, and reptiles. One percent of domestic cats excrete oocysts in their feces. Serologic evidence of infection is found in 5-30% of individuals aged 10-19, and in 10-67% over 50. The disease is commonly asymptomatic but may produce lymphadenopathy with or without fever and occasionally pneumonitis, myocarditis, pericarditis, hepatitis, polymyositis, or meningoencephalitis. It may be seen in the compromised host with lymphoproliferative or hematologic malignancy, where it usually produces a neurologic syndrome. It may be identified by IgM antibodies that appear and disappear earlier than the IgG antibodies identified by the Sabin-Feldman test.

Cat scratch fever. A small papule or vesicle with eschar and regional adenopathy may first occur up to 6 weeks after the scratch. The major problem is one of differential diagnosis, since the disease is usually mild and self-limited. Skin testing is sensitive and specific, but the antigen must be prepared from infected nodes and is difficult to obtain.

Specific serologic studies are available for other diseases producing fever and adenopathy. The heterophile antibody may be negative in up to 10% of adults with infectious mononucleosis, but IgM antibodies to Ebstein-Barr are present and provide a rapid diagnostic test. Cytomegalic disease and lymphogranuloma venereum (*C. trachomatis*) may be identified by complement fixation, syphilis by VDRL or specific treponema antibody studies (FTA-ABS).

FEVER AND SKIN RASH

Three life-threatening diseases—staphylococcal and meningococcal septicemia and Rocky Mountain spotted fever—may present with fever and a generalized skin rash consisting of macules or papules, vesicles or pustules, or purpura. Skin lesions may be aspirated and reveal staphylococci or meningococci; meningococci may be identified by cerebrospinal and blood culture or with counterimmunoelectrophoresis of body fluids. Microscopic examination of material scraped from the bottom of a surgically opened vesicle and stained with Wright stain (Tzanck preparation) demonstrates multinucleated giant cells in varicella-zoster and herpes simplex but not with vaccinia or variola. Dark field examination could reveal spirochetes, and a punch biopsy could identify rickettsiae with immunofluorescence techniques.

Staphylococcal bacteremia may present as generalized sepsis, but diagnostic confusion exists when phage group 2 strains produce an erythrodermal toxin without cultural evidence of bacteremia. The *scalded skin syndrome* with separation of epidermis from underlying dermis (epidermal necrolysis-Nikolsky's sign) and the *toxic shock syndrome* recently associated with tampon use and the presumed vaginal absorption of toxin may lead to death if untreated. The *Kawasaki disease* mucocutaneous lymph node syndrome, involving children under 2 years of age, may also be caused by elaboration of staphylococcal toxin.

Rocky Mountain spotted fever. This can occur in any area of the United States but should be particularly suspected in south Atlantic and south central states. A tick bite history is given in 75% of cases. The rash is initially macular but becomes maculopapular and hemorrhagic, beginning on the wrists, ankles, palms, and soles and spreading centripetally. Disseminated intravascular coagulation, thrombocytopenia, nonpitting edema, muscle tenderness, hepatosplenomegaly, and neurologic complications are found. Agglutinins to the OX-2 and OX-19 strains of proteus (Weil-Felix reaction) and the complement-fixation test become positive in 8-12 days; the latter is more specific but remains negative if antibiotics are administered. Since mortality is 20-25% without treatment, the diagnosis must be made clinically and therapy initiated. Two regimens appear effective: chloramphenicol, 50 mg/kg or tetracycline 25 mg/kg as a loading dose followed by the same amount in divided doses every 6-8 hours on subsequent days until the patient is afebrile for 24 hours.

Other causes of rash and fever. Other causes are (1) *viral* (measles, rubella, enterovirus, arbovirus, hepatitis, EB and CM viruses, roseola infantum), (2) *bacterial* (gonococcal), (3) *rickettsial* (murine and scrub typhus), (4) *parasitic* (toxoplasmosis and trichinosis), (5) *drug reactions*, and (6) connective tissue diseases.

EXOTIC DISEASES IN A MOBILE POPULATION

The major causes of human illness worldwide are protozoan and viral diseases that are unusual in the United States. The worldwide death rate from malaria, for example, is more than 50% of the total U.S. death rate. Fever, rash, diarrhea, abdominal pain, or neurologic symptoms in anyone with a history of foreign travel should raise the suspicion of an exotic disease. Symptoms within the first month of return are usually due to viral diseases;

protozoan diseases may occur many months or years after exposure.

A small group of protozoan diseases account for most morbidity and mortality. *Malaria* is endemic in a wide band between the Tropics of Cancer and Capricorn (but not limited there), is characterized by rigors, fever, anemia, hepatosplenomegaly, and a relapsing course, and is diagnosed by examination of blood smear or by an indirect fluorescent antibody test. *Amebiasis* occurs in the same distribution but is also endemic in the United States. It may be asymptomatic, may produce a severe intestinal syndrome, and causes a group of extraintestinal syndromes including hepatic, right pleuropulmonary, cardiac, and other abscesses. Diagnosis is made by identification of organisms in stool or tissue, sigmoidoscopy when intestinal syndromes are present, serologic tests such as indirect hemagglutination, and therapeutic trial with agents like chloroquine, metronidazole (Flagyl) and emetine. *Leishmaniasis*, transmitted by the bite of the phlebotomine sandfly, produces a visceral disease (kala azar) characterized by recurrent fever, splenomegaly, pancytopenia, weight loss, and high mortality. The cutaneous form produces destructive mucocutaneous lesions. Diagnosis is made by inspection of stained material or culture from blood, marrow, lymph nodes, or spleen; a complement-fixation test is sensitive but lacks specificity. *Trypanosomiasis* exists as an African form (sleeping sickness) and an American form (Chagas' disease), transmitted by the tsetse fly (African) or assassin and kissing bugs (American). African sleeping sickness presents with high fever, headache, insomnia, inability to concentrate, and an erythema resembling erythema marginatum (especially in Caucasians); a marked elevation of IgM immunoglobulins, anemia, and appearance of trypanosomes in body fluids are diagnostic points. The American trypanosome, *T. cruzei*, produces Chagas' disease and affects more than 7 million people from Chile to Mexico, with a few documented cases in the the southern United States. An acute febrile illness with lymphadenopathy, hepatosplenomegaly, and urticaria with meningoencephalitis and myocarditis may be followed by a chronic form; 10% of people in some populations have Chagas' myocarditis. The Machado-Guerreiro complement-fixation test supplements isolation of the flagella; xenodiagnosis is the exposure of parasite-free insect vectors to patients with suspected illness and then the examination of insect intestinal contents for parasites.

A variety of viral diseases can produce illness in travelers to foreign lands. Arthropod-borne or arboviruses may present with several syndromes:

1. *Fever, malaise, myalgia,* and *headache*—phlebotomus fever, Colorado tick fever, Rift Valley fever.
2. *Fever, malaise, arthralgia,* and *rash*—Chikungunya, O'nyong-nyong fever.
3. *Fever, malaise, lymphadenopathy,* and *rash*—dengue fever (endemic in the tropics and Caribbean, including Puerto Rico and the U.S. Virgin Islands), West Nile fever.
4. *Predominantly CNS involvement*—St. Louis, eastern, and western encephalitides.
5. *Hemorrhagic syndromes*—yellow fever, hemorrhagic chikungunya or dengue (all from *Aedes aegypti* mosquito), tick-borne hemorrhagic fevers (Crimean, Omsk, Kyasanur Forest). Diagnosis is usually by serologic evaluation.

Rickettsial diseases. These are endemic in the United States but may also be seen in travelers from other countries. *Rocky Mountain spotted fever* is limited to the Western hemisphere, with many patients contracting the tick-borne illness in the United States (see page 497). *Murine or endemic typhus* presents with fever, headache, myalgia, and a maculopapular rash. It is a self-limiting disease transmitted by fleas and found in harbor towns or other areas where rats and fleas are common. *Epidemic typhus*, a historically significant disease transmitted by the body louse and still found in areas of poor hygeine, produces a similar but much more severe syndrome. It occurs in the U.S. as *Brill-Zinsser disease* (recrudescent typhus) in individuals who had earlier contracted the epidemic form in areas where prevalent. (Typhus infected 30 million in Poland and Russia between 1915 and 1922, causing 3 million deaths.) *Rickettsialpox* is a mild, nonfatal disease transmitted by mice to humans via a mite bite. An initial skin lesion, covered by a black scab with regional lymphadenopathy, is followed by a papulovesicular rash. First discovered in New York City, it has been reported elsewhere. *Q fever* is the only rickettsial disease without rash; it presents with a febrile syndrome and interstitial pneumonitis.

Agglutinins to proteus OX-19 and OX-2 are found by the tenth day in Rocky Mountain spotted fever and murine typhus; they are positive to OX-19 alone in epidemic typhus; neither agglutinin is found in rickettsialpox or Q fever. Specific antigens for complement-fixation testing are available for all rickettsial diseases; titers become elevated in 2-3 weeks. *Treatment* for all is either tetracycline or chloramphenicol. Treatment is effective, but diagnosis is almost always difficult.

TETANUS

Almost all wounds can produce tetanus; 8% of tetanus during one year developed in the absence of antecedent injury. Tetanus is extremely rare in the immunized individual, so that immunization programs are essential.

Patients need to be given tetanus toxoid following injury only if they have not received a complete three-dose immunization program or a booster injection of tetanus toxoid within the preceding 5 years. This may be extended to 10 years for minor cuts. Toxoid must be administered if a booster has not been previously administered. If the patient has not been immunized or has had less than three doses, human tetanus immune globulin, 250 units I.M., is indicated. If unavailable, equine antitoxin, 3,000-6,000 units, may be used, but sensitivity reactions are common. Treatment may be limited to a toxoid booster in individuals who have received only two previous toxoid injections if wounds are minor and clean. All nonimmunized or inadequately immunized individuals should receive tetanus toxoid in addition to immune globulin to promote active immunity.

ACTIVE IMMUNIZATION OF CHILDREN AND ADULTS

Immunizations presently recommended for individuals living in the United States are given in Table 9-1. Physicians must evaluate the immunization status of their patients and immunize when deficiencies are observered. Additional immunization may be necessary for foreign travel. (See page 502.)

REFERENCES
Unexplained Fever

Vickery DM, Quinnell RK: Fever of unknown origin. An algorithmic approach. JAMA 238:2183, 1977.

Jacoby GA, Swartz MN: Fever of undetermined origin. N Engl J Med 289:1407, 1973.

Williams DM, Krick JA, Remington JS: Pulmonary infection in the compromised host. Part I. Am Rev Respir Dis 114:359, 1976.

Williams DM, Krick JA, Remington JS: Pulmonary infection in the compromised host. Part II. Am Rev Respir Dis 114:593, 1976.

Aduan RP, Fauci AS, Dale DC, Herzberg JH, Wolff SM: Factitious fever and self-induced infection. A report of 32 cases and review of the literature. Ann Intern Med 90:230, 1979.

Petersdorf RG, Beeson PB: Fever of unexplained origin. Medicine 40:1, 1961.

Wolff SM, Fauci AS, Dale DC: Unusual etiologies of fever and their evaluation. Ann Rev Med 26:277, 1975.

Selection of an Antimicrobial Agent

Murray BE, Moellering RC Jr: Antimicrobial agents in pulmonary infections. Med Clin North Am 64:319, 1980.

Guss D, Wang RIH: Therapy of gram-negative meningitis. Drug Therapy (Hosp), December 1977, pp 38-41.

Kaiser AB, McGee ZA: Aminoglycoside therapy of gram-negative bacillary meningitis. N Engl J Med 293:1215, 1975.

Gerding DN, Hall WH, Schierl EA: Antibiotic concentrations in ascitic fluid of patients with ascites and bacterial peritonitis. Ann Intern Med 86:708, 1976.

Center for Disease Control: Legionnaires' disease: diagnosis and management. Ann Intern Med 88:363, 1978.

Hirsch MS, Swartz MN: Antiviral agents. N Engl J Med 302:903, 1980.

Hirsch MS, Swartz MN: Antiviral agents. N Engl J Med 302:949, 1980.

Green GR: Evaluating penicillin hypersensitivity. Drug Therapy, October 1978, pp 155-158.

Cook FV, Farrar WE: Vancomycin revisited. Ann Intern Med 88:813, 1978.

Sanders WE Jr: Rifampin. Ann Intern Med 85:82, 1976.

TABLE 9-1—THE ADEQUATELY IMMUNIZED ADULT*

Immunizing Agent	Ideal Age for Administration	Basic Course
Diphtheria toxoid *B. pertussis* extract Tetanus toxoid	2 mo to 5 yr	0.5 ml at 4 to 6 week intervals for 3 doses
Tetanus toxoid	After 6 yr	0.5 ml each month for 2 doses
Mumps (attenuated, live)	1 yr or older	1 dose
Measles (attenuated, live)	1 yr or older	0.5 ml
Rubella (attenuated, live)	1 yr to puberty	1 dose
Small pox (live vaccinia)	After 6 mo	1 drop
Poliomyelitis	2 mo or older	1 dose at 8 wk intervals for 2 doses; third dose 8 to 12 mo later

* Patients travelling outside of the United States require additional immunoprophylaxis. Since the distribution of disease changes frequently, physicians or patients should call their local public health service office prior to foreign travel.
† Three years is the period of protection following vaccination. Since the disease is rare in the United States, three-year revaccination is frequently not advised. Post-vaccinal encephalitis occurs about 1 per 100,000 vaccinations with a mortality of 10%. It is much less common in individuals who have once been vaccinated.

Wormser GP, Keusch GT: Trimethoprim-sulfamethoxazole in the United States. Ann Intern Med 91:420, 1979.

Young LS, Armstrong D, Blevins A, et al.: Nocardia asteroides infection complicating neoplastic disease. Am J Med 50:356, 1971.

Booster	Efficacy	Side Effects
0.5 ml 1 yr after basic and at age 4 or entry into school	85 to 90%	Local discomfort
0.5 ml 1 yr after basic and every 10 yr thereafter	Almost 100%	Allergic reactions rare
None	95%	Mild induration
None	95%	Mild fever and rash in 15%
None	95%	Mild, local fever, rash, arthralgia
Every 3 yrs†	90%	Fever, malaise, local reaction
1 dose at six mo	95%	None

Walzer PD, Perl DP, Krogstad DJ, et al.: *Pneumocystis carinii* pneumonia in the United States: epidemiologic, diagnostic, and clinical features. Ann Intern Med 80:83, 1974.

Finland M (ed): Gentamicin. J Infect Dis 124(Suppl), December, 1971.

Finland M, Neu H (ed): Tobramycin. J Infect Dis 134(Suppl), August 1976.

Finland M, et al. (ed): Amikacin. J Infect Dis 134(Suppl), November 1976.

Neu HC: The penicillins. I. Overview of microbiology. NY State J Med 77:768, 1977.

Neu HC: The penicillins. II. Overview of pharmacology, toxicology, and clinical use. NY State J Med 77:962, 1977.

Moellering RC Jr, Swartz MN: The newer cephalosporins. N Engl J Med 294:24, 1976.

Moellering RC Jr: Cefamandole—a new member of the cephalosporin family. J Infect Dis, May 1978.

Weinstein L, Schlesinger JJ: Pathoanatomic, pathophysiologic and clinical correlations in endocarditis. N Engl J Med 291:832, 1122, 1974.

Garvey GJ, Neu HC: Infective endocarditis—an evolving disease. Medicine 57:105, 1978.

Menda KB, Gorbach SL: Favorable experience with bacterial endocarditis in heroin addicts. Ann Intern Med 78:25, 1973.

Hoppes WL: Treatment of bacterial endocarditis caused by penicillin-sensitive streptococci. Arch Intern Med 137:1122, 1977.

Bayer AS, Theofilopoulos AN, Tillman D, et al.: Use of circulating immune complex levels in serodifferentiation of endocarditic and nonendocarditic septicemias. Am J Med 66:58, 1979.

Byrd et al.: Treatment of pulmonary tuberculosis. Chest 66:560, 1974.

Doster B, et al.: Ethambutol in the initial treatment of pulmonary tuberculosis. Am Rev Respir Dis 107:177, 1973.

Johnson RF, Wildrick KH: State of the art review. The impact of chemotherapy in the care of patients with tuberculosis. Am Rev Respir Dis 109:636, 1974.

Symposium on Rifampin. Chest 61, volume 6 (special issue), 1972.

Treatment of Unexplained Fever of Bacterial Disease
Due to Unidentified Agents

Schimpff S, Satterle W, Young VM, et al.: Empiric therapy with carbenicillin and gentamicin for febrile patients with cancer and granulocytopenia. N Engl J Med 284:1061, 1971.

Lau WK, Young LS, Black RE, et al.: Comparative efficacy and toxicity of amikacin/carbenicillin versus gentamicin/carbenicillin in leukopenic patients. A randomized prospective trial. Am J Med 62:959, 1977.

Rahal JJ Jr: Antibiotic combinations: the clinical relevance of synergy and antagonism. Medicine (Baltimore) 57:179, 1978.

Esposito AL, Gleckman RA: Vancomycin: a second look. JAMA 238:1756, 1977.

Pollock , Berger SA, Richmond AS, et al.: Amikacin therapy for serious gram-negative infection. JAMA 237:562, 1977.

Local Collections of Pus

Weinstein MP, Iannini PB, Stratton CW, Eickhoff TC: Spontaneous bacterial peritonitis. A review of 28 cases with emphasis on improved survival and factors influencing prognosis. Am J Med 64:592, 1978.

Koehler PR, Moss : Diagnosis of intra-abdominal and pelvic abscesses by computerized tomography. JAMA 244:49, 1980.

Altemeier WA, Culbertson WR, Fullen WD, et al.: Intra-abdominal abscesses. Am J Surg 125:70, 1973.

Haaga JR, Alfidi RJ, Havrilla TR, et al.: CT detection and aspiration of abdominal abscesses. Am J Roentgenol 128:465, 1977.

Brewer NS, MacCarty CS, Wellman WE: Brain abscess: a review of recent experience. Ann Intern Med 82:571, 1975.

Crocker EF, McLaughlin AF, Morris JG, et al.: Technetium brain scanning in the diagnosis and management of cerebral abscess. Am J Med 56:192, 1974.

Sexually Transmitted Diseases

Keiser H, Ruben FL, Wolinsky E, Kushner I: Clinical forms of gonococcal arthritis. N Engl J Med 279:234, 1968.

Jacobs NF Jr: Suppurative gonococcal arthritis. JAMA 235:1357, 1976.

Holmes K, Counts G, Beatty H: Disseminated gonococcal infection. Ann Intern Med 74:979, 1971.

McCormack WM, Alpert S, McComb DE, et al.: Fifteen-month followup study of women infected with *Chlamydia trachomatis.* N Engl J Med 300:123, 1979.

Fever with Lymphadenopathy

Carey RM, Kimball AC, Armstrong D, et al.: Toxoplasmosis: clinical experience in a cancer transplant. Am J Med 54:30, 1973.

Ruskin J, Remington JS: Toxoplasmosis in the compromised host. Ann Intern Med 84:193, 1976.

Fever and Skin Rash

Toxic-shock syndrome—United States. Morbidity and Mortality Weekly Report 29:229, 1980.

Todd J, Fishaut M, Kapral F, Welch T: Toxic-shock syndrome associated with phage-group-I staphylococci. Lancet, November 25, 1978, pp 1116-1118.

Follow-up on toxic-shock syndrome—United States. Morbidity and Mortality Weekly Report 29:297, 1980.

Follow-up on toxic-shock syndrome. Morbidity and Mortality Weekly Report 29:441, 1980.

Barrett-Connor E: Latent and chronic infections imported from Southeast Asia. JAMA 239:1901, 1978.

Kean BH, Reilly PC Jr: Malaria—the mime: recent lessons from a group of civilian travellers. Am J Med 61:159, 1976.

Krogstad DJ, Spencer HC Jr, Healy SR: Current concepts in parasitology. Amebiasis. N Engl J Med 298:262, 1978.

Sanford JP: Arbovirus infections. In Isselbacher KJ, Adams RD, Braunwald E, Petersdorf RG, Wilson JD (eds): Principles of Internal Medicine, 9th ed. New York McGraw-Hill, 1980, pp 823-839.

10

The Nervous System

THE COMATOSE PATIENT

Coma implies an absence of response to external stimuli. The varying degrees of coma are best documented by listing the clinical signs, as these are more definitive than abstractions such as "semicoma," etc. Normal consciousness requires the integrated action of the ascending reticular activating system (ARAS) and the cerebral hemispheres: interruption of the former and diffuse disease of the latter is normally required for loss of consciousness.

Mechanisms Producing Coma

Space-occupying lesions in the supratentorial compartment. These only rarely cause enough destruction of the cerebral cortex to result in coma. Invariably, space-occupying lesions in this area produce loss of consciousness by herniation through the tentorial notch with compression of the diencephalon and brain stem. Initially, there are localizing signs referrable to the site of the lesion in one of the hemispheres, (headache, aphasia, etc.) but as distal pressure effects and herniation occur, the patient develops brain-stem signs, usually in a sequential manner rostral to caudal as coma develops.

Lesions in the subtentorial compartment. Such lesions directly compress or destroy the ARAS in the upper brain stem. They reveal themselves with asymmetrical involvement of pupillary and vestibular reflexes as well as long tract signs.

Metabolic derangements. Both cortical and brain stem abnormalities are produced, so that coma is frequently preceded by delirium or extrapyramidal abnormalities such as the flapping tremor (asterixis) of liver failure (the basal ganglia seem particularly sensitive to metabolic abnormalities). In many patients, however, loss of higher functions of intellect may be more evident. Pupillary reflexes are usually preserved.

1. *Mechanical causes:* Vascular lesions, hemorrhage (cerebral, cerebellar, pontine, subarachnoid), infarction (cerebral, brain stem), hematoma (epidural, subdural), abscess (cerebral, cerebellar), tumor (supratentorial, subtentorial), infections (meningitis, encephalitis), trauma (concussion, subdural hematoma).

2. *Metabolic abnormalities:* Anoxia (respiratory failure, severe anemia, carbon monoxide poisoning, methemoglobinemia), ischemia (cardiac factors—Stokes-Adams, etc., vascular factors—DIC, SLE), CO_2 narcosis in respiratory failure, hypoglycemia, uremic coma, hepatic coma, diabetes (hyperosmolar coma, ketoacidosis), thyroid disease (myxedema coma), adrenal failure (Addisonian crisis), nutritional deficiency (especially thiamine in alcoholics).

3. *Postictal coma:* Look for evidence of seizure—tongue biting, incontinence, etc.

4. *Drug-induced coma:* Barbiturates, alcohol, tranquilizers, opiates, antidepressants, anticholinergics, bromides, etc.

Management

Preservation of brain perfusion must be assured by maintenance of a patent airway to permit mechanical ventilation and prevent aspiration and by measures designed to augment cardiac output and peripheral circulation. An intravenous line should be inserted and blood drawn for baseline biochemical, hematologic, and toxicologic determinations. Dextrose, 50 ml of a 50% solution, should be administered if there is any chance of hypoglycemia.

This solution is nontoxic, but a baseline glucose determination must be obtained to evaluate any effects of therapy. Carbohydrate administration can precipitate Wernicke's encephalopathy so that thiamine, 50 mg I.M., should be given if there appears to be a history of alcoholism. Diagnosis is critical to management; certain historical clues from friends or family may guide therapy: (1) personality change suggesting space-occupying lesion, (2) seizures, (3) use of drugs of any type, and (4) illnesses such as diabetes or heart disease.

The neurologic examination should emphasize cause and attempt localization; the skull must be carefully evaluated for evidence of trauma. Mydriatics should not be administered for retinal visualization, because pupillary changes are important clues to diagnosis. Unilateral miosis, ptosis, enophthalmos, and reduced sweating suggest a Horner's syndrome due to a central lesion. Large fixed pupils with spontaneous constriction and dilatation suggest tectal lesions, fixed midposition pupils suggest midbrain lesions with damage to both sympathetic and parasympathetic fibers, pontine (and also midbrain) lesions may produce miotic pupils that react but slightly to light. Metabolic brain disease and drug overdose may make pupillary reflexes sluggish but does not obliterate them. Exceptions are glutethimide (Doriden), which produces medium-sized or large unreactive pupils, and heroin or morphine, which produces pinpoint pupils with reduced light reflex. Oculocephalic and oculovestibular reflexes also assist in localization; loss of movement of eyes conjugately to opposite side when the head is briskly turned (doll's eye movements) indicates brain-stem disease with loss of cortical integration.

In many respects, computed tomography has revolutionized the diagnosis of coma and headache. It does not replace a careful clinical evaluation and must be interpreted in conjunction with historical and other information. *Lumbar puncture* is contraindicated in the presence of increased intracranial pressure because of the danger of fatal herniation; a computed tomographic examination *before* lumbar puncture is a useful way of identifying space-occupying lesions and avoiding potential herniation. Ex-

amination of cerebrospinal fluid is mandatory, however, if meningitis is suspected as a cause for coma. Precautions include the
use of a sharp #20 needle, prior filling of the manometer with
normal saline, and refraining from dynamic studies.

HEADACHE

Headache may arise from extracranial or intracranial pain-sensitive structures. All extracranial structures, especially skin, muscle,
and arteries, are pain-sensitive; the venous sinuses, arteries at the
base of the brain, the basal dura, and the trigeminal, facial,
glossopharyngeal, vagal, and first three cervical nerves are pain-
sensitive intracranial structures.

Most headaches are caused by stimulation of extracranial
areas.

Muscle contraction headaches. These are common, tend to be
constant, and are occipital or encircle the entire head. They have
variable but limited duration and are found in association with
stress, emotion, and at times with faulty posture. Heat, aspirin,
muscle relaxants, and reassurance are usually adequate treatment.

Vascular headaches. There are two types, migraine and cluster.
Migraine is a genetically determined lability of cranial blood
vessels, perhaps related to increased sensitivity to catecholamines,
serotonin, bradykinin, or other vasoactive substances. The syndrome begins with a vasoconstrictor phase that may produce
visual scotomata, hemianopsia, sensory loss, speech disturbances,
vertigo, ataxia, or hemiplegia. These phenomena are transient
but an obvious source of anxiety, and are soon replaced by the
vasodilator phase, which produces the typical headache. The
headache is usually throbbing, unilateral, and located in the
temporal area or elsewhere in the head including the face and
neck. Photophobia, nausea, vomiting, and general malaise are
common. The severity and duration vary; headaches are frequently intense enough to require bed rest in a dark and quiet
room.

The precise pathogenesis is not known, but precipitation by
emotional stress, foods containing tyramine or phenylethylamine,
and use of reserpine, and relief by a serotonin antagonist,

methysergide, implicate serotonin. A metabolite, 5-HIAA as well as catecholamine metabolites (VMA), may be found in the urine of some patients during a migraine attack.

The most effective therapy for the individual attack is ergotamine tartrate. The earlier it is given, the more efficient its result. It may be given by almost any route, depending on the intensity of the attack and the history of prior effect. Minor analgesics may also be used; occasionally opiates or steroids are necessary. Methysergide, propranolol, and cyproheptadine may prevent attacks; fibroproliferation has been seen with methysergide limiting its use.

Cluster or "histamine" headaches differ from migraine in that they: (1) more commonly affect males and older individuals, (2) affect the eye and nasal areas where they also produce lacrimation, nasal stuffiness, and ipsilateral Horner's syndrome, (3) are severe and rapidly reach maximum severity, (4) frequently occur at night and may awaken the patient from sleep, (5) occur in clusters with symptom-free intervals, (6) do not exhibit neurologic defects (except for Horner's syndrome), nausea, vomiting, (7) require little psychologic management, and (8) do not have serotonic abnormalities.

Like migraine, cluster headaches respond to ergotamine. Since the attacks are predictable it may be given prophylactically an hour before the anticipated occurrence. Methysergide or corticosteroids may occasionally be necessary.

Lumbar puncture headache. Caused by traction on intracranial structures, this is a self-limiting condition, is probably due to lowering of pressure, and is exacerbated by standing and leakage of fluid at the site of puncture. The headache is generally occipital and throbbing, comes on soon after the procedure, lasts a few hours but occasionally may last for a number of weeks. It responds to lying down, staying in bed for 24 hours after lumbar puncture, and the precautions mentioned above.

Temporal arteritis. This may involve any cranial vessel, occurs in older individuals, and is a potentially treatable cause of blindness. There may be tenderness over the involved temporal artery (but not always), and a high sedimentation rate is usual. Biopsy of the affected vessel will show giant cell arteritis; malaise, weight loss, and fever may also be present. There is a good response to corticosteroids.

Trigeminal neuralgia. (Tic Douloureux). Severe jabs of pain occur in one of the divisions of the trigeminal nerve, usually the maxillary or mandibular division. The duration of the pain is variable, but usually brief. A trigger zone may be stimulated by shaving, brushing the teeth, or eating. Spontaneous recovery is the norm, but it may recur. In the primary (idiopathic) variety, no cause is found and neurologic exam is normal. The presence of laboratory or neurologic abnormalities suggests an underlying cause, such as cerebellopontine angle tumor or multiple sclerosis. The idiopathic variety usually responds to carbamazepine or phenytoin, although surgical section of the nerve root proximal to the ganglion may be necessary.

Brain tumors. These are not a common cause for headache, although patients frequently consider this possiblity when they experience severe pain. The pain is usually described as being a dull ache and not throbbing. It tends to be worse in the morning and is increased by coughing, laughing, or straining. It may be associated with nausea and vomiting.

Cerebral aneurysm. Headache of sudden onset may be accompanied by localizing sensory or motor disturbances. Subarachnoid hemorrhage produces sudden severe occipital headache.

NEUROLOGIC INFECTIONS

Bacterial Infections

MENINGITIS

Three agents account for more than 80% of bacterial meningitis: (1) pneumococcus, (2) influenza bacillus, and (3) meningococcus. All three infections have their highest incidence in spring and winter. The pneumococcus, which occurs in both children and older adults, accounts for the majority of cases of bacterial meningitis in adults. Meningococcal meningitis, which may occur in epidemics in populations living closely together (military personnel in barracks), has a peak incidence in adolescence and young adulthood. *H. influenzae* infections rarely occur beyond adolescence but may cause meningitis in adult patients with head trauma or compromised immunologic defenses. Of increasing importance as a cause of meningitis is *Listeria monocytogenes*, a gram-positive rod. In a patient with recurrent meningitis, pneumococcus is the most common cause. The occurrence of pneumococcal meningitis suggests an anatomic defect, usually around the cribiform plate. Neurosurgical repair of defects rather than prolonged antibiotic prophylaxis is recommended. Special attention should be made initially and after recovery for the presence of CSF rhinorrhea. In a patient with recurrent bacterial meningitis, computed tomography, polytomography, and radionuclide scanning (radioiodine labelled serum albumin—RISA) are useful in localizing the defect.

Meningitis usually occurs in association with pneumonia, bacteremia, or from an ear infection in the paranasal sinuses or middle ear. Meningitis most commonly occurs in infants when immunologic defense mechanisms are immature and in adults with compromised immune systems (diseases of the reticuloendothelial system or iatrogenic immunosuppression). Patients with diabetes, sickle cell anemia, and cirrhosis are also at risk. The dura and arachnoid space are natural barriers to disease. When the barrier is disrupted (trauma, lumbar puncture) there is increased risk of meningitis.

Patients present with headache, fever, and stiff neck. Symptoms of a middle ear or respiratory infection often precede the principal symptoms. Cerebritis or elevated cerebral spinal fluid pressure may produce lethergy, stupor and coma, seizures, cranial nerve palsies, and other focal neurologic findings.

Physical findings include nuchal rigidity with flexion of the head with Kernig's and Brudzinski's signs in adult patients. These latter signs of meningeal irritation may be absent in elderly patients and infants or masked in patients partially treated with antibiotics.

Although clinical features and findings are generally the same in all forms of meningitis, certain circumstances suggest specific bacteria. Meningitis that develops following a penetrating wound of the skull or spine is probably due to a mixed infection, the most common agents being *Staphylococcus* and gram-negative organisms such as *Proteus, E. coli,* and *Pseudomonas.* If the patient has a closed head injury, meningitis is probably pneumococcal, as is meningitis associated with chronic otitis, mastoiditis, or sinusitis. Streptococcal infections may occasionally account for meningitis in the latter cases. Meningococcal infections often present with a petechial or purpuric skin rash or a shocklike state. Opportunistic bacteria, such as *E. coli, Pseudomonas, Listeria,* and *Staphylococcus,* will cause infection in patients with leukemia or lymphoma or those treated with immunosuppressant drugs. If the infection is hospital-acquired, it is probably due to gram-negative bacilli. *Staphylococcus* or gram-negative rods account for the majority of cases of meningitis in patients who have a neurosurgical procedure or an infected ventriculoatrial shunt.

Mortality depends on several features, including the status of the patient on admission and the duration of the illness before diagnosis and institution of treatment. Poor prognostic features include advanced age, coma, cerebral edema, and delay in instituting treatment. Mortality rates approach 20% for pneumococcus, 10-15% for meningococcus, and 5% for *H. influenzae.*

LABORATORY EXAMINATION
The diagnosis of meningitis is made by examination of the cerebral spinal fluid (CSF) with cell count, differential, smear, Gram stain, and culture. The spinal fluid may appear normal in early meningitis, but becomes purulent with thousands of polymorphonuclear cells, elevated protein concentration, and low glucose concentration. A blood sugar should always be drawn at the same time as the lumbar puncture. A CSF sugar below 60% of the blood sugar is abnormal. Cultures of CSF should be done directly from the lumbar puncture needle. This is especially important in recovering meningococcus. Cultures for anaerobes, tuberculosis, and fungi should also be done routinely.

Bacterial typing of CSF sediment is done with Quelling antisera, immunofluorescent staining, or countercurrent immunoelectrophoresis (CIE). CIE will detect bacterial polysaccharide antigens in CSF and in concentrated urine. CIE is especially useful in detecting the antigens of *H. influenzae* type b, *S. pneumoniae, N. meningitidis, E. coli,* and the meningococcus (except group B). The greatest use of CIE is in detecting hemophilus meningitis, particularly if the patient has had prior antibiotic therapy. Results of a CIE are usually available in a few hours. Blood cultures and radiographs of the chest, sinuses, and mastoids are also indicated.

TREATMENT
Most otherwise healthy patients have meningitis caused by gram-positive organisms; treatment is with penicillin (penicillin G, 12-20 million units I.V. daily in 4-6 divided doses). If the CSF examination indicates gram-negative organisms, the treatment of choice is chloramphenicol and gentamicin. Any alteration of therapy will depend on clinical response and results of culture and sensitivity. Treatment of gram-negative infections should be for a minimum of 3 weeks. Uncomplicated pneumococcal or meningococcal infections should be treated for 10 days (1 week without fever).

Tuberculous Meningitis
Evidence of active infection in other organs is often minimal, but tuberculous meningitis generally occurs with either pulmonary or genitourinary tuberculosis. Meningitis presenting with a subacute or chronic picture suggests either fungal or tuberculous mening-itis. Nuchal rigidity, confusion and low-grade fever, headache, malaise, and vomiting develop over a course of 2-4 weeks. Suppurative infection of the basilar meninges, occlusive arteritis of vessels at the base of the brain, cranial nerve palsies, commu-nicating hydrocephalus, and multifocal signs from cerebral in-farction suggest tuberculous meningitis. The CSF pressure is elevated, and the CSF fluids contain 25-200 cells per cu ml, which are predominantly lymphocytes. The protein concentration is generally over 250 mg/dl. The CSF fluid should be stained for acid-fast bacilli. The CSF sugar will be low but not as depressed as in pyogenic meningitis.

Triple antibiotic therapy is indicated and consists of isoniazid 300 mg p.o. per day, streptomycin 1 gm p.o. per day, and ethambutol 25 mg/kg p.o. per day. After 3 months, streptomycin is reduced to twice weekly doses. The entire regimen is continued for 18-24 months. To prevent peripheral neuropathy, pyridoxine is given in a dose of 100 mg p.o. per day.

HEAT SYNDROMES

Young individuals exercising vigorously in hot environments become salt and water depleted and may develop muscle or *heat cramps*; rarely, cramps in the abdominal musculature may simulate an acute abdomen. The hematocrit is elevated, sodium and chloride concentrations reduced. Treatment is the oral replacement of salt and water.

Failure of the cardiovascular system to keep pace with the increased requirements produced by exposure to high temperatures produces *heat exhaustion*. It occurs commonly in the adult and produces weakness, vertigo, headache, dizziness, anorexia, nausea, and vomiting. The skin is clammy and may show peripheral cyanosis. Rest in a cool environment is usually sufficient treatment.

Heat stroke (or more properly *heat pyrexia*, since fever is the hallmark of the condition) occurs in the elderly individual with diminished circulation or in the younger person engaging in extremely vigorous activity during periods of great heat (roofers, or soldiers during forced marches, for example). It is more frequent in diabetics and alcoholics and in individuals taking diuretics, antihypertensive drugs, tranquilizers, and atropine-like agents. A hot and dry skin due to the failure of sweating, CNS symptoms, and a temperature greater than 106° rectally are diagnostic. Serious neurologic signs including a decorticate-like appearance are seen, but reverse with immediate and vigorous cooling. Myocardial necrosis, coagulation disturbances, particularly intravascular coagulation, and hepatic damage with jaundice have been reported.

Treatment is drastic but effective. Immersion in an ice water bath reduces temperature quickly and does not produce cutaneous vasoconstriction. Skin massage improves the redistribution of cooled blood, and phenothiazines may be given to reduce shivering (even though phenothiazines themselves may predispose to the condition). Fluids should be carefully administered, with central venous pressure monitoring to avoid overhydration or heart failure; fluid deficits are ordinarily modest.

Stroke

Cerebrovascular stroke is caused by hemorrhage, thrombosis, or embolism and may be categorized by its evolutionary pattern: (1) transient ischemic attack (TIA), (2) stroke in evolution, and (3) completed stroke.

Transient Ischemic Attack. The deficit lasts less than 24 hours and is frequently less than 2 hours, so that symptoms may disappear before medical advice is obtained. TIA may involve either the middle cerebral or vertebrobasilar arterial systems. Separation is important since the two types differ in pathogenesis and in prognosis. *Carotid-middle cerebral TIA* is thought to be more frequently embolic, with platelet or cholesterol emboli arising from atheromatous plaques at the origin of the internal carotid. Altered coagulability due to thrombocytosis, polycythemia, or macroglobulinemia, and cardiac emboli due to SBE or atrial myxoma must also be considered. Prolapsing mitral valve may be a factor, especially in younger patients. Such patients are at high risk of developing a completed stroke (up to 20% within the first 4 weeks). Amaurosis fugax, aphasia, or hemiplegia are more frequent symptoms.

Vertebrobasilar TIA. This may produce drop attacks, vertigo, ataxia, tinnitus, diplopia, or bilateral visual loss. These are frequently hemodynamic (arrhythmias, cervical bony disease or arterial narrowing) and less commonly due to emboli. In the *subclavian steal syndrome*, retrograde flow to the arm at the expense of the vertebral circulation occurs when there is a constriction proximal to the origin of the vertebral artery. Attacks are provoked by exercising the arms. Vertebrobasilar TIAs are much less likely to result in completed stroke than the carotid variety.

Investigation. Arteriography, radionucleotide scanning (measurement of blood flow using rapid sequence scintigraphy) and cardiac studies such as echocardiography or Holter monitoring may be involved. There is general agreement that these studies should be undertaken where neurologic skills are readily available for prompt intervention.

Management involves anticoagulation, especially during the initial high-risk period. Platelet modification with aspirin, sulfinpyrazone, and dipyridamole is under study; carotid endarterectomy is best used for unilateral localized disease of the proximal internal carotid. Conservative management is indicated with vertebrobasilar disease, since surgical approaches are usually ineffective.

ALCOHOL AND DISEASE

Besides the obvious effects of alcohol on social and family life, excessive quantities of alcohol affect the entire body. A measurable deterioration of concentration and coordination occurs with even small quantities of alcohol. With larger quantities, the classic picture of drunkenness with its well-known clinical and social picture emerges. Alcoholism, the chronic overconsumption of ethanol, is a very common disorder affecting 5-10% of the average population. It has important psychologic, psychiatric, and social as well as medical implications.

Alcohol is well absorbed in an unaltered state from the stomach and small intestine. The removal of alcohol from the system depends principally on hepatic oxidation by the enzyme alcohol dehydrogenase to form acetaldehyde and subsequent metabolism by acetyl-coenzyme A to form carbon dioxide and water; less than 10% is eliminated through the lungs and kidneys. This oxidization of alcohol proceeds at a constant rate independent of the serum levels; the rate is accelerated in regular drinkers.

The most common deleterious effects of alcohol are on the gut, liver and pancreas, central and peripheral nervous system, and the myocardium.

Alcohol increases the secretion of gastrin, thereby increasing acid production by the stomach. This, together with its effect on the mucosal barrier, results in the frequent complication of *alcoholic gastritis*. There is a much higher incidence of both gastric and duodenal *ulcers* in alcoholics, and vigorous vomiting can sometimes produce serious hemorrhage with laceration of the gastroesophageal junction (*Mallory-Weiss syndrome*). Alcohol also seriously interferes with the absorption of various nutrients such as the B vitamins, folic acid, and amino acids. This *malabsorption* is complicated by the poor dietary habits of chronic alcoholics. The effects on the liver are both acute and chronic. Acute poisoning of the liver with alcohol produces fatty infiltration and *alcoholic hepatitis*, both of which are reversible if drinking is discontinued. It is generally agreed that a combination of alcoholic excess and poor nutrition contribute to the development of alcoholic hepatitis. Repeated attacks of alcoholic hepatitis are an important predisposing factor to the chronic liver problem of *cirrhosis*. An important effect of alcohol on the liver is the blocking of gluconeogenesis, with resultant *hypoglycemia*. Acute and chronic *pancreatitis* are important causes of abdominal pain in the alcoholic. This can sometimes result in *steatorrhea*.

Chronic alcohol excess has *hematologic effects*, with global depression of the bone marrow, affecting red cell, white cell, and platelet production and function.

Alcohol has an important effect on the *metabolism of various drugs*, which can seriously alter the control of anticoagulants and hypoglycemic agents. Recent work has highlighted the beneficial effect of moderate alcohol intake on the levels of high-density lipoprotein (HDL), with possible benefits in the prevention of degenerative vascular disease.

The effects of alcohol on the nervous system range from the acute phenomenon of alcoholic intoxication, the important withdrawal syndromes, and the chronic neurologic syndromes. *Withdrawal syndrome* in its mildest forms may be manifested by the nausea and vomiting on the morning following an alcoholic debauch. On such occasions, a moderate degree of tremulousness and irritability is present. It is well known that alcohol itself can relieve such symptoms, as they are the mildest manifestations of withdrawal syndrome. With larger quantities of alcohol intake over a longer period, more serious withdrawal symptoms develop. These include marked tremulousness with "the shakes," auditory and visual hallucinations, or withdrawal seizures ("rum fits"). *Withdrawal seizures* produce epilepsy of the grand mal variety and occur in the early withdrawal phase, having their maximal incidence about 12-24 hours after discontinuation of drinking. The seizures are usually single, though a number may occur in quick sequence and status epilepticus may sometimes develop. Some of these patients go on to develop delirium tremens. Rum fits are an acute withdrawal phase phenomenon and are usually self-limiting. The EEG is abnormal during the seizures, but becomes normal between episodes. The seizures are invariably the grand mal type, and a focal type seizure should alert one to the presence of localized brain disease such as might occur following a head injury in the alcoholic patient. (Note that small amounts of alcohol can induce seizures in patients with chronic idiopathic epilepsy, so that alcohol use is generally not permitted.) Rum fits are generally self-limiting and do not require specific anticonvulsive therapy. Where they are persistent, phenobarbital or other anticonvulsant therapy may be required. The long-term use of anticonvulsants is not indicated, as alcohol is the provoking factor and treatment of that problem is more pertinent.

Delirium tremens is one of the most serious and potentially fatal manifestations of alcoholic withdrawal. The mortality is about 10%. In this condition, the patient is totally confused with frightening hallucinations, insomnia, and severe tremulousness. There is gross overactivity of the autonomic nervous system with tachycardia, profuse sweating, and dilated pupils. These patients are generally incontinent. It is important to rule out intercurrent infections such as aspiration pneumonia and gram-negative sepsis, as well as the coexistence of subdural hematoma and cerebral lacerations. The delirium may subside after a very short period or may have a protracted course, depending on the duration and severity of alcoholic excess. Hyperthermia and circulatory collapse may cause death. Therapy includes close attention to fluid and electrolyte balance and sedation usually using either paraldahyde, phenobarbital, chloradiazepoxide (Librium), or diazepam (Valium). The phenothiazines are not beneficial because of their seizure-provoking potential. Other neurologic complications of chronic alcoholism include cerebellar degeneration, cerebral atrophy, and central pontine myelinolysis. The latter condition may be asymptomatic, or it may produce a variety of neurologic syndromes including coma, quadriplegia, or pseudobulbar palsy. Peripheral neuropathy and a nonspecific alcoholic myopathy are other important complications.

Wernicke's syndrome and Korsakoff's psychosis are believed to be due to the severe B vitamin deficiency, particularly thiamine, seen in alcoholics. *Wernicke's syndrome* is characterized by abnormalities of conjugate gaze, horizontal and vertical nystagmus, occasional ptosis, bilateral VIth nerve paralysis, and truncal ataxia affecting gait and the ability to stand unaided. Rarely, there is complete paralysis of extraocular movement. *Korsakoff's psychosis* consists of amnesia with confabulation, which may not become apparent until the patient is able to speak. Tachycardia and high output failure, further evidence of thiamine deficiency, are frequently present. Infection or cardiovascular collapse contribute to the mortality rate of about 10%. Management includes the immediate administration of thiamine and the withholding of glucose solutions, which may exacerbate the thiamine deficiency until this vitamin has been given. Particular caution should be exercised in administering dextrose solutions to alcoholic patients; B vitamins should always be given first. Full recovery, especially of the amnestic syndrome, may take many months, and in some a degree of impairment is permanent.

Other important complications of chronic alcoholism include cardiomyopathy and the fetal alcohol syndrome. It has for a long time been known that the offspring of chronic alcoholic mothers tend to be of lower birth weight than other children. Recently, a wide-ranging group of abnormalities have been listed, including deformities of the head and neck and cardiac abnormalities.

DRUG OVERDOSE

Accidental and suicidal drug overdose is a very common problem. Every effort should be made to obtain the name and quantity of the substance involved. This facilitates management and the obtaining of information from the local poison control center. Multiple drugs are frequently involved.

General principles of management involve symptomatic and support therapy, prevention of further absorption of the compound, hastening and removal of the compound from the body, and specific antidotes. Supportive therapy should obviously begin immediately, and one should not delay this while trying to ascertain the exact nature and quantity of the substance involved.

General supportive measures involve the maintenance of a clear airway, adequate respiration, and support of the cardiovascular system. Arterial blood gases should be obtained to ascertain the adequacy of respiration. When the patient is comatose and ventilatory function is inadequate, a cuffed endotracheal tube should be inserted before lavage. Where perfusion is inadequate, the addition of intravenous volume expanders or of vasoactive drugs may be necessary. (A number of agents, including the phenothiazines and the tricyclic antidepressants, can produce alpha sympathetic blockade, which is aggravated by the use of dopamine. Levarterenol is the agent of choice in these cases.) Tachyarrhythmias are particularly common in overdoses of the tricyclic antidepressants, and these will require cardiac monitoring and prompt treatment.

If the patient is conscious, vomiting may be induced using ipecac; vomiting usually occurs after a delay of about 15 minutes. The dose is 15-30 ml of syrup of ipecac accompanied by large volumes of water. Vomiting should not be induced if the patient is unconscious, if the gag reflex is absent, or if the substance is a strong acid, alkali, or petroleum product. Gastric lavage using a large nasogastric tube produces excellent results. This should be preceded by the institution of a cuffed endotracheal tube if the patient is unconscious. Absorption from the gut may also be decreased by the administration of charcoal. Ten to 40 gm of activated charcoal should be administered in 100-200 ml of water after the stomach has been emptied of earlier contents. In the case of substances excreted by the kidneys, a forced diuresis using large volumes of fluids or the administration of diuretics may be very useful. The alkalinization of the urine greatly increases the loss of salicylates and phenobarbital; the clearance of salicylate, for example, may be increased 10-20 fold by keeping the urine pH between 7 and 8. Weak organic acids such as salicylate and phenobarbital diffuse passively back out of the tubular fluid only in their ionized forms. Alteration of the pH keeps them in the ionized form and prevents their reabsorption. Dialysis, especially hemodialysis, is very effective for the removal of many agents. Recently, the utilization of charcoal hemoperfusion, whereby the blood is made to come in contact with activated charcoal, has produced extremely good results and will become increasingly utilized.

The use of specific antidotes where these are available produces very impressive results. In the case of narcotic overdose, however, one has to guard against development of an acute withdrawal syndrome when naloxone is given.

Table 10-1 describes manifestations and management of some of the more common drugs involved in overdose.

SEIZURE DISORDERS

Epilepsy, one of the most common problems in neurology, is a symptomatic expression of neurologic malfunctioning rather than a disease. Approximately 0.5% of the population have recurrent episodes, while many others have single convulsive attacks (febrile episode in children). Seizure may be associated with any brain disease, tumor, or injury. If no definitive pathology is identified, the condition is called idiopathic epilepsy. There is a prevalence rate of seizures three times greater among close relatives of patients with idiopathic epilepsy than in the general population.

A seizure is the result of synchronous depolarization of a neuron group. Abnormalities (defective functioning of glial cells, disturbances in synaptic transmission, neuronal membrane abnormalities) have been suggested as causing the paroxysmal depolarization that leads to a clinical seizure. Seizures will be focal if the area of neuronal hyperexcitability remains localized, or generalized if there is a massive synchronous discharge in the cortex with spread to the thalamus and brain stem. A deficiency of an inhibitory transmitter (a-aminobutyric acid) or an overabundance of excitatory transmitter are suggested but yet unproved theories for a biochemical explanation of seizures. Evi-

TABLE 10-1—DRUG OVERDOSE

Drug	Manifestations
Acetyl salicylic acid (aspirin)	Vomiting, tinnitus, diaphoresis, hyperpnea; respiratory—alkalosis; pyrexia, hypoglycemia, hypokalemia; bleeding; acidosis (children)
Acetaminophen (Tylenol)	Few early signs Liver necrosis after 3-6 days
Amphetamines	Convulsions, coma, pyrexia; arrhythmias, vascular collapse, coagulopathy, renal failure, abdominal cramps
Barbiturates	Sedation—coma, respiratory depression, diminished reflexes, pulmonary edema, hypotension, reactive pupils
Benzodiazepines (Valium, Librium, Dalmane)	Drowsiness, coma, ataxia, hypotension
Glutethimide (Doriden)	Coma, hypothermia, fever; absent reflexes, dilated pupils, papilledema
Methaqualone (Quaalude)	Delerium, coma, hyperreflexia, convulsions, pulmonary edema, vomiting, increased salivation
Methyprylon (Noludar)	Confusion—coma, constricted pupils, apnea, hypotension

Management	Remarks
Lavage, alkaline diuresis, vitamin K, charcoal hemoperfusion in severe cases	Frequent—worse in children
Early n-acetyl cysteine hemodialysis, charcoal hemoperfusion	Fatal dose more than 12 gm
Symptomatic, lavage, sedation, acidify urine, dialysis	Delayed gastric emptying, so lavage is worthwhile
Supportive, lavage, alkaline diuresis for long-acting, dialysis, charcoal hemoperfusion	Common. Fatality higher with long-acting barbiturates
Symptomatic, levarterenol for hypotension (rarely)	Generally nonfatal
Lavage with alkaline solution, support BP—try steroids, dialysis	More than 10 gm may be fatal. Watch for sudden apnea during lavage
Support, lavage, charcoal hemoperfusion	More than 8 gm may be fatal
Supportive, levarterenol for hypotension, hemodialysis	Convulsions may occur during recovery

TABLE 10-1—DRUG OVERDOSE (Cont'd)

Drug	Manifestations
Narcotics (heroin, methadone, meperidine [Demerol], Darvon)	Respiratory depression, stupor—coma, flaccidity, meiosis, bradycardia, hypotension
Phenothiazines (Thorazine, Compazine, etc.)	Confusion, stupor, coma, convulsions, increased reflexes, dyskinesias (extrapyramidal), tachycardia, hypotension
Tricyclic antidepressants (Tofranil, Sinequan, Elavil)	Drowsy—coma, dilated pupils, increased reflexes, convulsions, clonic/athetoid movements, respiratory depression, arrhythmias—hypotension, vomiting

dence of focal onset of the seizure is helpful in localizing and characterizing lesions.

The generalized convulsion is the most common type of convulsive disorder and includes tonic-clonic (grand mal), absence (petit mal), akinetic (drop attacks), and myoclonic episodes. Generally, idiopathic epilepsy begins in childhood. If the onset of seizures is in adult life or if there is a change in the pattern or loss of seizure control, a search for focal brain disease is imperative.

Grand mal seizures are characterized by loss of consciousness, tonic followed by clonic movements of muscles, and occasional sphincteric incontinence. Once the seizure activity ceases, the patient remains comatose for several minutes. As the patient arouses, mental confusion, drowsiness, and headache (postictal depression of cerebral functions) become evident.

Petit mal or absence seizures begin between age 4 and adoles-

Management	Remarks
Airway/ventilatory, Naloxone (may produce acute withdrawal syndrome)	Look for associated infections—endocarditis, septicemia, etc.
Supportive, levarterenol (Levophed). See text—for hypotension. Diphenhydramine for extrapyramidal signs, phenytoin for seizures	Emesis may be dangerous with dystonia of head/neck
Lavage (repeat), charcoal slurry, cardiac monitor, Levophed for hypotension, physostigmine slowly (1-3 mg I.V.)	Dialysis poor—charcoal hemoperfusion better; blood levels poor guide

cence, and are characterized by brief losses of awareness with little or no motor activity. The loss of consciousness lasts a few seconds and may be accompanied by staring or blinking episodes. The EEG shows a three-per-second spike-and-wave pattern. Akinetic (drop attacks) are characterized by a brief loss of consciousness and postural muscle tone.

Myoclonic seizures are seen at certain stages of degenerative and metabolic brain disease. They are manifested by a loss of consciousness, stiffening, and clonic movements of the limbs. Often evoked by sensory stimuli, these seizures may be focal so that the tonic-clonic spasm may involve only one side of the body. These seizures may precede grand mal episodes.

Partial convulsive disorders include psychomotor epilepsy and localized motor seizures. Psychomotor epilepsy, the most frequent type of focal seizure pattern, may be preceded by an aura, which has the form of an hallucination or perceptual illusion. Heughlings Jackson coined the term "dreamy state" to describe these psychic disturbances. Behavior patterns may be bizzare; if convulsive movements are present, they usually consist of chewing, smacking and licking of lips, tonic spasms of limbs, and head turning.

The other major type of partial seizure disorders are localized motor seizures which accompany frontal lobe lesions and may produce a generalized seizure without aura. The *Jacksonian motor seizure* is characterized by a tonic contraction or a clonic twitching of the fingers of one hand, one side of the face, or one foot. This disorder spreads from the part originally affected to involve other muscles on the same side of the body. The lesions are usually confined to the premotor cortex.

Status epilepticus is a grand mal seizure with major motor convulsions which are continuous or interrupted by brief periods of incomplete recovery. It is a medical emergency, which results in death if untreated.

Even though the electroencephalogram (EEG) is an important item in the initial evaluation and periodic follow-up of seizure disorders, the final diagnosis must always be clinical, because an abnormal tracing does not prove the existence of a seizure disorder nor does a normal tracing exclude the possibility of a seizure. The EEG should include recordings while the patient is asleep, awake, hyperventilating, and during photic stimulation. Nasopharyngeal leads should also be used to record activity from the medial temporal regions, which are a common site of focal discharge in psychomotor epilepsy.

TREATMENT

Phenobarbital is the drug of first choice in treatment of seizure, except for petit mal, which is treated with ethosuximide (Zarontin), trimethadione (Tridone), or valproic acid (Depakene). Phenytoin or another agent is added if the seizures are not fully controlled with the first drug. Three or more drugs may be necessary to control difficult cases. The half-life of phenobarbital is long (120 hours), so care must be taken when giving it to patients with renal failure. Phenytoin, which is detoxified in the liver, also has a long half-life (24 hours) and so may be given as a single daily dose. It takes approximately 1 week to achieve therapeutic levels. Side effects of phenytoin include skin rash, leukopenia, megaloblastic anemia, gingival hypertrophy, ataxia, and mental confusion.

Primidone given in two or three divided doses is the drug of choice for control of psychomotor seizures. Phenobarbital is a primidone metabolite produced in the liver, so it is not advisable to use both phenobarbital and primidone. Patients with status epilepticus require special care. It is imperative that an adequate airway be assured and an I.V. started. Phenytoin in a dose of 1000 mg I.V. should be administered at a rate of 50 mg/minute. Phenytoin will form a precipitate, so it should not be mixed with the intravenous solutions. If seizures persist, phenobarbital should be administered (500-1,000 mg slowly I.V.), repeated in 4-6 hours if necessary. Respiratory depression may occur, requiring mechanical ventilation; general anesthesia may occasionally be necessary.

PARKINSON'S DISEASE
(PARALYSIS AGITANS)

Parkinson's disease, a disorder of middle or late life, is classified as a degenerative disease of the nervous system. The incidence is usually sporadic, but there is a strong positive family history in approximately 5%. Men are afflicted twice as often as women. The epidemic encephalitis of von Economo following World War I was followed by a syndrome (postencephalitic parkinsonism) clinically similar to true paralysis agitans of unknown cause (Parkinson's disease).

Pathologic findings include degenerative changes in the substantia nigra with neuronal loss, neurofibrillary degeneration, gliosis, and loss of melanin. Other brain-stem nuclei, the locus ceruleus, and dorsal motor nerve of the vagus nerve, are also involved. Lewy bodies, which are eosinophilic intracytoplasmic inclusions, are found in degenerating neurons in most cases of Parkinson's disease, but less commonly in postencephalitic parkinsonism.

There is a substantial reduction in the amount of dopamine and its major metabolite, homovanillic acid, in the striatum and the substantia nigra.

Clinically, the disorder usually begins with an asymmetrical tremor of one hand or leg, but progresses to symmetric involvement in later stages. The clearly recognized signs include generalized slowness and poverty of spontaneous movement, stooped posture, fixed facial expression, and arrhythmic resting tremor, which subsides with active movements. Muscle rigidity and bradykinesia are the most disabling features for patients. The rigidity appears first in proximal limb and nuchal muscles. Passively moving the muscles of the limbs or head results in an increased muscle tone in the flexors, extensors, and rotators. This uniform increase in muscle tone is present throughout the range of motion, but when periodically interrupted, gives rise to the cogwheel phenomenon.

Facial findings include decreased emotional responses, infrequent blinking, and staring. Tremor, affecting the distal parts first, is an alternating flexion and extension of the thumb and digits at a rate of five movements per second (pill-rolling tremor). The tremor is usually not present in the feet, but may involve the lips and tongue. Other symptoms include diminutive handwriting, repetitive speech, mild dementia, depression, oculogyric crises, diaphragmatic spasms, seborrhea, and pupillary abnormalities. The differential diagnosis of parkinsonism includes the postencephalitic variety, diffuse cerebrovascular arteriosclerosis, and exposure to toxins and drugs (reserpine, phenothiazines, and butyrophenones) which may produce extrapyramidal signs.

L-dopa is the drug of choice in the treatment of paralysis agitans and postencephalitic and arteriosclerotic parkinsonism. Carbidopa, which inhibits peripheral aromatic amino acid decarboxylase, an enzyme which converts L-dopa into dopamine, is often added to the drug treatment for parkinsonism. The dosage schedule for L-dopa averages 4-6 gm/day, and increments are individualized depending on the side effects of nausea, vomiting, and postural hypotension. When carbidopa is combined with L-dopa, only 20-25% of the former dose of L-dopa is required. The hypotensive and gastrointestinal side effects are less common with this combination. The ratio of ten to one of L-dopa to carbidopa is usually the optimal dose.

In mild situations, anticholinergic drugs may be used: trihexyphenidyl, 2 mg three to four times a day by mouth; benztropine, 1 mg three or four times a day; and procyclidine, 5 mg three or four times a day. Antihistamines, (chlorphenoxamine 50 mg three times a day by mouth) are used to control the extrapyramidal movements caused by phenothiazines or butyrophenones. Amantadine (100 mg two or three times a day by mouth), used in conjunction with L-dopa, acts by stimulating the release of dopamine from nerve terminals.

Major adverse side effects of L-dopa include cardiac arrhythmias, gastrointestinal hemorrhage, and psychiatric symptoms, e.g., confusion, agitation, depression, and psychoses. The most serious problem is the emergence of an involuntary disorder, the most common being chorea, facial-lingual pharyngeal dystonia, and athetosis. Dyskinesias occur in 75-80% of patients after a year of treatment with L-dopa. Approximately 15-20% of patients will develop periods of hyperkinesia and hypokinesia. Treatment of L-dopa toxicity consists of a gradual reduction in dosage at a rate of 250 mg/month.

MYASTHENIA GRAVIS

Myasthenia gravis (incidence of five per 100,000) is characterized by weakness and easy fatigability. The muscles most frequently affected are the facial, oculomotor, laryngeal, pharyngeal, and respiratory. The female-to-male ratio is 6:4, with peak onset for women in the third decade and for men in the seventh decade.

The weakness found in myasthenia patients is the result of a failure of normal transmission across the neuromuscular junction. There is also a decrease in the number of acetylcholine (ACh) receptors on the postjunctional membrane. A high percentage of patients have anti-ACh receptor antibodies, which act by either blocking ACh receptors or leading to their degradation. Myasthenia is often associated with thymus gland abnormalities; thymomas are found in 10-15% of patients, with myasthenia and hyperplasia of germinal centers in 70%.

Rapid fatigability is the principal feature of the disease.

Myasthenia typically develops over weeks or months with transient attacks of weakness. Muscles that are innervated by the
cranial nerves are most commonly involved in the disease. The
most common initial complaints are diplopia for ocular muscle
weakness or unilateral or bilateral ptosis. Jaw muscles become
fatigued when food is chewed. If the facial muscles are involved,
there will be weakness or eye closure and an inability to retract
the corners of the mouth, resulting in a smile that is "snarling"
(myopathic facies). Choking and regurgitation of fluids through
the nose may result from pharyngeal and laryngeal muscle
involvement. The head may droop with involvement of nuchal
muscles; limb muscles are less frequently involved than the
cranial muscles.

Diagnosis is made by demonstrating muscle weakness with
repetitive or sustained contractions (ptosis or dysphonia). The
diagnosis is confirmed by administering Tensilon (edrophonium),
a cholinesterase inhibitor with a brief (5-10 minute) duration of
action. Two mg of edrophonium are injected intravenously, and
strength is retested in 30 seconds. An additional 8 mg are injected
if improvement is not observed. Marked improvement in muscle
power in 30-60 seconds and lasting 2-3 minutes supports the
diagnosis of myasthenia gravis. A double-blind comparison of
edrophonium with saline placebo is useful if functional weakness
is suspected. Electromyography with measurement of muscle
action potential during repetitive stimulation reveals progressive
decrement in voltage in myasthenia. Thyroid function tests are
important, because there is a 14% incidence of thyroid disease; a
chest x-ray may identify a thymoma.

The two anticholinesterases used in the treatment of myasthenia are neostigmine and pyridostigmine. These are quaternary
ammonium compounds, which inhibit cholinesterase and allow
an increased concentration of ACh at the neuromuscular junction, resulting in improved transmission. Neostigmine bromide
15 mg every 2-3 hours orally is effective but produces a high
incidence of muscarinsic side effects requiring atropine. A 180-
mg delayed-release capsule is useful for nighttime coverage.

Prednisone is also used in the treatment of myasthenia: (1)
alternate-day prednisone 100 mg orally, (2) high-dose daily

prednisone, 60-100 mg for 1 month with tapering to an alternate-day maintenance schedule, and (3), increasing doses of prednisone from 25 mg on alternate days to a final dose of 100 mg on alternate days. Prednisone is continued for 1-3 years. Thymectomy is an accepted procedure for treatment of myasthenia by transcervical or sternum-splitting techniques. Spontaneous remission of myasthenia is common in young women. Approximately 70-75% of patients will have a remission following thymectomy.

REFERENCES
The Comatose Patient
Posner JB, Plum F: Spinal-fluid pH and neurologic symptoms in systemic acidosis. N Engl J Med 277:605, 1967.

Raskin NH, Fishman RA: Neurologic disorders in renal failure (Part 1). N Engl J Med 294:143, 1976.

Alfrey AC, LeGendre GR, Kaehny WD: The dialysis encephalopathy syndrome: possible aluminum intoxication. N Engl J Med 294:184, 1976.

Bell JA, Hodgson HJF: Coma after cardiac arrest. Brain 97:361, 1974.

Beecher HK, et al.: A definition of irreversible coma: report of the Ad Hoc Committee of the Harvard Medical School to examine the definition of brain death. JAMA 205:337, 1968.

Plum F, Posner JB: The Diagnosis of Stupor and Coma. Philadelphia, Davis, 1972.

Sigsbee B, Plum F: The unresponsive patient. Diagnosis and early management. Med Clin North Am 63:813, 1979.

Headache
Waters WE, O'Connor PJ: Prevalence of migraine. J Neurol Neurosurg Psychiatry 38:613, 1975.

Leviton A, Malvea B, Graham JR: Vascular diseases, mortality, and migraine in the parents of migraine patients. Neurology (Minneap) 24:669, 1974.

Weber RB, Reinmuth OM: The treatment of migraine with propranolol. Neurology (Minneap) 22:366, 1972.

Friedman AP (ed): Symposium on headaches and related pain syndromes. Med Clin North Am 62:427, 1978.

Healey LA, Wilske KR: Manifestations of giant cell arteritis. Med Clin North Am 61:261, 1977.

Neurologic Infections

DeLouvois J, Gortval P, Hurley R: Antibiotic treatment of abscesses of the central nervous system. Br Med J 2:985, 1977.

Ellner JJ, Bennett JE: Chronic meningitis. Medicine (Baltimore) 55:341, 1976.

Finland M, Barnes MW: Acute bacterial meningitis at Boston City Hospital during 12 selected years, 1935-1972. J Infect Dis 136:400, 1977.

Heat Syndromes

Glowes GHA Jr, O'Donnell TF Jr: Heat stroke. N Engl J Med 291:564, 1974.

Costrini AM, Pitt HA, Gustafson AB, Uddin DE: Cardiovascular and metabolic manifestations of heat stroke and severe heat exhaustion. Am J Med 66:296, 1979.

Goldfrank L, Osborn H: Heat stroke. Hospital Physician, August, 1977.

Shapiro Y, Magazanik A, Udassin R, Ben-Baruch G, Shvartz E, Shoenfeld Y: Heat intolerance in former heatstroke patients. Ann Intern Med 90:913, 1979.

Stroke

The Canadian Cooperative Study Group: A randomized trial of aspirin and sulfinpyrazone in threatened stroke. N Engl J Med 299:53, 1978.

Jay SJ, Johanson WG, Pierce AK: Respiratory complications of overdose with sedative drugs. Am Rev Respir Dis 112:591, 1975.

Barnett HJM: The pathophysiology of transient cerebral ischemic attacks. Therapy with platelet antiaggregants. Med Clin North Am 63:649, 1979.

Kannel WB, Dawber TR, Sorlie P, Wolf PA: Components of blood pressure and risk of atherothrombotic brain infarction: the Framingham study. Stroke 7:327, 1976.

Kannel WB, Wolf PA, Verter J, et al.: Epidemiologic assessment of the role of blood pressure in stroke: the Framingham study. JAMA 214:301, 1970.

Oral contraception and increased risk of cerebral ischemia or thrombosis: Collaborative Group for the Study of Stroke in Young Women. N Engl J Med 288:871, 1973.

Ziegler DK, Zileli T, Dick A, et al.: Correlation of bruits over the carotid artery with angiographically demonstrated lesions. Neurology (Minneap) 21:860, 1971.

Heathfield KWG, Croft PB, Swash M: The syndrome of transient global amnesia. Brain 96:729, 1973.

Millikan CH, McDowell FH: Treatment of transient ischemic attacks. Stroke 9:299, 1978.

Easton JD, Sherman DG: Stroke and mortality rate in carotid endarterectomy: 228 consecutive operations. Stroke 8:565, 1977.

Cerebrovascular Diseases. In Scheinberg, P (ed.): Princeton Conference on Cerebrovascular Diseases (10th ed.). New York, Raven, 1976.

Alcohol and Disease

Thompson WL, Johnson AD, Maddrey WL, et al.: Diazepam and paraldehyde for treatment of severe delirium tremens. A controlled trial. Ann Intern Med 82:175, 1975.

Berry RE Jr: Estimating the economic costs of alcohol abuse. N Engl J Med 295:620, 1976.

Bennion LJ, Li T-K: Alcohol metabolism in American Indians and whites: lack of racial differences in metabolic rate and liver alcohol dehydrogenase. N Engl J Med 294:9, 1976.

Criteria Committee, National Council on Alcoholism: Criteria for the diagnosis of alcoholism. Ann Intern Med 77:249, 1972.

Davis CN: Early signs of alcoholism JAMA 238:161, 1977.

Sellers EM, Kalant H: Alcohol intoxication and withdrawal. N Engl J Med 294:757, 1976.

Victor M, Adams RD, Collins GH: The Wenicke-Korsakoff syndrome: a clinical and pathological study of 245 patients, 82 with post-mortem examinations. Philadelphia, Davis, 1971.

Williams KH: Medical consequences of alcoholism. Ann Intern Med 81:265, 1974.

Singer K, Lundberg WB: Ventricular arrhythmias associated with the ingestion of alcohol. Ann Intern Med 77:247, 1972.

Asokan SK, Frank MJ, Witham AJ: Cardiomyopathy without cardiomegaly in alcoholics. Am Heart J 84:13, 1972.

Demakis JG, Proskey A, Rahimtoola SH, et al.: The natural course of alcoholic cardiomyopathy. Ann Intern Med 80:293, 1974.

Orlando J, Aronow WS, Cassidy J, et al.: Effect of ethanol on angina pectoris. Ann Intern Med 84:652, 1976.

Isselbacher KJ: Metabolic and hepatic effects of alcohol. N Engl J Med 296:612, 1977.

Miller PD, Heinig RE, Waterhouse C: Treatment of alcoholic acidosis: the role of dextrose and phosphorus. Arch Intern Med 138:67, 1978.

Ouellette EM, Rosett HL, Rosman NP, et al.: Adverse effects on offspring of maternal alcohol abuse during pregnancy. N Engl J Med 297:528, 1977.

Drug Overdose

Liden CB, Lovejoy FH Jr, Costello CE: Phencyclidine: nine cases of poisoning. JAMA 234:513, 1975.

Newton RW: Physostigmine salicylete in the treatment of tricyclic antidepressant overdose. JAMA 231:941, 1975.

Spiker DG, Biggs JT: Tricyclic antidepressants: prolonged plasma levels after overdose. JAMA 236:1711, 1976.

Jay SJ, Johanson WG, Pierce AK: Respiratory complications of overdose with sedative drugs. Am Rev Respir Dis 112:591, 1975.

Seizure Disorders

Penry JK, Newmark ME: The use of antiepileptic drugs. Ann Intern Med 90:207, 1979.

Simon D, Penry JK: Sodium di-N-propylacetate (DPA) in the treatment of epilepsy. A review. Epilepsia 16:549, 1975.

Schmidt RP, Wider BJ: Epilepsy. Philadephia, Davis, 1968.

Tharp BR: Recent progress in epilepsy—diagnostic procedures and treatment. Calif Med 119:19, 1973.

Woodbury DM, Penry JK, Schmidt RP (eds): Antiepileptic Drugs. New York, Raven, 1972.

Glazer GH: Epilepsy. In WB Matthews (ed): Recent Advances in Clinical Neurology. Edinburgh, Churchill, Lorngstone, 1975, pp 23-68.

Parkinson's Disease

Caline DB, Kebabian J, Silbergeld E, Evarts E: Advances in the neuropharmacology of Parkinsonism. Ann Intern Med 90:219, 1979.

Pollock M, Hornabrooke RW: The prevalence, natural history and dementia of Parkinson's disease. Brain 89:429, 1966.

Forno LS, Alvord EC Jr: The pathology of parkinsonism (Part 1). Some new observations and correlations. In McDowell FH, Markham CH (eds): Recent Advances in Parkinson's Disease. Philadelphia, Davis, 1971, p 120.

Barbeau A: The clinical physiology of side effects in long-term L-dopa therapy. Second Canadian-American Conference on Parkinson's Disease, Advances in Neurology Series, Vol 5, McDowell F, Barbeau A, eds., New York, Raven, 1974, p 347.

Teychenne PF, Pfeiffer RF, Bern SM, et al.: Comparison between lergotrile and bromocriptine in parkinsonism. Ann Neurol 3:319, 1978.

Myasthenia Gravis

Drachman DB: Myasthenia gravis. N Engl J Med 298:136, 186, 1978.

Osserman KE, Genkins G: Studies in myasthenia gravis: review of a twenty-year experience in over 1200 patients. Mt Sinai J Med NY 38:497, 1971.

Engel WK, Festoff BW, Pattern BM, et al.: Myasthenia gravis. Ann Intern Med 81:225, 1974.

Dau PC, Lindstrom JM, Cassel CK, et al.: Plasmapheresis and immuno-suppressive drug therapy in myasthenia gravis. N Engl J Med 297:1134, 1977.

Warmolts JR, Engel WK: Benefit from alternate-day prednisone in myasthenia gravis. N Engl J Med 286:17, 1972.

Mann JD, Hohns TR, Campa JF: Long-term administration of cortico-steroids in myasthenia gravis. Neurology (Minneap) 26:729, 1976.

Seybold ME, Drachman DB: Gradually increasing doses of prednisone in myasthenia gravis: reducing the hazards of treatment. N Engl J Med 290:81, 1974.

Genkins G, Papatestas AE, Horowitz SH, et al.: Studies in myasthenia gravis: early thymectomy. Electrophysiologic and pathologic correla-tions. Am J Med 58:517, 1975.

APPENDICES

A Note on Units

Systems of units change periodically as methods of analysis change and as the desire for standardization leads to new approaches. At one time, most analyses were made on a large volume of blood so that the volume 100 ml percent (per centum) was used. The newer standardized international unit for that volume is deciliter (dl). While dl is used in the text, the older expression per 100 ml is used in the following table.

Improved analysis has led to the use of smaller volumes so that many constituents are expressed per ml of blood. The amounts analyzed have also decreased and the following units are each 1/1000 of the preceding unit:

Milligram (mg)	10^{-3} gm
Microgram (μg)	10^{-6} gm
Nanogram (ng)	10^{-9} gm
Picogram (pg)	10^{-12}

THE NORMAL LUNG

	Men		Women	
	40 YEARS	70 YEARS	40 YEARS	70 YEARS
Vital capacity (VC, liters)	4.4	3.8	3.9	3.2
Functional residual capacity (FRC, liters)	3.5	3.5	3.1	3.1
1st second VC ($FEV_{1.0}$ liters)	3.6	2.7	3.1	2.4
Maximum midexpiratory flow rate (MMFR) (liters)	3.8	2.6	3.3	2.3
Single breath diffusing capacity ($D_{L_{CO}}$) ml/co/min/mmHg (liters)	28	19	25	17
Residual Volume/total lung Capacity (percent)	30	40	32	38
Arterial PO_2 (mm Hg)	85	75	85	75

Average values from various sources calculated for an individual 170 cm (5'7'') tall.

ELECTROCARDIOGRAPHIC DIAGNOSIS OF HYPERTROPHY

LEFT VENTRICULAR HYPERTROPHY: VOLTAGE CRITERIA

	18-25 yrs	Over 45 yrs
$S_{V1} + R_{V5}$ or R_{V6}	50 mm	35 mm
R_I	16 mm	13 mm
R_{aVF}	17 mm	9 mm
$R_I + S_{III}$		25 mm
R_{aVL}		11 mm

LEFT VENTRICULAR HYPERTROPHY:
Estes Scoring System (Am Heart J 75:754, 1968)

Largest R or S in limb lead: 20 mm or more	
S in $V_{1,2}$ or $_3$: 25 mm or more R in $V_{4,5}$ or $_6$: 25 mm or more if any present	3 points
Any ST shift without digitalis	3
Typical "strain" with digitalis	1
Left axis deviation more than $-15°$	2
QRS greater than 0.09 second	1
Intrinsicoid deflection in V_{5-6} more than 0.04 seconds	1
5 of available 10 points means LVH; 4 means probably LVH	

RIGHT VENTRICULAR HYPERTROPHY

In adult, RVH suggested when:

1. Right axis deviation greater than 110°
2. RV_1 greater than 7 mm
3. R/S ratio in V_1 greater than 1
4. $R_{V1} + S_{V5,6}$ greater than 10.5
5. RV strain pattern
6. Intrinsicoid defection in V_1 greater than 0.04

ATRIAL HYPERTROPHY

Right   Tall, peaked P wave (greater than 2.5 mm in height)
Left   P wave broader than 0.12 sec, notched in I, II and
            aVL; terminal negativity in V_1 more than 11 mm
            deep and 0.04 sec wide

TABLES OF NORMAL VALUES

BLOOD

HEMATCLOGIC VALUES
- Hemoglobin
  - Males — 14-18 g/100 ml whole blood
  - Females — 12-16 g/100 ml whole blood
- Hematocrit
  - Males — 40-54%
  - Females — 37-47%
- Erythrocytes
  - Males — 5.4 ± 0.8 million/mm^3
  - Females — 4.8 ± 0.6 million/mm^3
- Leukocytes — 5,000-10,000/mm^3
  - Segmented neutrophils — 54-62%
  - Bands — 3-5%
  - Basophils — 0-0.75%
  - Eosinophils — 1-3%
  - Monocytes — 3-7%
  - Lymphocytes — 25-33%
- Platelets — 150,000-450,000/mm^3
- Reticulocytes — 0.5-1.5%
- Erythrocyte sedimentation rate — 20 mm or less per hour (Westergren)
  - Male: 1-13 mm/hr
  - Female: 1-20 mm/hr
- Bleeding time (Template) — 3-8.5 min (IVY)
- Whole blood clotting time — 6-12 min (Lee-White)
- Clot retraction — >45% in 1 hr
- Recalcification time — 80-180 seconds (Quick's)
- One-stage prothrombin time — 11-13.5 seconds
- Activated partial thromboplastin time — 27-39 seconds
- Fibrinogen — 275 mg/100 ml
- Fibrin split products — Less than 8 µg/ml
- Euglobulin lysis time — More than 2 hours
- Haptoglobin — 75-150 mg/100 ml

BLOOD CONSTITUENTS
- Acetone — 0.3-2.0 mg per 100 ml
- Albumin — 3.5-5.5 g per 100 ml
- Ammonia — 30-100µg/100ml
- Amylase — 40-180 Somogyi units/100 ml

BLOOD (Cont.)

Antistreptolysin-O titer	Less than 200 Todd units (serial titers suggested)
Ascorbic acid	0.4-1.5 mg per 100 ml
Bilirubin	
Total	Up to 1.1 mg%
Direct	Up to 0.4 mg%
Indirect	Up to 0.6 mg%
Blood volume	Approx. 8% of body weight
Bromsulphalein (BSP)	Less than 5% retention/45 min
Blood urea nitrogen (BUN)	10-20 mg per 100 ml
C-reactive protein	0
Calcium	8.5-10.5 mg/100 ml
Ionized calcium	5.6 mg/100 ml
Carbon dioxide (CO_2)	
Content	22-31 mEq/liter
Carotene	70-200μ per 100 ml
Catecholamines	
Norepinephrine	80-250 picograms/ml
Epinephrine	15-80 picograms/ml
Chloride	100-106 mEq/liter
Copper	70-140 μg/100 ml
Cholesterol	120-250 mg/100 ml
Cholinesterase	0.5 pH units/hr or more
Creatinine	0.5-1.5 mg/100 ml
Digoxin	Toxicity suspected when >2.0 ng/ml
Ethanol (medicolegal)	0.15% unfit to drive
	0.3-0.4% marked intoxication
	0.45-0.6% coma
Ferritin	10-200 ng/ml
Iron deficiency	0-20 ng/ml
Iron excess	> 300 g/ml
Folic acid	7-16 ng/ml
Glucose	70-110 mg/100 ml
Iron	50-150μg/100 ml
Iron-binding capacity	150-300 μg/100 ml
Lactic acid	<1.2 mM/liter

(continued)

BLOOD (Cont.)

Lead	Less than 30 µg/100 ml
Lipase	Less than 2 units
Lipids, total/serum	450-850 mg/100 ml
Magnesium	1.5-2.5 mEq/liter
Methemoglobin (adults)	Approx. 0.1 g per 100 ml
5' Nucleotidase	0.3-3.2 Bodansky U/100 ml
Osmolality	280-300 mOsm/kg
Phenytoin (Dilantin)	Therapeutic level 10-20 µg/ml
Phosphatase, acid	0.5-2.0 units total
Phosphatase, alkaline	30-115 IU/liter
Phosphorus	3.0-4.5 mg/100 ml
Potassium	3.5-5.5 m Eq/liter
Protein	6-8 g per 100 ml (total)
Albumin	3.5-5.5 g per 100 ml
Globulin	2.0-3.5 g per 100 ml
paper electrophoresis	
alpha 1	0.2-0.4 g/100 ml
alpha 2	0.5-0.9 g/100 ml
beta	0.6-1.1 g/100 ml
gamma	0.7-1.7 g/100 ml
Pyruvic acid	<.15 mM/liter
Quinidine	4-8 mg/liter
Salicylate	
Therapeutic	20-25 mg/100 ml
Toxic	Over 30 mg/100 ml
Serotonin	0.08-0.22 µg/ml of serum
Sodium	132-144 mEq/liter
Transaminase	
SGOT	8-40 IU/liter
SGPT	5-30 units
Urea nitrogen	5-25 mg/100 ml
Uric acid	
Male:	3.9-9.0 mg/100 ml
Female:	2.2-7.7 mg/100 ml

CARDIOPULMONARY

	Pressure	O₂ Saturation % of normal
Right atrium	2-5 mm Hg	74 ± 4
Right ventricle	25/2 mm Hg	74 ± 4
Pulmonary artery	25/10 mm Hg	74 ± 4
Pulmonary capillary	5-14 mm Hg	
Left atrium	2-12 mm Hg	97 ± 1

1 mm Hg = 1.36 cm H_2O

CEREBROSPINAL FLUID

Cells	0-5 mononuclear cells/mm³
Character	Clear, colorless
specific gravity	1.005-1.009
Chloride	120-130 mEq/liter
Gammaglobulin	<12% of total protein
Glucose	45-80 mg per 100 ml (approx. ½ of blood sugar)
Pressure (reclining)	70-200 mm H_2O
Protein	15-45 mg/100 ml

Note: Usually, grossly bloody CSF will not clot in the test tube.

GASTROINTESTINAL: GASTRIC ACIDITY

Average Values—12 Hours Overnight Collection	Volume	Free HCl mEq/liter (or clinical units)
Normals	600	29
Duodenal ulcer	1,000	61
Gastric ulcer	600	21
Zollinger-Ellison syndrome	1,000+	100+

Average Values— Hourly Collection.	Volume	pH	Free HCl mEq/liter
Normal	20-60	1.5-3.0	20-30
Duodenal ulcer	60-100	1.2-0.5	30-60

GASTROINTESTINAL: MALABSORPTION TESTS*

Serum carotene	70-200 µg/100 ml (best simple test for sprue)
d-xylose test	Fasting subject given 25 gm d-xylose; average 5 hr output over 4 gm
Idiopathic malabsorption	Output less than 2.5 gm/5 hr
Secondary malabsorption	Output 2.5-4 gm/5 hr
Triolein and oleic acid I¹³¹ normal	Compare blood and fecal counts
	4th, 5th, & 6th hr blood specimens average more than 10% of the administered dose; less than 5% of dose in stool during a 2-3 day period
Stool fat, total	Up to 6 gm/24 hr

*See Chapter 3

LIVER FUNCTION TESTS

Bromosulphalein	5% or less after 45 min
Cephalin flocculation	2+ or less in 48 hrs
Gammaglutamyl transpeptidase (GGT)	4-45 IU/liter
5' Nucleotidase	0.3-3.2 Bodansky units per 100 ml
Onithine carbamyl transferase (OCT)	0-500 sigma U/ml
Phosphatase, alkaline	30-115 IU/liter
Portal pressure (splenic pulp)	Under 280 mm H₂O
Prothrombin time	70-100% of normal control approx 13 seconds
Thymol turbidity	0-4 units
Transaminase (SGPT)	5-30 units
Urobilinogen	
Urine	1.3-3.5 mg/24 hr
Feces	50-280 mg/24 hr

RENAL FUNCTION TESTS

Clearance tests (corrected to 1.73 sq m body surface area)
    Glomerular filtration rate (GFR)
        Inulin clearance   100-150 ml/minute
        Mannitol clearance   120-130 ml/minute
        Endogenous creatinine   100-120 ml/minute
          clearance
        Endogenous urea   50-75 ml/minute
          clearance
    Renal plasma flow (RPF)
        Para-aminohippurate
        (PAH) clearance   400-600 ml/minute
    Filtration fraction (FF)   17-23%

$$FF = \frac{GFR}{RPF}$$

    Phenolsulfonphthalein Test
      (PSP)
      >25% of dye excreted in
      15 min
      >65% of dye excreted in
      60 min
    Maximum concentration
      (after 12 hr of dehydration)
      Specific gravity   >1.028
    Maximum dilution   < 1.003
    Maximal Diodrast excretory
      capacity TM_D
      Males   43-59 mg/minute
      Females   33-51 mg/minute
    Maximal glucose
      reabsorptive capacity
      TM_G
      Males   300-450 mg/minute
      Females   250-350 mg/minute
    Maximal PAH excretory   80-90 mg/minute
      capacity TM_{PAH}

URINE

Albumin	< 100 mg/24 hr
Aldosterone	
In urine	6-16 μg/24 hr
Total adrenal production	100-300 μg/24 hr (isotope dilution)
Bacterial count	Over 10,000 colonies/ml usually due to infection, less than 10,000 to contamination
Calcium	150 mg/day or less
Casts	0-400/12 hr
Cathecholamines	
Epinephrine	Under 20 μg/day
Norepinephrine	Under 100 μg/day
Copper	0-100 μg/day
Corticosteroids	
17-hydroxy	Male 5-15 mg/24 hr
	Female 4-10 mg/24 hr
17-keto	Male 8-25 mg/24 hr
	Female 5-15 mg/24 hr
Creatine	Less than 100 mg/24 hr
Creatinine	1.0-1.7 g/24 hr
Epithelial and white blood cells	32,000-1,000,000/12 hr
Erythrocytes	0-425,000/12 hr
5-Hydroxyindoleacetic acid	2-9 mg/24 hr
Lead	Up to 120 μg/24 hr
Phosphorus	Approx. 1gm/24 hr
Porphobilinogen	0/24 hr
Potassium	25-100mEq/24 hrs
Serotonin	60-160 gm/24 hr
Sodium	180-220mEq/24 hrs
Sugar	0/24 hr
Uric acid	250-750 mg/24 hrs
Urobilinogen	Up to 1.0 Ehrlich units/2 hr or 1-3.5 mg in 24 hrs
Vanillyl mandelic acid (VMA)	1.8-8.4 mg/24 hr
Volume	800-1,600 ml/24 hr

ENDOCRINE FUNCTION TESTS (PLASMA VALUES)

Adrenocorticotropin (ACTH)	15-70 pg/ml		
Aldosterone	levels vary with Na^+ and K^+ intake and posture; follow laboratory protocol (range 40-500 pg/ml)		
Angiotensin II (100 mEq Na 50-100 mEq K), supine	10-20 pg/ml		
	10-30 pg/ml		
Cortisol			
8:00 A.M.	8-24 µg/100 ml		
8:00 P.M.	3-10 µg/100 ml		
11-deoxycortisol	Less than 1 µg/100 ml		
Estradiol (women)	20-55 pg/ml		
Growth hormone (fasting, at rest)	Less than 5 ng/ml		
Serum insulin (fasting)	6-26 µIUml		

Gonadotropins	EARLY CYCLE	MID CYCLE	MEN
FSH (mIU/ml)	5-30	5-20	5-25
LH (mIU/ml)	5-20	15-40	6-18

Parathyroid hormone	150-300 pg/ml
Prolactin	2-15 ng/ml
TSH (RIA)	0.5-5 µU/ml
Thyroxine (T_4) (radioimmunoassay)	4-12 µg/100 ml
Triiodothyronine (T_3) (radioimmunoassay)	80-180 ng/100 ml
T_3 resin uptake	25-40%
Serum testosterone	
(adult male)	300-1000 ng/100 ml
(adult female)	20-80 ng/100 ml

ANTIBIOTICS

PENICILLINS AND CEPHALOSPORINS

Name	Properties
PENICILLIN G (CRYSTALLINE PEN)	Parenteral only (acid labile), penicillinase-sensitive. CSF—10% serum concentration. Rapid renal clearance. Bactericidal
PROCAINE PENICILLIN G	Same
BENZATHINE PENICILLIN G	Same
PENICILLIN V (PHENOXY-METHYL PEN)	Acid stable Active orally especially as potassium salt
AMPICILLIN	Well-absorbed; excreted in urine and bile. Skin rashes common, especially in patients with infectious mononucleosis
CARBENICILLIN	Chemically similar to ampicillin with substitution of a carboxyl group. Excreted in urine
OXACILLIN CLOXACILLIN DICLOXACILLIN	Acid-stable, well-absorbed (especially dicloxicillin); Oxacillin may be given parenterally
CEPHALOTHIN	Bactericidal; 100% excreted in urine. Not present in CSF; some nephrotoxicity

Spectrum	Administration
Gram-positive and gram-negative; anaerobes; spirocetes	I.V. bolus 2-6 million units every 4 hours; I.V. infusion 2-6 million units/day. Probenecid 500 mg b.i.d.; can double levels
Same	300,000-600,000 units I.M. every 12 hours
Same	1.2 million units I.M. every 2-4 weeks
Same as Penicillin G	1-2 million units orally in 4 doses/day (125 mg = 200,000 units)
Broad-spectrum; active against many gram-negative organisms; *H. influenzae, E. coli, Shigella, Salmonella, Proteus mirabilis*	1-2 gm/day, q6h, orally I.V.: 2-12 gm/day at 6 hr intervals
As with ampicillin but also active against *Pseudomonas, Proteus*, and *Enterobacter*	4-30 gm/day I.V. High doses needed, except for urinary infections, as 80% is excreted over 6 hours
Active against penicillinase-producing staphylococci. Not active against gram-negative organisms	2-4 gm/day orally; give 6 hourly
Broad-spectrum including penicillinase-producing *Staphylococcus*. Inactive against *Pseudomonas, Enterobacter*	1-2 gm every 4-6 hours *(continued)*

PENICILLINS AND CEPHALOSPORINS (Cont.)

Name	Properties
CEPHALEXIN	Well-absorbed orally; good blood levels; low serum binding; high renal excretion
CEFOXITIN	Resistant to beta lactamases of gram-negative bacilli; 85% excreted unchanged by kidneys
CEFAMANDOLE	Similar to cefoxitin, 60-80% excreted unchanged by kidneys
VANCOMYCIN	Bactericidal, not absorbed orally; most is excreted in urine exchanged

Spectrum	Administration
Broad-spectrum. Less active against *Staphylococcus* than parenteral cephalosporins	1-4 gm/day, given 6-hourly
Broader spectrum, especially against *Bacteroides* and *Serratia*	3-12 gm/day given 6-8 hourly. I.M. or I.V. Reduce dose in renal impairment
Broad-spectrum with good activity against *Proteus* (indole-positive) and *Enterobacter*	2-12 gm/daily given 4-8 hourly. I.M. or I.V. Reduce dose in renal impairment.
Major use is against severe septicemia from penicillin-resistant gram-positive cocci and in antibiotic-associated (pseudomembranous) colitis due to *Clostridium difficile*	0.5-1 gm/6 hours I.V.; 125-500 mg orally for 5-10 days in cases of pseudomembranous colitis

AMINOGLYCOSIDES

Name	Properties
STREPTOMYCIN	Bactericidal Parenteral only Ototoxicity; renal toxicity. Rapid onset of resistance if used alone.
NEOMYCIN	Not used systemically because of toxicity
KANAMYCIN	Similar to neomycin but less toxic. Effective parenterally. Excreted by kidneys
GENTAMICIN	Good gram-negative spectrum. Excreted by kidneys. Urine levels increased by alkaline urine. Nephrotoxicity. Use with care in presence of renal disease.
TOBRAMYCIN	Similar to gentamicin; may be less toxic to kidneys
AMIKACIN	Similar to kanamycin, broader antibacterial activity

Spectrum	Administration
Broad-spectrum Gram-positive gram-negative organisms and *Mycobacteria*, especially *tuberculosis*	2-4 gm/day I.M. q 12°
Oral use only to "sterilize" bowel, preoperatively or in liver failure. Ointments	4 gm daily orally. q 6°
Serious gram-negative infections, except *Pseudomonas*	1-2 gm daily Max: 7.5 mg/kg/12 hourly Adjust for renal function
Most gram-negative organisms including *Pseudomonas* and *Proteus*. Also against gram-positive, but less toxic antibiotics should be used if possible	1-2 mg/kg every 8 hours I.M./I.V. Adjust for renal function
More active against *Pseudomonas* than is gentamicin	1-2 mg/kg every 8 hours I.M./I.V. Adjust for renal function
Active against gram-negative and gram-positive organisms and *Pseudomonas and* other organisms resistant to gentamicin	5 mg/kg 8 hourly I.M./I.V. Adjust for renal function

TETRACYCLINES

Name	Properties
TETRACYCLINE (OXYTETRACYCLINE, CHLORTETRACYCLINE)	Bacteriostatic Resistance develops Liver and renal toxicity Staining of teeth in children GI upset; candidiasis
DOXYCYCLINE	High protein binding, long half-life. Levels do not increase in renal insufficiency

MACROLIDES

ERYTHROMYCIN	Bacteriostatic at usual concentrations. Estolate ester is better absorbed but causes cholestatic hepatitis
CLINDAMYCIN	Similar to erythromycin but more potent. Danger of pseudomembranous colitis
VANCOMYCIN	Bactericidal not absorbed orally; most is excreted in urine unchanged

SULFONAMIDES

SULFISOXAZOLE (Gantrisin)	Bacteriostatic; well absorbed orally; acts by preventing conversion of PABA to folic acid in bacteria. CSF—30-55% of serum level; over 50% excreted unchanged in urine
SULFADIAZINE	Good absorption, slow excretion, good blood levels. Tends to produce crystalluria

Spectrum	Administration
Broad-spectrum; gram-positive and negative bacteria, *Mycoplasma*, rickettsia, Legionnaire's disease	250-500 mg 6 hourly orally or I.V. Do not use in renal failure
Also active against *B fragilis*	100 mg orally once/twice daily. May be given I.V. 100 mg, q 12 hr or 200 mg QD

Similar spectrum to penicillin. Active against penicillin-resistant staphylococci and *Mycoplasma*. Used in persons allergic to penicillin and in Legionnaire's disease	Oral 250-500 mg q.i.d. Rarely given I.V.; I.M. is painful
Similar spectrum to erythromycin Effective against *B fragilis*	Oral 150-300 mg q.i.d. I.V.: 300-600 mg q6h
Major use is against severe septicemia from penicillin-resistant gram-positive cocci	0.5-1 gm I.V. 6 hourly

Broad-spectrum. Common uses: *E. coli*, urinary infections, nocardiosis, trachoma, toxoplasmosis	Oral 2-4 gm stat. 0.5-1.0 gm q 6 hourly I.M. 25 mg/kg q.i.d. Alkalinize urine
Same as sulfisoxazole. Used in meningococcal meningitis	Same as sulfisoxazole

OTHER ANTIMICROBIALS

Name	Properties
TRIMETHOPRIM-SULFAME-THOXAZOLE (Septra, Bactrim)	Fixed dose combination which acts synergistically, bactericidal
AMPHOTERICIN B	Antifungal; inactive against bacteria. Not absorbed orally. Does not enter CSF. Metabolized. Very toxic to kidney, liver, marrow, and heart.
FLUCYTOSINE	Less toxic; oral drug; not as effective in some infections; synergistic with amphotericin B in cryptococcal meningitis
MICONAZOLE	Imidazole derivative; metabolized in liver; less toxic than amphotericin B. Parenteral only; no serious renal or liver toxicity
CHLORAMPHENICOL	Bacteriostatic Inhibits RNA synthesis in bacteria. Well-absorbed orally. Metabolized by liver. Aplastic anemia rare but may be fatal

Spectrum	Administration
Urinary infections; *Pneumocystis carinii;* chronic bronchitis, *Shigella* dysentry	Oral only 2 tab q 12° Dose higher for pneumocystis, 4 tabs QID.
Used in systemic fungal infections. Broad antifungal spectrum including histoplasmosis, cryptococcal meningitis, blastomycosis, systemic candidiasis	Incremental dosage with monitoring of renal function—e.g. 0.25 mg/kg/day gradually increased to 1 mg/kg/day I.V. Intrathecal 0.5 mg in 5 mg of CSF twice weekly
Cryptococcal meningitis, candidiasis	100-150 mg/kg/day given 6 hourly
Good alternative to amphotericin in cryptococcal and candidal infections. Meningitis requires intrathecal injections	I.V. 300-1,000 mg t.i.d. May need to be prolonged
Broad-spectrum; especially effective against *Bacteroides*, acute typhoid fever, *H. influenzae* meningitis (good CSF levels obtained)	Oral 0.5-1 gm q 6* May be given I.V. also (I.M. is erratic)

CARDIAC MEDICATIONS

Name	Properties
DIGITALIS	Positive inotropic agent Slows conduction in A-V node Increases vagal tone
DIGOXIN	Well-absorbed orally (80%); excreted by kidneys, both by glomerular filtration and tubular secretion in unchanged form (85%). Half-life in plasma of 1½ days
DIGITOXIN	Well-absorbed (close to 100%); long acting—half-life about 5 days. Metabolized in liver 85% with remainder excreted unchanged in urine
OUABAIN	Rapid action, short duration when given I.V. Not reliable orally. Excreted by kidney
PROCAINAMIDE (PRONES-TYL)	Decreases cardiac automaticity and conduction velocity. Increases duration of action potentials and refractory period. Peripheral hypotension; vagolytic. Well-absorbed orally. Half is metabolized by liver; half is excreted unchanged by kidney. Toxicity: marrow; lupus syndrome

Indications	Administration
Heart failure; supraventricular tachyarrhythmias. Atrial fibrillation; paroxysmal atrial tachycardia.	Dose affected by age, renal function, liver function, K^+, Mg^+, calcium levels. Digitalization may be rapid or slow
As for digitalis	Adjust for creatinine clearance. *Maintenance*—0.125 to 0.25 mg daily p.o Intravenous dose is less *Rapid digitalization:* IV 0.25 mg I.V. stat (over 3 min.). Repeat q 4* with same dose or 0.125 mg up to max of 0.5-1.0 mg
As for digitalis	*Oral maintenance* 0.1 mg/ daily. May take up to 3 weeks to reach steady levels (less than 1 week with digoxin)
Rapid I.V. digitalization only	I.V. Digitalizing dose: 0.2-0.5 mg Onset 5 minutes Peak 1 hour
Treatment of atrial and ventricular arrhythmias. (in atrial flutter or fibrillation use digitalis or propranol first to control rate of impulses through A-V node). Prevention of recurrences of supraventricular or ventricular tachyarrhythmias	*Oral* 1 gm initially, 250-500 mg q 3h (initial dose may be given I.M.) *Short half life (3 hours) is reason for q 3h schedule. *Adjust dose in renal failure

(continued)

CARDIAC MEDICATIONS (Cont.)

Name	Properties
QUINIDINE SULFATE	Cardiac actions same as procainamide; group I drug. Well-absorbed—80% bound by plasma proteins. Half-life 5-7 hours. 50% metabolized in liver; 50% excreted unchanged Toxicity: nausea, cinchonism, thrombocytopenia
DISOPYRAMIDE (NOR-PACE)	Cardiac action similar to quinidine and procainamide. Good oral absorption. 50% metabolized by liver; 50% excreted unchanged by kidney. Half-life $5\frac{1}{2}$ hrs. Side effects: Vomiting, diarrhea; urinary retention, dry mouth, blurred vision (anticholinergic effects)
LIDOCAINE (XYLOCAINE)	Diminishes automaticity in HIS-Purkinje conducting system, and in ventricular muscle. Not effective orally. Metabolized by liver. Rapid onset given IV; half-life about 15 minutes *Side effects:* Convulsions, coma
PHENYTOIN (DILANTIN)	Reduces automaticity in conducting system and raises threshold for spontaneous diastolic depolarization. Absorbed orally. Metabolized in liver. *Side effects:* Ataxia, nystagmus, vomiting; respiratory arrest, megaloblastic anemia, hyperplasia of the gums

Indications	Administration
Same as procainamide *Note:* Same precautions in treating atrial arrhythmias because of its vagolytic action	Oral (sulfate), loading dose 200-500 mg then 200-300 mg q 6° I.M. (gluconate), 200-300 mg q 6* I.V. (gluconate), 800 mg in 50 ml over 30-60 minutes
Same as quinidine and procainamide Used in patients who cannot tolerate quinidine or procainamide	Oral 200-300 mg stat; 100-200 mg q 6° Reduce in renal/liver disease
Ventricular extrasystoles or tachycardia. Contraindicated in S-A block	*I.V. bolus:* 1 mg/kg May repeat every 5 minutes to max of 5 mg/kg *Infusion:* 0.5-4 mg/minute
Arrhythmias due to digitalis intoxication—both atrial and ventricular arrhythmias	15-18 mg/kg start, then 300-500 mg daily

(continued)

CARDIAC MEDICATIONS (Cont.)

Name	Properties
PROPRANOLOL (INDERAL)	Beta adrenergic blockade. Slows conduction in AV node. Negative inotropic (may exacerbate failure). Exacerbation of asthma. Good oral absorption. First pass effect in liver. Metabolized by liver
BRETYLIUM	Antiadrenergic, decreases automaticity of ventricular conducting system and muscle. Transient release of catecholamines followed by blockade (↑BP-↓ BP); Accumulates in sympathetic ganglia and postsynaptic neurones. Majority excreted in urine. Parenteral use only

Indications	Administration
Supraventricular tachyar-rhythmias. Atrial fibrilla-tion, flutter; paroxysmal atrial tachycardia; Wolf-Parkinson-White syn-drome. Digitalis toxicity; IHSS. Angina pectoris; an-tihypertensive actions	*I.V.:* 1 mg q 5 minutes to 10 mg *Oral:* 10-400 mg q 6 hours NB—danger with sudden withdrawal
Refractory ventricular tachy-cardia or fibrillation Digitalis-induced ventricular arrhythmias	*I.V.:* 5 mg/kg bolus every 15 minutes up to 30 mg/kg *I.M.:* 5-10 mg/kg q 6-8 hours

DIURETICS: PREPARATIONS AND EFFECTS

	Tradename	Equivalent Dose
THIAZIDES		
Chlorothiazide	Diuril	500 mg
Hydrochlorothiazide	Hydrodiuril Esidrex	50 mg
Benzthiazide	Aquatag, Exna, Hydrex	50 mg
Hydroflumethiazide	Diucardin, Saluron	50 mg
Bendroflumethia-zide	Naturetin	5 mg
THIAZIDE DERIVATIVES		
Metolazone	Zaroxolyn	5 mg
Chlorthalidone	Hygroton	50 mg
DISTAL TUBULE (POSTASSIUM-SPARING) DIURETICS		
Triamterene	Dyrenium	100 mg
Spironolactone	Aldactone	50 mg
LOOP DIURECTICS		
Furosemide	Lasix	20 mg
Ethacrynic Acid	Edecrin	50 mg

Onset (hours)	Peak (hours)	Duration (hours)
1-2	4	6-12
2	4	12
2	4-6	12-18
1-2	3-4	24
1-2	6-12	18-24
$\frac{1}{2}$-1	2	12-24
2	6	24-72
2	6-8	12-16
Gradual	48-78	48-72
p.o. 1 hour	1-2	6
I.V. 5 minutes	$\frac{1}{2}$	6-8
p.o. 30 minutes	2	6-8
I.V. 15 minutes	$\frac{3}{4}$	3

ANTIHYPERTENSIVES

Name	Properties
METHYLDOPA (ALDOMET)	May act as a false transmitter at alpha receptors or an inhibitor of noradrenalin release. Dose does not lower renal blood flow
RESERPINE	Rauwolfia alkaloid. Decreases noradrenalin levels in heart and blood vessels. Decreases CNS serotonin levels
GUANETHIDINE (ISMELIN)	Blocks sympathetic nerves. Decreases cardiac output; does not enter CNS. Antagonized by tricyclic antidepressants
PROPRANOLOL (INDERAL)	Central and cardiac and renal adrenergic blockade. Lowers renin levels
HYDRALAZINE	Vasodilator; reflex tachycardia and sodium retention Good oral absorption. Metabolized in liver (over 95%)
PRAZOSIN (MINIPRESS)	Vasodilator by peripheral alpha sympathetic blockade. May be very effective with a beta blockade even in small doses

Toxicity	Dose
Depression, liver toxicity, Coombs + hemolytic anemia, impotence	250 mg t.i.d. up to 2 gm/day
Depression, parkinsonism, peptic ulcers, cardiac arrhythmias	0.125-0.25 mg once daily
Postural hypotension; impotence and ejaculatory disturbances; sodium retention. Diarrhea	Oral: 10-20 mg daily, increasing to 200 mg./day
Bronchospasm, bradycardia, heart failure; sudden discontinuation may produce arrhythmias or myocardial infarct	10 mg q.i.d. increasing to 320 mg or higher
Angina pectoris; GI symptoms, lupus syndrome, headache	Oral: 10 mg q.i.d. up to 200 mg/day
Initial hypotension prevented by commencing with small dosage	Initial: 0.5 mg orally at bedtime, then 1 mg b.i.d. or t.i.d. Range: 3-20 mg/day

(continued)

ANTIHYPERTENSIVES (Cont.)

Name	Properties
MINOXIDIL (LONITEN)	Very potent new agent. Vasodilator. Renal blood flow is preserved. Well absorbed. Metabolized by liver (greater than 90%). Reflex tachycardia and salt retention
DIAZOXIDE (HYPERSTAT)	Used in hypertensive emergencies intravenously; vasodilator
SODIUM NITROPRUSSIDE (NIPRIDE)	Vasodilator given by infusion and titrated to BP level, in hypertensive emergencies (and vasodilator therapy of heart failure)
TRIMETHAPHAN (Arfonad)	Ganglion blocker used in hypertensive emergencies

Toxicity	Dose
Pericardial effusion and tamponade. Sodium retention. Angina pectoris, hypertrichosis; reserved for resistant cases	5 mg orally initially, increase to 20 mg b.i.d. if necessary. Max: 100 mg/day
Hyperglycemia. Sodium retention; angina pectoris	I.V.: 5 mg/kg, repeat every 4-24 hours as needed
Too rapid infusion produces nausea, diaphoresis, anxiety, muscle twitching	50 mg dissolved in 250-1000 ml 5% dextrose and rate adjusted to BP level
Atropine action (parasympathetic blockade)	500 mg vial in 500 ml of 5% dextrose. Adjust rate to BP

ANTI-INFLAMMATORY ANALGESICS

Name	Actions
ASPIRIN (ACETYLSALICYLIC ACID)	Analgesic, antipyretic, antiinflammatory. Inhibits prostaglandin synthesis
ACETAMINOPHEN (TYLENOL)	Analgesic, antipyretic (not antiinflammatory)
IBUPROFEN (MOTRIN) NAPROXEN (NAPROSYN)	Analgesic, antipyretic, antiinflammatory
INDOMETHACIN (INDOCIN)	Antipyretic, analgesic, antiinflammatory. Inhibits prostaglandin E. Effective in many inflammatory situations
PHENYLBUTAZONE (BUTAZOLIDIN) OXYPHENBUTAZONE (TANDEARIL)	Analgesic, antiinflammatory. Completely metabolized by liver. Active metabolite is oxyphenbutazone
TOLMETIN (TOLECTIN)	Antiinflammatory analgesic. Related to Indocin
PENICILLAMINE	Good antiinflammatory in severe RA. Well absorbed. Excreted by kidneys. Delayed response

Interactions and Toxic Effects	Dose
Gastric bleeding, hypoprothrombinemia, platelet effects, tinnitus; vertigo	*Oral:* 3-6 gm/day Give 4-6 hourly. *Rectal:* suppositories 300 mg, 1-2 q4h
Liver toxin in high dosage. Methemoglobinemia, analgesic nephropathy	300-600 mg every 4-6 hours (over 3 gm/day is unsafe)
Displaces other drugs from plasma proteins. Less GI upset than aspirin	Max dosage 2.4 gm/day. Usual dose 300-600 mg every 6 hours. Naproxen 250-500 mg b.i.d.
Peptic ulcers and hemorrhage common. Anorexia, dyspepsia in up to 50%. CNS-vertigo, psychosis. Diminishes effects of furosemide. Marrow depression—rare. Headache	*Oral:* 25-50 mg t.i.d. Max 200 mg/day. Give after meals to lessen GI upset.
Serious marrow depression—all elements. Sodium retention is common. Gastric distress and ulcers. Potentiation of Warfarin and oral hypoglycemic agents	100 mg t.i.d., q.i.d. Higher doses for short intervals. Use only with blood counts and for short duration, e.g., 1 week
Mild GI upset and other side effects as for Indomethacin but tend to be milder	200-400 mg t.i.d. after meals
Skin rashes, pruritus, nephrotic syndrome, marrow suppression, careful monitoring needed. [Mild proteinuria is not a reason to discontinue.]	Incremental dosage schedule is best tolerated. 250 mg daily—1 month; 250 mg b.i.d.—1 month; 250 t.i.d. May need 3 months for response to occur

(continued)

ANTI-INFLAMMATORY ANALGESICS (Cont.)

Name	Actions
GOLD (MYOCHRYSINE)	Good in RA, which is resistant to first-line drugs; delayed response
CHLOROQUINE AND HYDROXYCHLOROQUINE	Effective in some cases of RA, SLE as second-line drug. Delayed response

Interactions and Toxic Effects	Dose
Skin rash may progress to exfoliative dermatitis; Renal—proteinuria, nephrotic syndrome. Marrow suppression	Blood counts before each injection. Test dose 10 mg I.M.—wait one week then 50 mg weekly I.M. to max of 1 gm
Blindness due to retinal degeneration with higher doses. GI disturbances and skin reactions are common. Bleaching of hair—rarely	Chloroquine—250 mg daily. Hydroxychloroquine—200 mg daily. May increase to 400 mg daily. See ophthalmologist at regular intervals

MEDICATIONS USED FOR MODERATE TO SEVERE PAIN

Name	Actions
PROPOXYPHENE (DARVON)	Mild to moderate pain; centrally acting non-narcotic; related to methadone. More potent combined with aspirin, acetaminophen, etc.
PENTAZOCINE (TALWIN)	Nonnarcotic; one-third potency of morphine; metabolized in liver; tolerance develops
CODEINE	Opium derivative; properties of morphine; about one-tenth potency of morphine; metabolized in liver; 10% converted to morphine
MEPERIDINE (DEMEROL)	Synthetic narcotic used for short-term analgesia. Less GI and biliary spasm than morphine. Metabolized in liver
MORPHINE	Narcotic derivative of opium. Depresses pain centrally and peripherally, cough reflex. Mental effects on mood and alertness. Metabolized in liver to glucuronide
HYDROMORPHONE (DILAU-DID)	Morphine derivative; less sedation; good analgesia
METHADONE	Synthetic opioid similar properties to morphine; metabolized in liver

APPENDICES   **579**

Toxic Effects	Dose
Psychic and physical dependence; dizziness, nausea, vomiting	65 mg p.o. q 4-6 hourly
Sedation; dizziness and vomiting; psychosis. It is a narcotic antagonist and may cause withdrawal in patients on narcotics; may be addictive	*Oral:* 50-100 mg q4h *I.M.:* 30-60 mg q4h
Dependence; tolerance; constipation; vomiting; dizziness; respiratory depression; mental changes; abdominal cramps; additive with other CNS depressants	*Pain:* 15-60 mg q4h orally or I.M. (more potent parenterally) *Cough suppression:* 15-30 mg p.o. q4h
Tolerance and addiction occurs quickly; nausea and vomiting; respiratory depression; dizziness	50-100 mg p.o. or I.M. q 2-3 hrs. May be given slowly I.V.
Addiction; constipation; spasm of bowel and biliary tract; respiratory and mental depression; hypotension; pinpoint pupils, coma	*I.M.:* 5-10 mg q4h *I.V.:* 1-4 mg slowly (watch for lowering of blood pressure)
Same as morphine	1-4 mg oral, I.M., or SQq4h
Dependence, etc., as for morphine (used in opiate withdrawal syndrome in drug programs)	5-20 mg I.V., I.M. or p.o. q4h

HYPOLIPOPROTEINEMIC AGENTS: PREPARATIONS AND EFFECTS

Drug	Initial Daily Dose	Usual Daily Dose	Mechanism of Action
Cholestyramine	12 gm	12.0-24.0 gm	↓Cholesterol absorption (through bile acid sequestration)
Cholestipol	15 gm	15-30 gm	↓Cholesterol absorption (through bile acid sequestration)
Clofibrate	1.5 gm	1.5-2.0 gm	↑Cholesterol excretion ↓Cholesterol synthesis ↓VLDL release
D-thyroxine	1 mg	4.0-8.0 mg	↑Cholesterol metabolism ↑Cholesterol excretion
Nicotinic acid	300 mg	1.5-5.0 gm	↓Lipolysis (↓LDL synthesis) ↓VLDL→LDL ↑Cholesterol metabolism
Neomycin		0.5-2.0 gm	↓Cholesterol absorption (through bile acid deconjugation)
Beta-sitosterol		12.0-24.0 gm	↓Cholesterol absorption

Use	Predominant Effects	Side effects
?IIb	LDL-cholesterol	Constipation; nausea; steatorrhea→↓ warfarin, thyroxine, digitalis absorption
	LDL-cholesterol	Constipation; nausea; steatorrhea→↓ warfarin, thryxoine, digitalis absorption
III	VLDL-triglycericles	Myositis; hepatotoxicity
IV IIb?	VLDL-cholesterol (LDL-cholesterol)	Nausea; alopecia; agranulocy tosis
II		↑Angina pectoris;
III	LDL-cholesterol	cardiotoxicity
III		Flushing; nausea; pruritis
IV V IIa IIb	LDL-cholesterol	Hyperuricema; glucose intolerance
	LDL-cholesterol	Nausea; diarrhea
	LDL-cholesterol	Nausea; diarrhea

THYROID HORMONES

Preparations	Approximate Equivalent Dose
Thyroid USP	1 gr (grain) (65 mg)
Thyroglobulin	65 mg
Thyroxine	100 µg
Tri-iodothyronine	25µg

REGULAR INSULIN

	Onset	Half-Life	Peak (hours)	Duration (hours)
INTRAVENOUS (BOLUS)	Immediate	2-6 minutes	Immediate	Dose-dependent
INTRAMUS-CULAR	10-30 minutes		1/2-1	1-3
SUBCUTA-NEOUS	15-60 minutes		2-4	5-8

INSULIN: PREPARATIONS AND EFFECTS*

Type	Onset (hours)	Peak (hours)	Duration (hours)
RAPID/SHORT			
Regular (crystalline)	1/4-1	2-4	5-8
Semilente (Insulin zinc susp., prompt)	1/2-2	4-8	12-16
INTERMEDIATE			
NPH (isophane)	1-4	8-12	18-24
Lente (insulin zinc susp.)	1-4	8-12	18-28
Globin (globin zinc insulin)	2-4	6-10	12-20
SLOW/SUSTAINED			
PZI (protamine zinc)	3-8	14-24	20-36
Ultralente (insulin zinc susp., extended)	3-8	16-24	24-36

* After s.c. administration; only regular insulin may be given I.M. or I.V.

ORAL HYPOGLYCEMIC AGENTS PREPARATIONS AND EFFECTS

	Tradename	Equivalent Dose
SULFONYLUREAS		
Short-acting		
Tolbutamide	Orinase	500
Intermediate-act-ing		
Acetohexamide	Dymelor	250
Tolazamide	Tolinase	100
Long-acting		
Chlorpropamide	Diabinese	100
BIGUANIDES		
Short-acting		
Phenformin*	DBI, Mel-trol	
Medium-acting		
Phenformin*-T.D.†	DBI, Mel-trol	

* Available only on I.N.D. status; removed from the general market by the F.D.A.
† Timed-disintegration capsule.
L = Liver
K = Kidney

Usual Daily Dosage (mg)	Doses per Day	Half Life (hours)	Duration	Metabolism
500-3000	2-3	5	6-12	L
250-1500	1-2	7	10-24	K,L
100-750	1-2	7	12-24	L,K
100-750	1	16-32	24-72	K
25-100	2-4	3-4	6-7	
50-200	2	4-7	8-14	

CORTICOSTEROID PREPARATIONS

	Approximate Equivalent Dose (mg)	Plasma Half-Life (minutes)
SHORT-ACTING		
Cortisone	25.0	30
Hydrocortisone (Cortisol)	20.0	90
Prednisone	5.0	60
INTERMEDIATE ACTING		
Prednisolone	5.0	≥200
Methylprednisolone	4.0	≥180
Meprednisone	4.0	
Triamcinolone	4.0	≥200-300
Paramethasone	2.0	
Methasone	1.5	
LONG-ACTING		
Dexamethasone	0.75	≥200-300
Betamethasone	0.6	≥300

Daily Dosages
Replacement: generally 1-2 times amount in first column.
Moderately severe illness: generally 4-8 times amount in first column.
Life-threatening illness: generally 10-20 times amount in first column.
Septic shock (or equivalent): generally 5-10 times (*per kilogram*) amount shown in first column.

Biological Half-Life (hours)	Relative Potency	
	GLUCOCORTICOID	MINERALOCORTICOID
2-8	0.8	0.8
8-12	1	1
6-24	4	0.8
12-36	4	0.8
12-36	5	0.5
	5	0.5
12-36	5	0
	10	0
	13	0
36-54	27	0
36-54	33	0

TREATMENT OF HYPERLIPOPROTEINEMIAS

	I	II A	II B	III	V	
	CHYLOMICRON	LDL (BETA-LIPOPROTEINS)		BROAD-BAND BETA-LIPOPROTEINS	VLDL (PREBETA-LIPOPROTEINS)	VLDL AND CHYLOMICRONS
DIET						
Calories	—	—	—	WR	WR	WR*
Carbohydrates	—	—	Controlled	Controlled	Controlled	Controlled
Fat	25-35 gm	Limited polyunsaturated preferred		40-50% of calories (Polyunsaturated preferred)	Polyunsaturated preferred	30% of calories, High (Polyunsaturated preferred)
Protein	—	—		High	—	High
Cholesterol	—	<300 mg.		<300 mg.	300-500 mg.	300-500 mg.
Ethanol	Avoid	Discretion		<3 oz. (as CHO Subs)	<3 oz. (as CHO Subs)	Avoid

588

DRUGS	None	Cholestyramine, Colestipol, Neomycin, Clofibrate, Nicotinic acid, Beta-sitosterol	Clofibrate	Clofibrate	Clofibrate
OTHER	—	Ileal bypass (? portacaval shunting)	—	—	(? Progestins)

*WR = weight reduction

ORAL IRON PREPARATIONS

Preparation	Strength (gm)	Iron Content (mg Fe)
Ferrous fumarate	0.20	66
Ferrous fumarate	0.32	104
Ferrous sulfate, dessicated	0.20	58
Ferrous sulfate, hydrated	0.32	64
Ferroglycine sulfate	0.25	40
Ferrous gluconate	0.32	38

DIAGNOSIS AND TREATMENT OF CANCER

The possibility of benign, premalignant, or malignant tumor must be considered with almost any sign or symptom. Survival is frequently linked to early diagnosis and selection of appropriate treatment. Cancer manifests itself by symptoms and signs related to its location, by distant spread or metastasis, and by a group of paraneoplastic syndromes not directly due to the tumor itself.

These paraneoplastic syndromes include (1) ectopic hormone production, (2) degeneration of cerebellum or spinal cord, (3) myasthenic syndromes (Eaton-Lambert syndrome), (4) phlebitis, purpura, flushing, urticaria, hyperpigmentation, acanthosis nigricans, pruritis, and other dermatologic syndromes, (5) leukemoid and polycythemic syndromes, (6) glomerular or tubular abnormalities, and (7) collagen diseases such as dermatomyositis, Sjögren's syndrome, systemic lupus, and others.

A number of ectopic hormone syndromes have been described (see index).

- *ACTH:* Lung (small cell especially), pancreas, thyroid, stomach, ovary
- *ADH:* Lung, pancreas, prostate
- *Parathormone:* Lung, breast, kidney, colon, parotid, lymphoma, gynecologic, pancreas, liver
- *Calcitonin:* Small cell lung, medullary of thyroid, carcinoid
- *Erythropoietin:* Kidney, cerebellum, liver, uterus, ovary
- *Insulin:* Pancreas, liver, adrenal
- *Chorionic gonadotropin:* liver, adrenal, stomach, ovary
- *Alkaline phosphatase:* lung, breast, colon, ovary, pancreas, lymphoma
- *Growth hormone:* lung, endometrium

It is likely that cancer begins in a single transformed cell, becoming a clone that divides in logarithmic fashion; a 1 cm tumor mass contains 10^9 cells while 10^{12} cells could be a lethal body dose for certain tumors. Chemotherapeutic agents are most effective against cells that are dividing; cells in the G_1 (first gap after division) or G_0 (quiescent phase) are much less sensitive. An increasingly larger proportion of tumor cells are inactive and not sensitive to chemotherapy as the tumor increases in size, emphasizing the advantage of early treatment. Chemotherapy generally acts in a logarithmic fashion, killing a percentage of active cells.

Surgical excision, once the cornerstone of cancer therapy, is useful for removing bulky tumors with regional manifestations but has no impact on disseminated disease. Radiation therapy has similar effects but may be used in some situations with generalized disease. Chemotherapy is best reserved for smaller primary lesions or for individuals with systemic dissemination. Multimodality therapy attempts to take advantage of each technique. Immunotherapy is still relatively investigative but by improving defense against cancer may become a useful preventive technique.

COMMON CHEMOTHERAPEUTIC AGENTS

Name and Class	Indications	Side effects
ALKYLATING AGENTS (Alkylate groups in DNA)		
Nitrogen Mustards		
Mechlorethamine ("nitrogen mustard")	Lymphomas as MOPP combination	Damages resting marrow cells
Cyclophosphamide (Cytoxan)	Lymphomas, leukemias, oat cell etc. Good immunosuppresive: Wegener's, rheumatoid, nephrosis	Nausea, alopecia, cystitis, marrow depression but less platelet effect
Phenylalanine mustard (Alkeran)	Myeloma, breast, ovary	Nausea, marrow suppression Little alopecia
Chlorambucil (Leukeran)	Lymphoma, lymphocytic leukemia, Ovarian, breast, testicular Vasculitis	Bone marrow suppression
Ethylenimine compounds		
Thio-TEPA	Lymphoma, breast, ovarian Malignant effusions	
Alkyl Sulfonates		
Busulfan (Myeleran)	Chonic granulocytic leukemia, polycythemia vera	Granulocyte suppression, pigmentation; interstitial pulmonary fibrosis
Nitrosoureas		
(BCNU, CCNU)	Similar to other alkylating agents	Bone marrow suppression delayed 4-6 weeks: pulmonary fibrosis

COMMON CHEMOTHERAPEUTIC AGENTS (Cont.)

Name and Class	Indications	Side effects
ANTIMETABOLITES Folate Antagonists		
Methotrexate (Amethopterin)	Lymphoblastic leukemia, breast, testicle, head and neck, female choriocarcinoma	Marrow suppression, alopecia, stomatitis, liver and kidney malfunction
Pyrimidine Analogs		
5-fluorouracil	Colon and breast. Frequently used in combinations	Similar to methotrexate; anorexia common
Purine Analogs		
6-mercapto-purine	Acute lymphoblastic and myeloblastic leukemia	Marrow suppression, hepatic dysfunction, cholestasis
Azathioprine (Imuran)	Inhibits DNA and RNA synthesis. Leading drug for immuno-suppression	Marrow suppression, jaundice, anemia alopecia
VINCA ALKALOIDS (Periwinkle plant) (inhibit cell cycle at metaphase)		
Vinblastine	Hodgkin's, lymphoma, female choriocarcinoma	Marrow suppression; mental changes, constipation, phlebitis
Vincristine	Common combination therapy for Hodgkin's, neuroblastoma, Wilm's Acute lymphoblastic leukemia	Marrow suppression minimal; peripheral neuropathy, alopecia

COMMON CHEMOTHERAPEUTIC AGENTS (Cont.)

Name and Class	Indications	Side effects
ANTIBIOTICS (untwisting of DNA helix)		
Bleomycin	Squamous cell carcinoma, lymphoma, testicular	Marrow suppression minimal; fever, alopecia, pulmonary edema and fibrosis, skin and nail changes
Dactinomycin (actinomycin-D)	Wilm's, testicular, sarcoma, female choriocarcinoma	Marrow suppression; nausea, vomiting
Adriamycin (doxorubicin)	Breast, lymphoma, leukemia	Marrow suppression, alopecia, cardiomyopathy, GI disturbances
Daunomycin (daunorubicin)	Acute leukemias	Marrow suppression, alopecia, GI disturbances

Index

The index is constructed primarily as a guide to analysis of signs, and symptoms, although drugs, disease processes, and other information are also alphabetized. Signs, symptoms, and laboratory abnormalities are identified by bold type. A variety of causes for each manifestation is presented, but the list is not meant to be exhaustive; occasionally entries are not discussed in the text.

Quick bedside differential diagnosis is facilitated by use of the mnemonic *TIMID:*

> *T*umor, *T*oxin or *T*rauma
> *I*nflammatory
> *M*etabolic
> *I*mmunologic
> *D*rug or *D*egenerative

RNA virus
  and leukemia, 433
  in hepatitis A, 179
Rotor syndrome, 178
Rubella
  and thrombocytopenia, 449
Rum fits, 519, 520

Salicylates, 574
Salivary gland swelling
  drug causes
    bretylium
    clonidine, 67
    guanethidine
    iodides, 334
    phenylbutazone, 574
  sarcoid, 106
  Sjogren's, 287
Salmonella
  infectious diarrhea, 199
  sickle cell disease, 417
Sarcoidosis, 105, 474
  arthritis, 290
  cardiomyopathy, 33
  hepatosplenomegaly, 183
  neuropathy, 237
  pleural effusion, 92
Scan, radioisotope, 196
Scarlet fever, 84
Schilling test, 407, 410
Schirmer test, 288
Schmidt's syndrome, 350
Sclerodactyly, 189, 274
Scleroderma, 274
  bronchogenic carcinoma, 120
  interstitial fibrosis, 112
  interstitial stasis syndrome, 156
  nephropathy, 238
  pleural effusion in, 92
Sclerosing cholangitis and ulcera-
    tive colitis, 167
Scurvy, 453
Secretin, 142
Sedimentation rate
  psoriatic arthritis, 298
  relapsing polychondritis, 290
  scleroderma, 276

Sedimentation rate *(cont.)*
  temporal arteritis, 284
Seizure disorder, 523
  alcohol, 520
  meningitis, 513
  pathophysiology, 523
  treatment, 528
  types, 527
Sella turcica
  empty, 330
  evaluation, 325, 356
Septicemia
  and alcohol, 520
  arthritis, 300
Seronegative spondylarthritides,
    294
Serotonin
  carcinoid syndrome, 161
  hemostasis, 446
  migraine headache, 510
Serum sickness, 472
Sexual abnormalities, 385
Sexual disturbances
  Cushing's, 354
  delayed maturity, 330
  diabetes, 376
  loss of libido, 329
Sexual malfunction
  drug causes
    clonidine, 67
    guanethidine, 570
    lithium
    methyldopa, 570
    most tranquilizers
    oral contraceptives, 387
Sezary syndrome, 444
Sheehan's syndrome, 326, 351
Short bowel syndrome, 156
Shock
  kidney, 229
  lung, 134
  treatment, 9
Shoulder-hand syndrome, 24
Shulman's syndrome, 277
Sicca syndrome, 286
Sick sinus syndrome, 49
Sickle C syndrome, 417